BIOCHEMICAL ASPECTS OF NUTRITION

BIOCHEMICAL ASPECTS OF NUTRITION

The Proceedings of the First Congress of The Federation of Asian and Oceanian Biochemists

edited by
KUNIO YAGI
Institute of Biochemistry, Faculty of Medicine
University of Nagoya, Nagoya (Japan)

JAPAN SCIENTIFIC SOCIETIES PRESS, Tokyo
UNIVERSITY PARK PRESS, Baltimore

JSSP No. 01592–1104

Printed in Japan

Published jointly by
JAPAN SCIENTIFIC SOCIETIES PRESS
Tokyo
and
UNIVERSITY PARK PRESS
Baltimore

Library of Congress Cataloging in Publication Data

Federation of Asian Oceanian Biochemists.
Biochemical aspects of nutrition.

Held Oct. 10–12, 1977, at Nagoya Kanko Hotel, Nagoya, Japan.
Bibliography: p.
1. Metabolism—Congresses. 2. Nutrition—Congresses. 3. Biological chemistry—Congresses. I. Yagi, Kunio, 1919– II. Title. [DNLM: 1. Biochemistry—Congresses. 2. Nutrition—Congresses. QU145 F293b 1977]
QP171.F42 1979 599′.01′3 79-4865

ISBN 0-8391-1444-3

PREFACE

This book records, in principle, the proceedings of the symposium on "Biochemical Aspects of Nutrition", which was held on October 10–12, 1977 at the Nagoya Kanko Hotel, Nagoya, as a part of the First Congress of the Federation of Asian and Oceanian Biochemists. However, it is not the simple proceedings, but resembles a monograph written by experts for the following reasons. First, the program committee for the symposium carefully selected speakers from all over the world so as to cover the main topics in this field. Second, the speakers were asked to prepare their papers in the form of reviews in miniature. Accordingly, the book is expected to be useful for biochemists in wider areas than the specialists. The editor's thanks are due to Drs. S. Fukui, N. Hosoya, A. Ichihara, Y. Imai, and A. Yoshida, the members of the program committee, for their efforts in preparing the program.

By the way, it should be mentioned that since the Federation of Asian and Oceanian Biochemists started in 1972, five years passed until the first congress was held. This period was necessary for the Federation to accumulate the energy to hold such an event. Accordingly, this book is a testimony to the cooperation of the members of the Federation. In this respect, encouragement received from the delegates of the member countries, especially Dr. A. W. Linnane, the president of the Federation, is highly appreciated. The efforts of the members of the organizing committee of this congress, Drs. O. Hayaishi, K. Imahori, B. Maruo, Y. Miura, D. Mizuno, and T. Murachi are also greatly appreciated.

Kunio YAGI
The Congress President
First Congress of the
Federation of Asian and
Oceanian Biochemists

CONTENTS

Preface v

PROTEINS

UNSTABLE PROTEIN IN MAMMALIAN CELLS SYNTHESISED IN THE PRESENCE OF AMINO ACID ANALOGS OR UNDER CONDITIONS OF AMINO ACID IMBALANCE
F. J. BALLARD, C. S. CHANDLER, AND S. E. KNOWLES 1
Amino Acid Substitutions 1
Nutritional Significance of Analog Amino Acids 5
Imbalances of Normal Amino Acids 6
Regulation of the Breakdown of Labile Proteins 8

UTILIZATION OF LIMITING AMINO ACIDS FOR PROTEIN SYNTHESIS IN AMINO ACID IMBALANCE
A. YOSHIDA 13

THE BIOSYNTHESIS OF SECRETORY PROTEINS WITH SPECIAL REFERENCE TO MILK PROTEINS
P. N. CAMPBELL, R. K. CRAIG, AND A. P. BOULTON 17
Proproteins 18
The Primary Translation Products of Secretory Proteins 18
The Biosynthesis of Milk Proteins 21
Characterization of mRNA Associated with Free and Bound Polyribosomes . . . 25
Conclusions from Studies on Synthesis of Milk Proteins 28

FERRITIN BIOSYNTHESIS AND ITS RESPONSE TO IRON
H. N. MUNRO 31
Current Concepts of Ferritin Structure 31
Intracellular Sites of Synthesis of Ferritin 33
Response of Apoferritin Synthesis to Iron Administration 34
Role of Ferritin in Cell Metabolism 36

USE OF LIVER CELLS IN PRIMARY CULTURE FOR BIOCHEMICAL STUDIES OF LIVER FUNCTION
A. ICHIHARA, K. TANAKA, Y. TOMITA, AND M. SATO 41

AMPLIFICATION OF DIHYDROFOLATE REDUCTASE GENES IN METHOTREXATE-RESISTANT CULTURED MOUSE CELLS
R. T. SCHIMKE, F. W. ALT, R. E. KELLEMS, R. KAUFMAN, AND J. R. BERTINO 45
Synthesis of Dihydrofolate Reductase 45
Quantitation of DHFR mRNA and Gene Number 47

ROLE OF DIPEPTIDASES AND DIPEPTIDE ABSORPTION IN INTESTINAL DIGESTION OF PROTEINS
V. GANAPATHY AND A. N. RADHAKRISHNAN 55
Intestinal Dipeptidases 57
Intestinal Dipeptide Transport 57
Amino Acid Interaction with Dipeptide Transport and Dipeptide Hydrolysis . . 59
Harmaline and Dipeptide Transport 63
A General Scheme for Protein Digestion and Absorption 64

INTESTINAL ABSORPTION OF ENZYME PROTEINS
T. MURACHI 67
The *in Vitro* Experiments 67
The *in Situ* Experiments 69
Effect of Molecular Size and Concentration of Test Proteins 72
Mechanism of Absorption 73

LIPID

FATTY ACID SYNTHETASE OF YEAST AND 6-METHYLSALICYLATE SYNTHETASE OF *PENICILLIUM PATULUM*—TWO MULTIENZYME COMPLEXES
F. LYNEN, H. ENGESER, J. FRIEDRICH, W. SCHINDLBECK, R. SEYFFERT, F. WIELAND, AND E. SIESS 77
The Architecture of Fatty Acid Synthetase 79
6-Methylsalicylate Synthetase 84

MOLECULAR MECHANISMS FOR BIOLOGICAL REGULATION OF LIPOGENESIS
S. NUMA, T. KAMIRYO, M. MISHINA, S. TASHIRO, S. NAKANISHI, S. HORIKAWA, T. TANABE, S. YAMASHITA, K. HOSAKA, U. SCHIELE, AND Y. MIKI 91
Regulation of Acetyl-CoA Carboxylase Synthesis 91
Regulation of Fatty Acid Distribution in Glycerolipids 98

MECHANISM OF CHOLESTEROL-LOWERING EFFECTS OF POLYUNSATURATED FATS
J. GANGULY, R. PAUL, C. S. RAMESHA, AND P. BALARAM 105
Effect of Dietary Fats on the Biliary Excretion of Cholesterol 106
Absorption of Dietary Lecithin 108
Influence of Dietary Lecithin on Biliary Lecithin 109
Physico-chemical Studies of the Bile Micelle 110
Physiological Implications 111

MICROSOMAL ELECTRON TRANSFER SYSTEM IN LIPID METABOLISM
T. ONO, T. OKAYASU, K. KAMEDA, AND Y. IMAI 115

Desaturation of Fatty Acid 115
Lipid Peroxidation 118
Squalene Epoxidation 120

CARBOHYDRATE

SOME ASPECTS OF DIETARY STARCH UTILIZATION IN THE MAMMALIAN DIGESTIVE TRACT
J. J. MARSHALL AND W. J. WHELAN 125
Pancreatic α-Glucosidases 126
Breakdown of α-Limit Dextrins by Intestinal Mucosal α-Glucosidases 128

THE SUCRASE-ISOMALTASE COMPLEX, A LARGE DIMERIC AMPHIPATHIC PROTEIN FROM THE SMALL-INTESTINAL BRUSH BORDER MEMBRANE: ITS POSITIONING AND IMPLICATION AS TO ITS BIOSYNTHESIS
G. SEMENZA 131
Most or All of the Sucrase-Isomaltase Molecules Protrude towards the Luminal Side of the Brush Border Membranes 132
Is There Any Functional Interaction between the Catalytic Sites of the Sucrase-Isomaltase Complex and the Hydrophobic Layer of the Native Brush Border Membrane? 133
What Macromolecular Differences Exist between Triton-solubilized and Papain-solubilized Sucrase-Isomaltase Complex? 133
The Chemical Difference(s) between Triton-solubilized and Papain-solubilized Sucrase-Isomaltase 137
Some Questions on the Biosynthesis of the Sucrase-Isomaltase Complex 140

VITAMIN

UPTAKE AND UTILIZATION OF THIAMINE IN LIVING ORGANISMS
Y. NOSE, A. IWASHIMA, AND Y. WAKABAYASHI 143
General Properties of the Thiamine Uptake System in Microorganisms 144
Properties of Thiamine Uptake by Mammalian Systems 147
Thiamine Transport and Thiamine-binding Protein 152

METABOLISM OF FLAVINS
J. OKUDA AND K. YAGI 155
Biosynthesis of Flavin Nucleotides in Mammalian Tissues 155
Exchange of Flavins in Higher Animals 158

STRUCTURAL STUDIES OF FLAVOPROTEINS
K. T. YASUNOBU AND M. TANAKA 161
Group I and Group II Flavodoxins 161
Amino Acid Composition of *Azotobacter* Flavodoxin 161
Amino Acid Sequence of *Azotobacter* Flavodoxin 162
Calculated Conformation of the *Azotobacter* Flavodoxin 165
Active Site Comparison of the *Azotobacter* Flavodoxin 166
Distribution of Hydrophobic, Neutral, and Ionic Residues 168

Recent Progress with the *A. nidulans* Flavodoxin 169
Structural Studies of Other Flavoproteins 169
Concluding Remarks 169

METHIONINE SYNTHETASE: CHARACTERIZATION OF PROTEIN COMPONENTS AND MECHANISMS FOR ACTIVATION AND CATALYSIS
K. FUJII AND F. M. HUENNEKENS 173
Methionine Synthetase from *E. coli* K-12 174
Activation System in *E. coli* K-12 174
Transfer of Reducing Equivalents 176
B_{12} Intermediates of the Catalytic Cycle 179
Mechanisms for Activation and Catalysis 182

STRUCTURE-FUNCTION INTERRELATIONSHIP OF COENZYME B_{12} (ADENOSYLCOBALAMIN) IN DIOL DEHYDRASE SYSTEM
S. FUKUI AND T. TORAYA 185

ENZYMATIC MODIFICATION OF PROTEINS BY NICOTINAMIDE ADENINE DINUCLEOTIDE
K. UEDA, H. OKAYAMA, AND O. HAYAISHI 195

VITAMIN A TRANSPORT IN PLASMA AND CONTROL OF ITS METABOLISM BY THYROXINE
M. K. BHAT, K. SREEKRISHNA, AND H. R. CAMA 207
Mode of Vitamin A Transport for Embryonic Development: Characterization of RBP, PA, and PA-RBP from Duck Egg Yolk and Demonstration of Their Identity with the Plasma Counter Parts 208
Thyrodial Control of Vitamin A Metabolism 210

THE METABOLISM AND MECHANISM OF ACTION OF VITAMIN D
H. F. DELUCA 219
The Origin of Vitamin D in Skin 220
The Metabolism of Vitamin D to Its Active Hormone 1,25-$(OH)_2D_3$ 220
24-Hydroxylation and Its Significance 222
Regulation of 1,25-$(OH)_2D_3$ Production 223
Mechanism of Action of 1,25-$(OH)_2D_3$ 226

POSSIBLE ROLE OF VITAMIN D IN CALCIUM ABSORPTION IN INTESTINE
S. MORIUCHI AND N. HOSOYA 231

UNSTABLE PROTEIN IN MAMMALIAN CELLS SYNTHESISED IN THE PRESENCE OF AMINO ACID ANALOGS OR UNDER CONDITIONS OF AMINO ACID IMBALANCE

F. J. BALLARD, C. S. CHANDLER, AND S. E. KNOWLES
CSIRO Division of Human Nutrition, Adelaide (Australia)

Labile proteins can be produced in *E. coli* strains which have a requirement for an amino acid by the substitution of a structural analog for the amino acid in the growth medium.[1] The relative stability of proteins fromed by this procedure will depend on the extent to which the analog is substituted and thus the degree of structural abnormality produced in the protein. In general, only those analogs which can charge tRNA will be incorporated and produce modified protein chains. Recently, we and others have shown that mammalian cells incubated in media lacking an essential amino acid are also capable of synthesising labile proteins in the presence of an analog to the omitted amino acid.[2,3] Although amino acid analogs are a convenient way of producing abnormal proteins, it is quite likely that such proteins are more normal events arising from translational errors in protein synthesis as well as from post-translational modifications. This concept is well established in bacteria, where mutants with reduced fidelity in protein synthesis have been isolated. The situation is less definite in higher organisms. However, one experimental finding consistent with translational errors in mammalian cells is the rapid degradation of approximately 10% of protein synthesised after a brief labelling period. This result has been found with several cell types and may be indicative of errors in translation followed by a "proof-reading" mechanism which detects and degrades the error proteins.[2,4,5] The experiments described in the following sections summarise our approach to an understanding of mechanisms responsible for the synthesis and breakdown of several types of abnormal proteins.

AMINO ACID SUBSTITUTIONS

We have tested a wide range of naturally-occurring and synthetic analogs for their ability to alter protein breakdown in mammalian cells. Our aims in these studies were to (a) determine the extent to which analogs modified the degradation rate, (b) look for tissue-specific effects, and (c) provide indirect evidence for the insertion of the analog into proteins. The experimental procedure used was incubation of reticulocytes in a complete medium containing ^{3}H-leucine, with various concentrations of the analog replacing the normal amino acid. After labelling for 30 min, the cells were washed, transferred to fresh medium and degradation of ^{3}H-protein was followed for 2 hr. A similar

Abbreviations: PEPCK, phosphoenolpyruvate carboxykinase; L-DOPA, L-dihydroxyphenylalanine; TCA, trichloracetic acid.

TABLE I

EFFECTS OF AMINO ACID ANALOGS ON PROTEIN DEGRADATION AND PEPCK HEAT LABILITY

Labelled protein was synthesised in the presence of complete medium minus individual amino acids and with analogs added, usually at a concentration of 2mM. Those analogs which decreased protein labelling in comparison to controls with the normal amino acid omitted are indicated by superscript 1. Stimulation of protein synthesis is indicated by superscript 2. Although azetidine-2-carboxylic acid behaves as a proline analog in hepatoma cells, it competes with alanine and not proline in rat reticulocytes. Degradation of labelled protein was followed for 2 hr. Analogs which increased protein degradation above that occurring in controls are indicated by + (slight effect) or ++ (large effect). PEPCK heat lability was measured at 42° using cytosol fractions prepared from Reuber cells which had been incubated for 16 hr in the presence of analogs, usually at a concentration of 2 mM, with dibutyryl cyclic AMP, dexamethazone and theophylline added in order to induce the enzyme.[6] Small (+) or large (++) increases in lability are indicated.

	Effect on protein degradation in		*PEPCK lability*
	reticulocytes	*hepatoma*	
Proline analogs			
L-Thioproline	+[1]	0	0
4-Hydroxy-L-proline	0	0	0
L-Pipecolic acid	0	0	0
5-Hydroxy-L-pipecolic acid	+[1]	0	0
3,4-Dehydro-L-proline	0	0	++
L-Azetidine-2-carboxylic acid	++	++[1]	++
Tyrosine or phenylalanine analogs			
L-Mimosine	0	N.D.*	0
β-2-Thienyl-DL-alanine	0[2]	0	+
DL-2-Fluorophenylalanine	0[2]	+	+
DL-3-Fluorophenylalanine	0[2]	+	++
DL-4-Aminophenylalanine	0	0	0
DL-α-Aminophenyl-acetic acid	0	0	0
2-Thiazolyl-DL-alanine	++[2]	0	0
L-Dihydroxyphenylalanine	+[1]	0	+
Arginine analogs			
L-Canavanine	0[2]	++	++
L-Indospicine	0[2]	+	++
L-Homoarginine	0	N.D.	0
Histidine analogs			
L-Histidinol	+[1]	0[1]	+
DL-1,2,4-Triazol-3-alanine	+[2]	+[2]	+
1-Methyl-L-histidine	0	N.D.	0
3-Methyl-L-histidine	0	N.D.	0

*N.D., not determined.

procedure was used for the Reuber H35 hepatoma cells in monolayer culture except for an increase in the labelling period to 4 hr. Since the specific activity of ^{3}H-leucine in newly-synthesised protein was also measured, we were able to tell whether the analog replaced the normal amino acid in protein synthesis.

Of the analogs tested in Table I with reticulocytes, thienylalanine, 2- and 3-fluorophenylalanine and thiazolylalanine increased protein synthesis above that found when tyrosine and phenylalanine were omitted from the medium; canavanine and indospicine similarly increased labelling in arginine-deficient medium, and triazolalanine increased labelling in histidine-deficient medium. Only triazolalanine increased protein labelling in hepatoma cells.

Since PEPCK is present in hepatoma cells at a low basal activity and can be induced to a high activity by cyclic AMP, the heat lability of enzyme formed in the presence of an analog can be readily tested. Further, heat-labile enzyme would only be expected when analogs are actually incorporated into the enzyme. Thus, both this procedure and the stimulus of protein labelling by an analog provide indirect evidence for incorporation of the analog in place of the normal amino acid.

The amino acids which give rise to labile proteins or labile PEPCK are indicated in Table I. Several types of effect can be distinguished:

Type 1 analogs produce labile proteins after being incorporated. In this group we include all the analogs which affect PEPCK stability as well as those which increase protein labelling in either reticulocytes or hepatoma cells, *viz.*, dehydroproline, azetidine carboxylic acid, thienylalanine, 2- and 3-fluorophenylalanine, thiazolylalanine, L-DOPA, canavanine, indospicine, histidinol, and triazolalanine. Although most of these amino acids are known to be substrates of tRNA-acylating enzymes in bacterial or other systems, L-DOPA and histidinol are more difficult to explain. Some comments on histidinol are given in a later section. It should be noted that some analogs have large effects on reticulocytes but not in hepatoma cells (*e.g.*, thiazolylalanine), while several produce labile PEPCK or hepatoma protein but do not affect reticulocyte proteins.

Type 2 analogs produce labile reticulocyte or hepatoma protein without any evidence of incorporation. Analogs in this group do not affect PEPCK lability and usually inhibit protein labelling. Examples are thioproline and hydroxypipecolic acid. These analogs will be considered below in the section on amino acid omissions.

Type 3 analogs show evidence of incorporation into protein but do not produce labile proteins. These analogs presumably do not modify the structure of proteins in which they are incorporated to a sufficient extent to target the abnormal protein for rapid degradation. None of the analogs qualify for this category when data on both reticulocytes and hepatoma cells are considered, although thienylalanine and the fluorophenylalanines stimulate protein synthesis in reticulocytes without producing labile proteins.

Type 4 analogs show no effects on protein degradation or synthesis and must be considered as non-substrates for the tRNA acylation enzymes.

The most interesting analogs from a biochemical and nutritional standpoint are those type 1 analogs which are naturally occurring. Two such analogs, canavanine and indospicine (see Fig. 1) are present in legumes, plant species which are potentially useful foods. Indeed some legumes contain up to 5% of their dry weight as free canavanine.[7] Both arginine analogs are particularly toxic to liver cells because they can be present at very much higher concentration than arginine. This competitive situation arises because arginine is maintained at very low levels in liver by the high activity of arginase, while neither indospicine nor canavanine are good substrates for arginase. Feeding indospicine to rats leads to severe liver damage even when only small amounts are given.[8] The significance of this finding is also borne out by our heat lability measurements on hepatoma PEPCK. The enzyme has a heat inactivation rate up to 20 times more rapid than the normal enzyme, and even when indospicine is included in the culture medium at concentrations as low as 10 μM, a significant increase in lability is found (S. E. Knowles and F. J. Ballard, unpublished experiments). The lack of toxic effects found with canavanine or indospicine

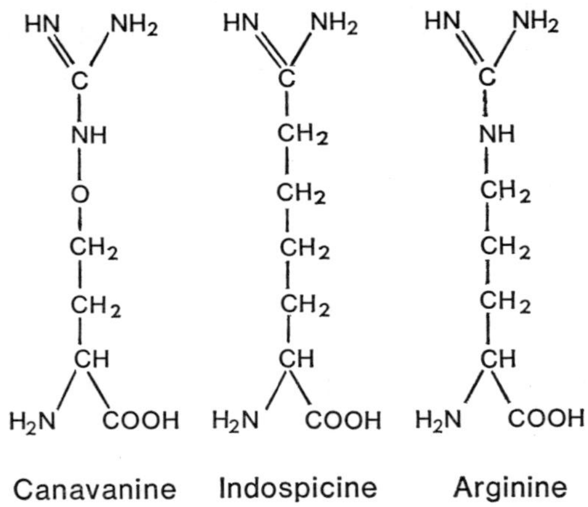

Fig. 1. Structures of the arginine analogs, canavanine and indospicine.

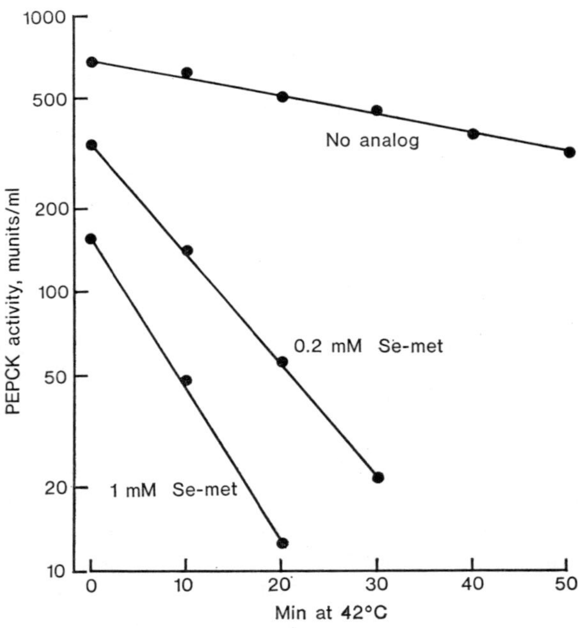

Fig. 2. Heat inactivation of normal and selenomethionyl-PEPCK in Reuber hepatoma cells. Enzyme was induced and the heat lability measured as described in the legend to Table I (see also 6). Se-met, selenomethionine.

in reticulocytes is presumably a result of the relatively high residual arginine concentrations in this cell type.

Canavanine is not incorporated into the protein of plant species which accumulate the analog, an adaptation resulting from a mutation in the tRNA synthetase in those species.[9] Indeed a similar mutation has been reported in the tRNA synthetase of bruchid beetles which live on seeds containing 13% canavanine by weight. In addition to their altered tRNA synthetase, the beetles have arginase together with an extraordinarily high activity of urease,[10] thus permitting the use of urea nitrogen. Clearly these adaptations offer a selective advantage to the insects.

Azetidine carboxylic acid, like canavanine, occurs as a free amino acid in substantial amounts. Again producer species such as lily-of-the-valley, cannot incorporate the analog in place of proline.[9] The analog leads to a large increase in haemoglobin degradation in reticulocytes, but surprisingly it behaves as an alanine analog rather than a proline analog (Table I). We have no evidence for the incorporation of azetidine carboxylic acid into reticulocyte protein in place of alanine, but the protein formed in its presence is extremely labile with up to 50% being degraded during a subsequent incubation of the cells. In the hepatoma cells azetidine carboxylic acid reacts as a proline analog and again produces large changes in protein lability.

Two analog amino acids not listed in Table I are the selenium derivatives selenocysteine and selenomethionine. These two amino acids are present at low concentrations in cells, are substrates for the cysteine-or methionine-specific tRNA synthetases respectively, and may be the means by which selenium is incorporated into proteins. Incorporation of both analogs occurs into reticulocyte protein and hepatoma protein to produce labile proteins. Thus PEPCK induced in the presence of either analog is extremely heat-labile, as illustrated for selenomethionine in Fig. 2. Yet selenomethionine does not change the degradation rate of total hepatoma protein even at concentrations which produce a 10-fold increase in the heat lability of PEPCK. Further, measurements of PEPCK degradation did not show that the heat-labile enzyme was selectively degraded by the intact cells. Presumably, therefore, the modifications to the enzyme structure resulting from selenomethionine incorporation do not lead to changes in conformation that can be detected by the proteolytic pathways of the cell.

NUTRITIONAL SIGNIFICANCE OF ANALOG AMINO ACIDS

Analog amino acids which either inhibit protein synthesis or can be incorporated into proteins might reduce the growth rate of organisms or lead to altered properties of enzymes and other cellular proteins. This could be a serious problem if the analog in question is present at high concentrations in feed and also if the analog is a good substrate or potent inhibitor of tRNA acylation. Incorporation into protein is explained since a tRNA molecule charged with an analog amino acid is not distinguished from correctly charged tRNA in subsequent reactions in protein synthesis. Accordingly any selection against the analog must occur at the tRNA acylation reaction, or at an earlier step in protein synthesis such as transport into the cell. The different types of antimetabolite actions by which analog amino acids can exert their effects have been reviewed recently.[9]

Even if a non-protein amino acid is a good substrate for tRNA acylation and is also present at high concentrations in the diet, deleterious effects on the animal may not be seen. Thus, unless some key enzymes or other proteins are modified to the extent that their functions are altered, an increase in degradation rate will remove the abnormal protein and permit the organism to synthesise new protein molecules. However, even this response would be nutritionally important because the increased rate of protein turnover would require an increased energy expenditure. Although we have no useful information on the magnitude of any increase in nutritional requirements, it could become significant when substantial amounts of an analog are incorporated.

A more drastic effect of analog amino acids than an increase in energy requirements is the production of toxic symptoms. Mention has already been made of the selective advantage which arginine analogs have in mammalian liver. Thus ingestion of food containing canavanine or indospicine leads to liver damage because the arginine in liver is maintained at very low levels.[7,8] Indeed the toxicity of plant species which contain the analogs, for example *Dioclea megacarpa* or *Indigofera spicata*, is largely caused by their canavanine or indospicine content respectively.

IMBALANCES OF NORMAL AMINO ACIDS

It is essential for optimal rates of protein synthesis that all amino acids are present at concentrations sufficiently high to maintain each tRNA in the charged form. Thus drastic reduction in the concentration of a single amino acid will reduce protein synthesis by an amount dependent on both the degree to which the tRNA is present in the uncharged state and also the proportion of the amino acid in the protein being synthesised. For example, omission of histidine or valine from the medium in which reticulocytes are incubated produces a marked reduction in haemoglobin synthesis, while isoleucine or arginine omission has little if any effect (see Table II).

In order to provide controls in studies with analogs, we labelled protein with ^{3}H-leucine with single amino acids left out of the reticulocyte labelling medium, and subsequently measured degradation. As well as an inhibition of protein synthesis when some amino acids were omitted, the reduced amount of protein formed was unstable, often to the extent seen with amino acid analogs. Further, a negative correlation is seen between protein labelling and protein degradation (Table II). This surprising result could possibly be explained if haemoglobin synthesis was preferentially inhibited when single amino acids

TABLE II

EFFECTS OF SINGLE AMINO ACID OMISSIONS ON PROTEIN SYNTHESIS AND BREAKDOWN IN RETICULOCYTES

Protein was labelled in rat reticulocytes in the presence of a complete medium with amino acids added at concentrations equivalent to those occurring in rat plasma. Single amino acids were omitted. Labelling for 30 min in the presence of ^{3}H-leucine was followed by rapid washing of the cells. Degradation in complete medium was then measured over a 2-hr period.

Amino acid omitted	*Protein synthesis (% of control)*	*Protein degradation (% in 2 hr)*
None	100	6.6
Isoleucine	91	7.1
Arginine	80	7.1
Phenylalanine	68	8.8
Lysine	53	11.0
Valine	27	18.9
Histidine	21	24.2

TABLE III

CHANGES IN PROTEIN SYNTHESIS AND PROTEIN BREAKDOWN CAUSED BY INHIBITION OF PROTEIN SYNTHESIS

These experiments were carried out as indicated in the legend to Table II. Inhibitors were added only during the labelling period.

Inhibitor	*Protein synthesis (% of control)*	*Protein degradation (% in 2 hr)*
None	100	3.3
His omission	17	14.0
Histidinol 3mM, his omission	8	27.6
Cycloheximide, 30 μM	7	8.0
Cycloheximide, 3 μM	22	5.7
NaF, 30 mM	10	5.6

were left out of the labelling medium, leaving a labile protein or proteins. However, chromatography of the labelled protein on Sephadex columns or electrophoresis in the presence of sodium dodecyl sulphate gave good evidence for the labelling of haemoglobin or slightly shortened haemoglobin molecules. Accordingly we believe that omission of certain amino acid leads to a modified haemoglobin.

There does not seem to be any obvious mechanism how an abnormal protein could be produced simply by reducing the content of a single amino acid. Reduction in the content of charged $tRNA_{his}$ as compared to uncharged $tRNA_{his}$ might be expected to lower protein synthesis rates, but mischarging of the tRNA with other amino acids or substitutions of other charged tRNA species at positions coded for by histidine triplets seems unlikely. Yet the fraction of labile protein formed when histidine is omitted is quite substantial and is further increased when histidinol, an inhibitor of histidine charging to tRNA, is included in the labelling medium (Table III).

One possible explanation for the production of labile haemoglobin is that inhibition of protein synthesis by any inhibitor, not just by reduction of the proportion of tRNA in the charged form, will lead to an accelerated protein degradation. Inhibition of reticulocyte protein synthesis by cycloheximide or fluoride does indeed give rise to labile protein (Table III), but the increase in lability is well below that found when protein synthesis is inhibited by the reduction of tRNA charging produced by histidine omission or addition of histidinol. Since histidinol is not an amino acid, it cannot be incorporated in place of histidine, even if it could be charged by $tRNA_{his}$. However, any resultant uncharged $tRNA_{his}$ could bind to the ribosome at the "A" site in place of charged $tRNA_{his}$. Protein synthesis would then be stopped until the uncharged $tRNA_{his}$ was replaced by charged $tRNA_{his}$. However, although this would reduce the rate of protein synthesis, it is hard to envisage how a labile protein could be formed. Perhaps the growing peptide might "skip" the histidine coding triplet and give rise to a protein shortened by the absence of a histidine residue; but there is no evidence for a reaction of this type.

Incubation of histidinol with hepatoma cells in the presence of cyclic AMP results in the induction of a labile form of PEPCK. This finding is also hard to reconcile unless histidinol produces a modification to PEPCK such as a substitution of an amino acid for histidine or a histidine deletion, as suggested above. An alternate possibility is for histidinol to have an effect unrelated to protein synthesis, perhaps a stimulation of the breakdown of cellular proteins not restricted to proteins being synthesized during the labelling period.

Should this occur, it would be analogous to the stringent response in bacteria, a process which gives rise to a number of effects including the breakdown of cell protein. We have tested whether a "stringent"-type of response occurs in reticulocytes starved of histidine, by prelabelling reticulocyte protein before addition of histidinol. Under these conditions the pre-existing protein remains stable, since only that protein made in the presence of histidinol is degraded. Therefore the mechanism by which histidine starvation produces labile protein remains obscure.

REGULATION OF THE BREAKDOWN OF LABILE PROTEINS

Lysosomes are thought to be a site for the breakdown of intracellular proteins, because of their high content of proteolytic enzymes, and also by analogy with the known involvement of lysosomes in the catabolism of proteins pinocytosed into cells.[3] Since direct evidence for this hypothesis has been elusive, more indirect approaches have been attempted.

We have quantified degradation of canavanine-containing protein and normal protein in hepatoma cells by a double label technique.[2] Normal proteins were first labelled with ^{14}C-leucine, after which the medium was changed to an arginine-free, canavanine-containing medium with ^{3}H-leucine added. Following the second labelling period, the cells were thoroughly washed and placed in a medium containing 2mM leucine to restrict

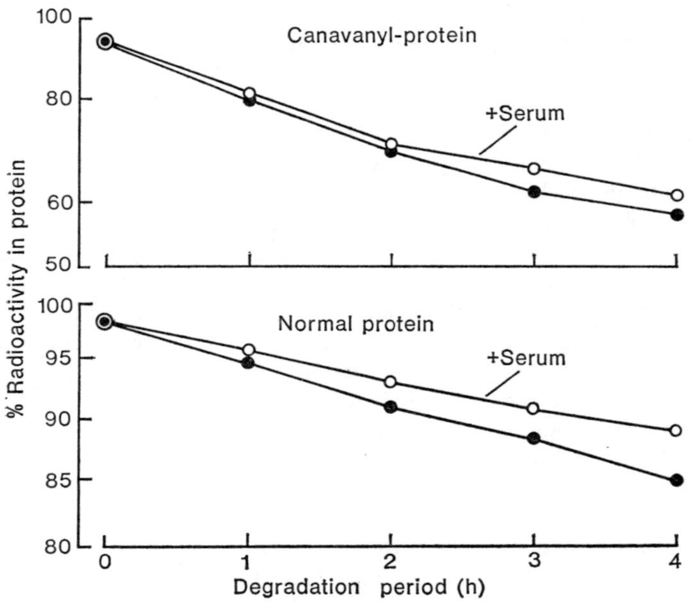

Fig. 3. Degradation of normal protein and canavanyl-protein in Reuber hepatoma cells. Normal and canavanyl-protein was labelled sequentially in hepatoma cells, after which the degradation of both protein types was followed in cells incubated in serum-free medium or medium with 10% fetal calf serum added.[2]

isotope reincorporation. Production of TCA-soluble radioactivity and loss of TCA-insoluble radioactivity was followed during the degradation period (see Fig. 3).

From the experiment shown in Fig. 3 and others similar, it was evident that the rapid degradation of canavanyl protein continued for approximately 2 hr. Accordingly we chose to compare the breakdown of normal and canavanyl protein over the initial 2 hr of degradation. The effects of various nutrients, hormones, and putative inhibitors were tested on the breakdown of both types of protein in the same cells.

The addition of fetal calf serum to the degradation medium reduced breakdown of normal proteins by approximately 25% at all time periods (Fig. 3), whereas no significant inhibition on the breakdown of canavanyl protein could be detected at least during the period of rapid catabolism. In order to see whether the lack of effect on the breakdown of abnormal protein is a general response to agents which reduce the degradation rate of normal proteins, a range of inhibitors have been tested (Table IV). With the exception of inhibitors of overall cellular metabolism, such as NaF or dinitrophenol, the compounds tested selectively reduce the degradation of normal proteins with little effect on canavanyl proteins. Further, none of the inhibitors were additive even though they would be expected to have quite different mechanisms of action. Thus hormones (*e.g.*, insulin), inhibitors of protein synthesis (*e.g.*, cycloheximide), and proteolytic inhibitors (*e.g.*, leupeptin) all reduced the breakdown rate of normal proteins by about 30% when added as single compounds or in combination. Slightly greater extents of inhibition were found when the weak base ammonia was present.

Although the evidence is by no means conclusive, it is probable that the four types of inhibitor act by preventing lysosomal protein breakdown *via* an inhibition of the autophagic engulfing process. In searching for mechanisms to explain the effects of such apparently diverse compounds, an effect on autophagy appears reasonable. Insulin is known to prevent the formation of autophagic vacuoles while glucagon has the opposite

TABLE IV

ACTION OF INHIBITORS ON THE BREAKDOWN OF NORMAL AND CANAVANYL-PROTEIN IN HEPATOMA CELLS

Normal proteins were labelled with ^{14}C-leucine for 16 hr, after which the hepatoma cells were transferred to an arginine-free medium with 0.5 mM canavanine and ^{3}H-leucine added for a further 3 hr. Degradation of both ^{3}H- and ^{14}C-labelled protein was then measured over a 2 hr-period in the presence of the various listed compounds. The percentage inhibition of degradation caused by each agent is indicated as the mean effect ± SEM.[11]

Additions	*% inhibition of the degradation of*	
	Normal proteins	*Canavanine-containing proteins*
Insulin, 7nM	28±2	5±1
Cycloheximide, 0.1 mM	27±3	9±2
Leupeptin, 50 μg/ml	33±3	9±2
NH_4Cl, 5mM	44±2	11±2
Insulin+cycloheximide	30±2	12±3
Leupeptin+insulin	34±1	7±2
Leupeptin+cycloheximide	34±2	11±2
NH_4Cl+insulin	43±3	14±3
NH_4Cl+cycloheximide	43±4	18±1
NaF, 2mM	19±3	18±1

effect.[12,13] A possible explanation is a prevention of synthesis of membrane proteins by insulin. Such a hypothesis would also account for the action of cycloheximide, since this inhibitor of protein synthesis has also been shown to lead to a reduction in lysosome activity.[14] Both leupeptin and ammonia reduce the proteolytic process itself. Leupeptin is effective because of its inhibitory action on cathepsin B, one of the principal proteases in lysosomes, while ammonia diffuses into lysosomes, where it is protonated to the non-diffusible ammonium ion. This increases the intralysosomal pH and prevents the action of the proteases which have acid pH optima. Our interpretation of the inhibitions noted in Table IV is that the autophagic lysosomal system accounts for 30–40% of the breakdown of normal proteins and is fully inhibited by each of the agents tested. By this mechanism additive effects would not be expected (see Fig. 4).

If 30% of protein breakdown occurs *via* the autophagic process, how can the other 70% be accounted for? A minimal hypothesis to explain the results is illustrated in Fig. 4. We envisage two distinct pathways of protein breakdown. In addition to autophagic proteolysis, which might not distinguish between abnormal and normal proteins, there must be a second pathway to account for the remaining degradation. What is the nature of this pathway? Unfortunately it is poorly characterised at present, although several non-lysosomal proteases have been identified. Yet some information on the pathway can be predicted. For example, it probably has an excess proteolytic capacity with the degradation rate of each protein being a property of the protein itself. Such a "substrate-regulated" pathway is needed to explain the heterogeneity of protein degradation rates. Thus analog-containing and other short-lived proteins would be good substrates while long-lived proteins would be poor substrates. Although the individual reactions of this pathway are not characterised, it is possible that initial steps are a denaturation-like process, followed by the binding of proteins to intracellular membranes.[15-17] The intracellular site of the actual proteolytic reactions may be the lysosome, but other proteases could also be involved.[18] Indeed recent experiments by Etlinger and Goldberg[19] and ourselves (C. S. Chandler and F. J. Ballard,

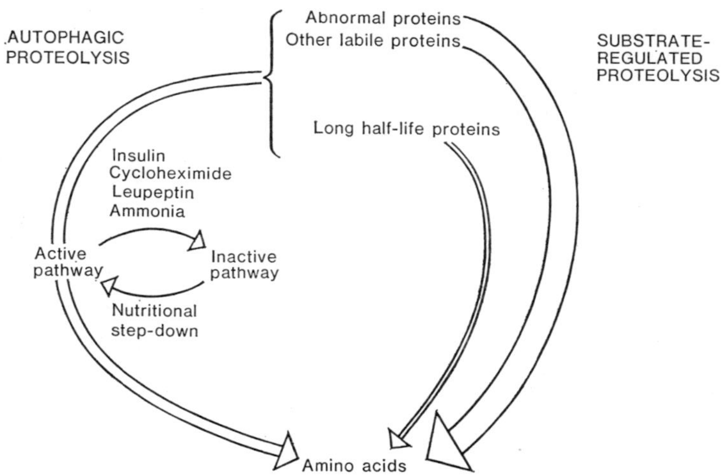

Fig. 4. A hypothesis to explain selective controls on the degradation of normal, long-lived proteins and not affecting abnormal protein or other short-lived proteins.[11]

unpublished experiments) suggest the existence of proteolytic enzymes with specificity towards analog-containing and other unstable proteins. These enzymes may be cytosolic or microsomal and may account for the substrate-regulated pathway. A major goal at the present time is the isolation and characterisation of degradative enzymes and the establishment of a function independent from the lysosomal autophagic process.

REFERENCES

1 A. L. GOLDBERG and J. F. DICE, *Annu. Rev. Biochem.*, 43 (1974) 835.
2 S. E. KNOWLES, J. M. GUNN, R. W. HANSON, and F. J. BALLARD, *Biochem. J.*, 146 (1975) 595.
3 A. L. GOLDBERG and A. C. ST. JOHN, *Annu. Rev. Biochem.*, 45 (1976) 747.
4 B. POOLE and M. WIBO, *J. Biol. Chem.*, 248 (1973) 6221.
5 M. O. BRADLEY, L. HAYFLICK, and R. T. SCHIMKE, *J. Biol. Chem.*, 251 (1976) 3521.
6 S. E. KNOWLES, J. M. GUNN, L. RESHEF, R. W. HANSON, and F. J. BALLARD, *Biochem. J.*, 146 (1975) 585.
7 E. A. BELL, *FEBS Lett.*, 64 (1976) 29.
8 G. S. CHRISTIE, M. WILSON, and M. P. HEGARTY, *J. Pathol.*, 117 (1975) 195.
9 L. FOWDEN, *Res. Adv. Phytochem.*, 8 (1974) 95.
10 G. A. ROSENTHAL, D. H. JANZEN, D. L. DAHLMAN, *Science*, 196 (1977) 658.
11 S. E. KNOWLES and F. J. BALLARD, *Biochem. J.*, 156 (1976) 609.
12 A. U. ARSTILA, J. D. SHELBURNE, and B. F. TRUMP, *Lab. Invest.*, 27 (1972) 317.
13 A. N. NEELY, P. B. NELSON, and G. E. MORTIMORE, *Biochem. Biophys. Acta*, 338 (1974) 458.
14 K. WILDENTHAL and E. E. GRIFFIN, *Biochim. Biophys. Acta*, 444 (1976) 519.
15 F. J. BALLARD, M. F. HOPGOOD, L. RESHEF, and R. W. HANSON, *Biochem. J.*, 140 (1974) 521.
16 M. F. HOPGOOD and F. J. BALLARD, *Biochem. J.*, 144 (1974) 371.
17 F. J. BALLARD and M. F. HOPGOOD, *Biochem. J.*, 154 (1976) 717.
18 E. Kominami and N. KATUNUMA, *Eur. J. Bioclem.*, 62 (1976) 425.
19 J. D. ETLINGER and A. L. GOLDBERG, *Proc. Natl. Acad. Sci. U.S.*, 74 (1977) 54.

UTILIZATION OF LIMITING AMINO ACIDS FOR PROTEIN SYNTHESIS IN AMINO ACID IMBALANCE

AKIRA YOSHIDA
Department of Agricultural Chemistry, Nagoya University, Nagoya (Japan)

The elucidation of the mechanisms of amino acid imbalances is important for the nutritional evaluation of food proteins and also as the basis for amino acid supplementation. According to Elvehjem and Harper,[1,2] amino acid imbalance is generally defined as adverse effects produced by an addition of amino acids, and the effects can be recovered by a supplementation of the limiting amino acid. Adverse effects may be growth depression, liver fat accumulation, or in some cases vitamin deficiency. Depression of body protein synthesis, inhibition of absorption of a limiting amino acid or increased catabolism of a limiting amino acid are easily expected from the word "amino acid imbalance." However, the fact is not so simple.

Amino acid imbalance is created by adding to a low protein diet an essential amino acid mixture lacking one. Altered plasma and tissue amino acid patterns, especially a significant reduction in the concentration of the most limiting amino acid accompanying the reduction of food intake and growth retardation, are observed in one type of amino acid imbalance. The rapid decrease in the plasma concentration in rats fed the amino acid imbalanced diet may be produced by decreased rate of absorption, increased degradation, or increased utilization of limiting amino acid for body protein synthesis.

To test these possibilities trained rats were fed a single meal of basal low casein diet or imbalanced diets which are the basal diet supplemented with essential amino acid mixture lacking threonine or histidine, and the tracer amount of ^{14}C-threonine or ^{14}C-histidine was included. Animals took about 10 g of the diet within a short time.[3] In both the control group and the imbalanced group, the absorption of ^{14}C-threonine or ^{14}C-histidine were almost the same; there was no indication of inhibition of intestinal absorption of the amino acid by imbalanced composition of amino acids.

Plasma level of ^{14}C-free threonine increased after feeding the basal diet or threonine imbalanced diet similarly, reaching the maximum level 2 to 3 hr after feeding diets, and then gradually decreased. The disappearance of ^{14}C-threonine from plasma was more rapid in the imbalanced group.

Expired carbon dioxide was collected for 48 hr after feeding diets. ^{14}C in expired carbondioxide was rather less for the imbalanced group indicating no increase in threonine degradation in the imbalanced group.

Unexpectedly, the incorporation of ^{14}C-threonine into liver protein for the imbalanced group was increased as compared with the control group. In the histidine imbalance, this increase in the ^{14}C-histidine incorporation into liver protein was more significant, and the ^{14}C in acid-soluble fraction was inversely reduced in the imbalanced group. These results may indicate of the increased utilization of threonine for protein synthesis in the liver for the imbalanced group at the initial stage of the intake of the imbalanced diet.

On the other hand, incorporation of ^{14}C-threonine or ^{14}C-histidine into whole muscle tissue was reduced in the imbalanced groups, while the incorporation into protein fraction was rather increased for both threonine-imbalanced and histidine-imbalanced groups. Thus, the supplies of the limiting amino acid increased in the liver and decreased in muscle, while the utilization of the limiting amino acid for protein synthesis were rather increased in both tissues accompanying the significant decrease in plasma level of free threonine or histidine, and this may relate to the depression of food intake as Harper suggested.[4]

Liver polysome aggregation in rats fed an amino acid-imbalanced diet were studied by Pronczuk *et al.*[5] and also by Ip and Harper.[6] When the tissue pool of a limiting amino acid had not been depleted prior to feeding of the experimental diets, ingestion of the imbalanced diet stimulated polysome aggregation and ^{14}C-leucine incorporation into liver protein more than did the ingestion of the basal diet.

We further studied the utilization of the limiting amino acid using other type of amino acid-imbalanced diet. In this case, rats were fed either an 8% casein basal diet or the methionine-supplemented imbalanced diet for 1 week. Diets were supplied *ad libitum.*

Body weight gain of the imbalanced group was higher than that of the basal diet group. However, liver fat began to accumulate within 1 week. Highest accumulation of liver fat was observed after 2–3 weeks on the imbalanced diet. This liver fat accumulation can be protected by the supplementation of threonine to the imbalanced diet. Plasma level of free threonine—that is, the limiting amino acid—is significantly reduced by feeding the imbalanced diet. Accompanying this decrease in the level of threonine, free serine and glycine were also reduced.

Rats were administered ^{14}C-threonine orally or by intraperitoneally injection after 1 week on the experimental diets, and were killed 5 hr after the oral administration. Distribution of ^{14}C-threonine in various tissues and tissue proteins was studied. When ^{14}C-threonine was administered orally, the content of ^{14}C-threonine in the tissue of small intestine was higher and that in muscle was lower in the imbalanced group. Incorporation of ^{14}C-threonine into protein fraction was significantly higher for the imbalanced group in small intestine, spleen, liver, and plasma, and the ratios of ^{14}C in protein and free amino acid were also significantly higher in all tissues tested, indicating more exhaustive utilization of limiting amino acid for the imbalanced group.

Distribution of ^{14}C-threonine in subcellular fractions of liver homogenates was also examined. The relative ^{14}C contents in microsomal protein and cytosol proteins were higher for the imbalanced group accompanying the reduction of ^{14}C in free amino acid fraction.

Polyacrylamide gel electrophoresis of liver cytosol proteins was carried out and the patterns of the peaks of proteins indicated the differences between the control and the imbalanced group.

Similar results were obtained when ^{14}C-threonine was intraperitoneally administered. These results indicate the disturbances of limiting amino acid metabolism might occur in various proteins. Fatty liver may be only an example of these metabolic disturbances.

In connection with this type of amino acid imbalance we realized the significant reduction of urinary excretion of nitrogen in rats fed a nonprotein diet supplemented with methionine and threonine, this effect was more significant than methionine alone.[7,8] It is usually assumed that when animals were fed a nonprotein diet, all essential amino acids are equally deficient. However, the supplementation of only methionine or methionine and threonine significantly improved the nitrogen balance. When nonessential amino acids were previously added to a nonprotein diet, the addition of valine, isoleucine, and tryptophan in addition to methionine and threonine further improved the nitrogen balance. These would indicate the sequence of limiting amino acids among the endogenous amino acids.

Finally, I should like to describe one more example of unbalanced utilization of limiting amino acid(tryptophan) for protein synthesis and for niacin formation. This type of amino acid imbalance was originally reported by Krehl *et al*[10]. They indicated niacin deficiency in rats fed a low casein diet supplemented with gelatin or corn grit and two hypotheses were proposed. One is an increased degradation of the limiting amino acid tryptophan by a supplement of tryptophan-deficient protein. Another is the increased tryptophan utilization for protein synthesis leading to niacin deficiency, and the definite answer has not been obtained yet. These hypotheses were examined with other experimental dietary system.[9] We used a basal diet containing an amino acid mixture stimulating the amino acid composition of rice protein in which lysine and threonine are the limiting amino acids followed by tryptophan. Niacin was omitted from the basal diet. On this basal diet, animals could continue to grow. When the limiting amino acids including lysine and threonine were supplemented to the basal diet, animals grew faster than the basal diet group for the first 5 to 6 days. During this period nitrogen balance was also improved by the addition of amino acid mixture. But later, the body weight began to decrease accompanying the reduction of urinary excretion of niacin metabolites. By addition of niacin or tryptophan to this imbalanced diet, the body weight gain was rapidly recovered. These results support the hypothesis that the addition of limiting amino acids except tryptophan to a low protein diet stimulated the utilization tryptophan for protein synthesis leading to its shortage for niacin synthesis. In this type of amino acid imbalance, therefore, unbalanced utilization of tryptophan occurred between protein synthesis and niacin formation.

Thus, in amino acid imbalances, addition of amino acid or amino acid mixture partially stimulates the tissue protein synthesis using the limiting amino acid more exhaustively. This exhaustion of the limiting amino acid may lead to the shortage of tha amino acid in some tissues or tissue proteins and may disturb the normal physiological functions.

REFERENCES

1 C. A. Elvehjem, *Fed. Proc.*, 15 (1956) 965.
2 A. E. Harper, N. J. Benevenga, and R. M. Wohlheuter, *Physiol. Rev.*, 50 (1970) 428.
3 A. Yoshida, P. Leung, Q. R. Rogers, and A. E. Harper, *J. Nutr.*, 89 (1970) 80.
4 A. E. Harper, P. Leung, A. Yoshida, and Q. R. Rogers, *Fed. Proc.*, 23 (1964) 1087.
5 A. W. Pronczuk, Q. R. Rogers, and H. N. Munro, *J. Nutr.*, 100 (1970) 1249.
6 C. C. Y. Ip and A. E. Harper, *J. Nutr.*, 104 (1974) 252.
7 A. Yoshida and K. Moritoki, *Nutr. Rep. Int.*, 9 (1974) 159.
8 H. Yokogoshi, K. Hayase, and A. Yoshida, *J. Nutr.*, 107 (1977) 783.
9 A. Yoshida, *Agric. Biol. Chem.*, 35 (1971) 1943.
10 W. A. Krehl, L. J. Taply, and C. A. Elvehjem, *Science*, 101 (1945) 408.

THE BIOSYNTHESIS OF SECRETORY PROTEINS WITH SPECIAL REFERENCE TO MILK PROTEINS

P. N. CAMPBELL, R. K. CRAIG, AND A. P. BOULTON
Courtauld Institute of Biochemistry, The Middlesex Hospital Medical School, London (England)

In a symposium dealing with the biochemical aspects of nutrition it is appropriate to consider the biosynthesis of proteins and especially the synthesis of secretory proteins. In the case of milk and egg proteins the animal provides these proteins for the young, but man has diverted the proteins for his own use and hence we have the major industries of dairy and poultry. First we will review in general terms some current ideas on the way that proteins come to be secreted from cells and then consider the synthesis of milk proteins in the mammary gland.

A cell such as the hepatocyte synthesizes protein for many different physiological functions as listed in Table I. The purpose of this table is to show that at one end of the spectrum we have secreted proteins and at the other end the soluble proteins of, for example, the glycolytic pathway. Between these extremes we see that proteins are synthesized for many different functions, such as the membrane of the endoplasmic reticulum and the proteins that are packaged in organelles such as the lysosomes. There are also the soluble proteins of the mitochondria which are made on the endoplasmic reticulum and then transported to the mitochondria. It now seems likely that there are certain common characteristics in the way in which proteins are synthesized which are subsequently packaged within membranes, irrespective of whether the protein eventually leaves the cell or whether it is transported within the cell from one organelle to another. Figure 1 shows the pathway for the synthesis and package of secreted proteins in the acinar cell of the pancreas. We see here the role of the rough endoplasmic reticulum and of the Golgi complex in the formation of secretory granules. Although there are certainly differences of detail

TABLE I

PHYSIOLOGICAL FUNCTIONS OF PROTEINS SYNTHESIZED BY EXTRA-MITOCHONDRIAL RIBOSOMES OF PARENCHYMAL LIVER CELL

a)	Export, *e.g.*, plasma protein
b)	Membrane of endoplasmic reticulum
c)	Packaged proteins, *e.g.*, microbodies, lysosomes
d)	Soluble protein for other organelles
e)	Soluble protein for soluble cytoplasm

Abbreviations: ER, endoplasmic reticulum; ATA, aurin tricarboxylic acid; α-LA, α-lactalbumin; CNBr, cyanogen bromide; PTH, parathyroid hormone.

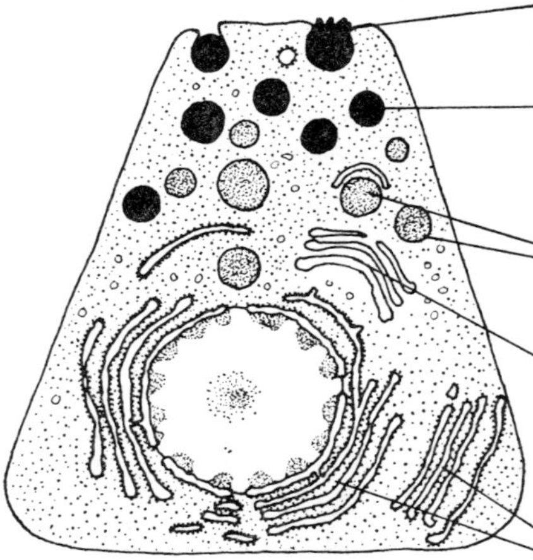

Fig. 1. Pathway for the synthesis and package of secreted proteins in the acinar cell of the pancreas. RER, rough-surfaced endoplasmic reticulum. (Published with permission of Longmans from *Companion to Biochemistry*, vol. 2).

in the way in which proteins are secreted from different kinds of cells, the acinar cell has been taken as a model in this respect.

PROPROTEINS

The discovery of proinsulin showed that a protein may be synthesized in the cell in the form of a precursor and that such a protein is converted from its precursor to the authentic protein during its passage through the Golgi complex. Other examples of proproteins have been discovered since, in particular pro PTH and more recently proalbumin. As shown in Fig. 2 the two latter proproteins involve an extension of the chain at the N-terminus and this extension contains six amino acids of which four are basic. At the present time we do not understand the function of the precursor proteins in the case of pro PTH and proalbumin but it seems likely that their conversion to authentic proteins is an important event in secretion.

THE PRIMARY TRANSLATION PRODUCTS OF SECRETORY PROTEINS

It seems generally accepted that a cell such as the hepatocyte contains two functionally different forms of polyribosomes. On the one hand there are the polyribosomes which are bound to the membrane of the ER (bound polyribosomes) and which are responsible for the synthesis of secreted proteins, and on the other hand there are the

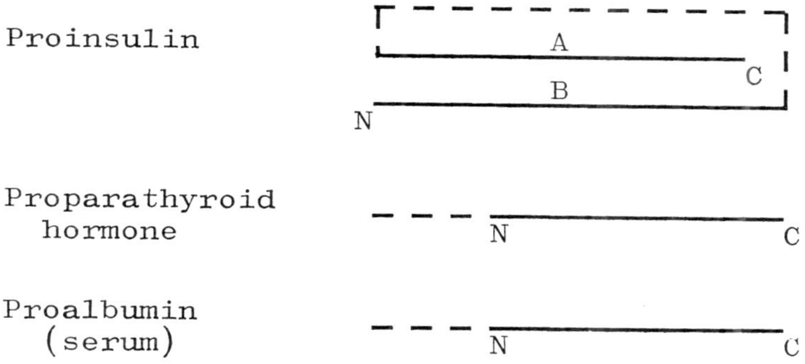

Fig. 2. The structure of some proproteins. N, N-terminus of the polypeptide chains; C, C-terminus of the polypeptide chains.

polyribosomes which are not associated with membrane (free polyribosmes) and which are responsible for the synthesis of the proteins of the cytosol which are retained by the cell. For many years now the problem has been to understand how these two types of polyribosomes arise in the cell. It is possible, following disruption of the cell, to isolate fractions enriched in either free polyribosomes or bound polyribosomes and to examine the ribosomes associated with each of them. Analysis has indicated that there is no major difference between the ribosomes from the free and bound polyribosomes so that the idea has now been accepted that bound polyribosomes can be derived from free polyribosomes.

The larger of the two subunits of the ribosomes is directly associated with the membrane of the ER and three different forms of linkage have been considered to account for this ribosome-membrane interaction. Certainly ionic forces are important for we know that if magnesium ions are removed by treatment of the rough ER with EDTA then the linkage is disrupted; others have suggested that mRNA is important; while others have advanced the role of the nascent polypeptide chain which of course is associated with the larger of the subunits. Our interest is centred on the role of the nascent polypeptide chain.

Most of the mRNA in eukaryotic cells possesses a tail of poly (A) at the 3′ end which allows for poly (A) containing mRNA to be readily isolated from animal cells by affinity chromatography. A number of *in vitro* systems have been devised for the translation of isolated mRNA. These are listed in Table II. The first four are strictly cell-free systems while the *Xenopus* oocyte is of course rather different. You will see that the constituents of these systems with respect to membrane is also indicated. Thus the wheat germ system contains no membrane whereas that from ascites tumour cells does and the *Xenopus* oocyte also contains many membranous vesicles. The endogenous activity of the systems with respect to mRNA varies and you will see that in this respect the reticulocyte system which has been treated with ribonuclease[1] is particularly low. Indeed this is now the favoured system for the translation of heterologous mRNA.

From the results of the isolation of mRNA containing a poly (A) tail from a variety of different animal cells and its subsequent translation in heterologous systems it has become apparent that the primary translation product is in many cases larger than the authentic protein. Some of the recent results are summarized in Table III. You will see that proPTH (for a review see ref. 2) to which we have already referred, is synthesized on the ribosomes

TABLE II

HETEROLOGOUS SYSTEMS FOR THE TRANSLATION OF mRNA

	Endogenous activity	*Membranes*
Wheat germ	Low	None
Ascites tumour	Low	Plenty
Reticulocytes	High	Negligible
Retic. + RNase	Low	Negligible
Xenopus oocyte	Some	Many

TABLE III

THE STRUCTURE OF SOME PROPROTEINS

1)	pre 25 aa	Proparathyroidhormone
2)	pre 23 aa	Proinsulin
3)	pre 15 aa	Myeloma IgG light chain
4)	pre 20–25 aa	Zymogens of pancreas
5)	pre 7–10 aa	α-Lactalbumin
6)	pre	Proalbumin (serum)

as a precursor, preproPTH, with a 23 amino acid extension at the N-terminus. Similarly proinsulin is synthesized as a precursor, preproinsulin. The first protein to be shown to be synthesized as a precursor was the light chain of IgG by Milstein *et al.*[3] Recently several groups have shown that serum albumin is synthesized as preproalbumin.[4] Considerable progress has been made in the determination of the sequence of amino acids in the precursor peptides and these have been shown to be rich in hydrophobic amino acids. The precursor proteins are the sole product of translation in the heterologous systems which contain no membranes; whereas translation in systems which contain membranes will produce both precursor proteins and the proproteins or authentic proteins.

The finding of precursor proteins as the primary translation products of secretory proteins has enabled Blobel and Dobberstein[5] to elaborate a hypothesis which was originally formulated by Blobel and Sabatini[6] and independently by Milstein *et al.*,[3] as to the role of these precursor peptides in the synthesis of secretory proteins. This hypothesis which is known as the "signal hypothesis" is depicted in Fig. 3. The hypothesis predicts that ribosmes in the cell are able to associate with any mRNA in the cytoplasm. Under appropriate conditions the polyribosomes will then be the site of translation of the mRNA and in the case of a secretory protein the nascent polypeptide chain will contain a "signal" peptide. This signal peptide has a particular affinity for the membrane of the ER and hence the polyribosome becomes attached through the signal peptide to the membrane and becomes a bound polyribosome. The mRNA for proteins which are not to be secreted have no signal peptide and are, therefore, synthesized by polyribosomes which remain free. As translation of the mRNA for secretory proteins proceeds so the signal peptide emerges

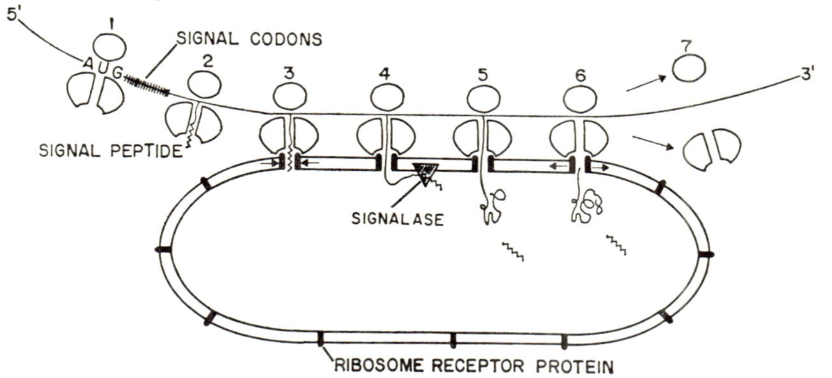

Fig. 3. Blobel's signal hypothesis. A schematic representation of the translation of mRNA for secretory proteins on membrane bound ribosomes and the transfer of the translation products across the microsomal membrane. (From Campbell and Blobel[2] with permisson of *FEBS Lett.*).

TABLE IV

THE BIOSYNTHESIS OF PROTEINS OF EGG-WHITE*

Protein	*% total*	*Mol. wt.*	*Signal peptide*
Ovalbumin	55	42,000	None
Conalbumin	10	26,000	19
Ovomucoid	10	20,000	23
Lysozyme	2	14,500	18

*From the work of Palmiter *et al.*, ref. 7.

into the cisternae of the ER and as it emerges so it is cleaved from the chain. The end result, therefore, is that either the authentic protein or the proprotein appears within the cisternal vesicles of the ER. The enzyme which effects the selective cleavage of the signal peptide has not been fully characterized and the designation "signalase" given in Fig. 3 is preliminary. The hydrophobic nature of the amino acid residues of the signal peptides of the proteins, which have so far been studied, certainly is consistent with the signal hypothesis.

Recently Palmiter *et al.*,[7] have studied the synthesis of egg-white proteins. Their results are summarized in Table IV. This shows that whereas three of the proteins in egg-white are synthesized as precursors, ovalbumin has no signal peptide. The reason for this is not clear although the authors have suggested that the N-acetylation of the N-terminal amino acid and/or glycosylation of the polypeptide chain may be relevant.

THE BIOSYNTHESIS OF MILK PROTEINS

We have been concerned with the synthesis of guinea-pig milk proteins.[8] Figure 4 shows that guinea-pig milk contains only one whey protein, α-LA together with three major caseins which we have designated A, B, and C. Following isolation of mRNA with a poly (A) tail from the lactating mammary gland of the guinea-pig three bands may be demonstrated on polyacrylamide gel electrophoresis in formamide. When this mRNA is

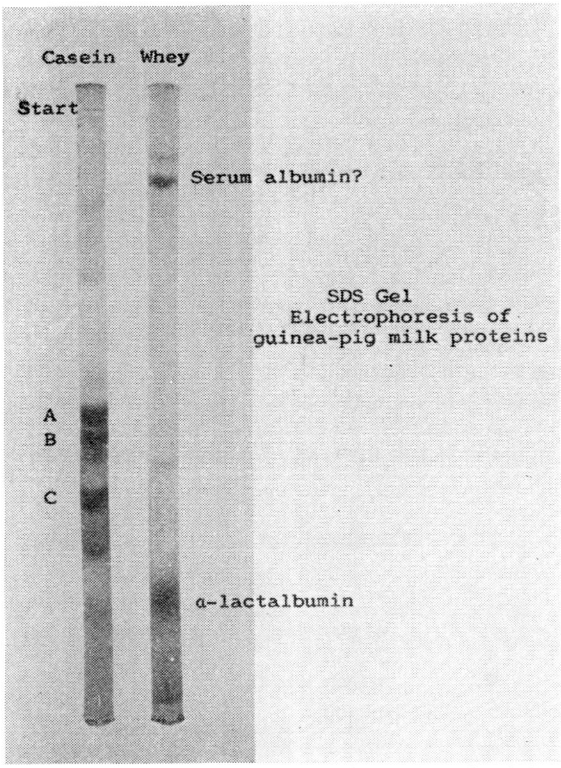

Fig. 4. SDS-polyacrylamide-gel electrophoresis of the proteins of guinea-pig milk. (From Craig *et al.*[8]).

translated in a wheat-germ system and the product is precipitated with an antibody to guinea-pig α-LA, the product is shown to be larger than authentic α-LA. This is demonstrated in Fig. 5. On the other hand if the translation takes place in a system based on ascites tumour cells then both the larger product and the authentic product are produced (Fig. 6). We have demonstrated, following CNBr cleavage of the radioactive protein, that the larger product is accounted for by a peptide extension at the N-terminus. From the change in mobility on polyacrylamide gels we estimate that the extra peptide has a mol. wt. of approximately 1,000. In summary α-LA appears to be synthesized as a precursor in the wheat germ and ascites tumour cell systems, and is partially cleaved to the authentic α-LA by the membranes of the ascites cell system during on-going translation.

By similar means the synthesis of casein has also been studied using antibodies specific for guinea-pig caseins. The results are summarized in Fig. 7 which shows that, in contrast to α-LA, the products that have the antigenic properties of casein are apparently smaller than the authentic milk caseins. The caseins of milk are both phosphorylated and glycosylated and it is known that these secondary modifications affect the mobility of polypeptides on SDS-polyacrylamide gels. Hence the significance of the difference in mobility of the primary translation products and the authentic casein is not at present clear. The primary structure of the three caseins is at present being studied. So far there is little

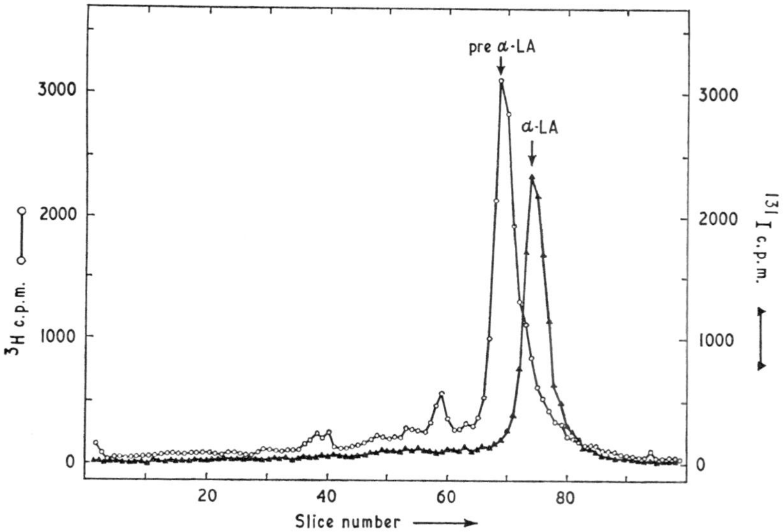

Fig. 5. SDS-polyacrylamide-gel electrophoresis of a ^{3}H-labelled amino acid-labelled α-LA immunoprecipitate, derived from a wheat-germ cell-free system directed by lactating-mammary gland mRNA species. (From Craig *et al.*[8]). ▲ ^{131}I-labelled marker α-LA; ○ ^{3}H-labelled product of translation.

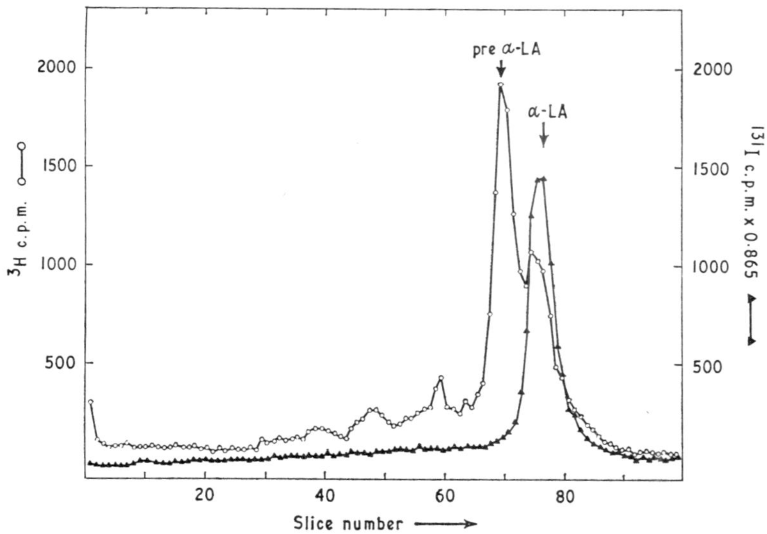

Fig. 6. As for Fig. 5 but the labelled α-LA was derived from a Krebs II ascites cell-free system. ▲ ^{131}I-labelled marker α-LA; ○ ^{3}H-labelled product of translation.

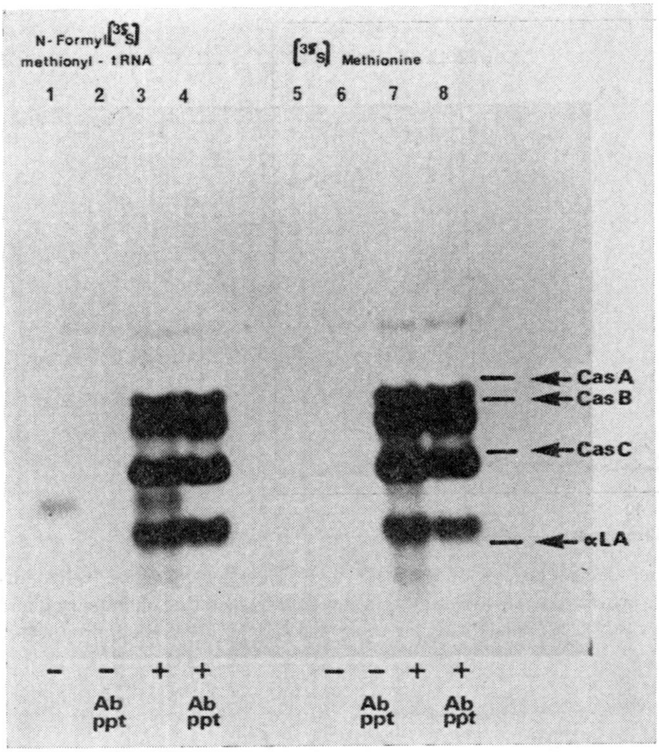

Fig. 7. A radioautograph of SDS-polyacrylamide-gel electrophoresis of the products of translation of lactating-gland mRNA in a wheat-germ cell-free protein synthesizing system using either N-formyl[^{35}S]methionine-tRNA or [^{35}S]methionine. The products were either subjected to electrophoresis without treatment or were first precipitated with combined antisera to casein and α-LA (Ab ppt.).

evidence for homology among them so that it is unlikely that they are derived merely by secondary modifications of a common polypeptide chain. It seems probable that it will not be possible to come to a firm conclusion concerning the presence or absence of signal peptide in the synthesis of casein until the completion of structural studies on authentic milk caseins and the primary translation products. These studies are proceeding.

Another idea that has been discussed concerning the presence in milk of various casein components is that they may be derived from the "big" casein by subsequent proteolytic cleavage. In order to test this hypothesis we have studied the incorporation of [^{35}S]-methionine into casein in the mRNA-directed wheat-germ system using either the free amino acid or formyl-[^{35}S]methionine attached to the appropriate tRNA. Under these circumstances the formyl-methionine is not cleaved from the product of synthesis. Figure 7 also indicates the results of such an experiment and shows that the synthesis of all three caseins is initiated under these conditions. Hence it would appear unlikely that the "big" casein hypothesis is correct.

As indicated in Table II the *Xenopus* oocyte contains membranous components. Zehavi-Willner and Lane[9] have recently studied the synthesis of various proteins by mRNA-directed oocytes and the association of the resulting protein with the membrane's The light membrane fraction of the oocyte indeed appears to function in a similar manner to the rough ER of secretory cells. Figure 8 shows the results for the synthesis of guinea-pig milk protein. After injection of the oocytes and their incubation with [^{35}S]methionine the light membrane fraction was isolated from the disrupted oocytes and then treated with either detergent alone (0.2% deoxycholate+1.5% Triton X-100, labelled D) or proteolytic enzymes (chymotrypsin+trypsin, labelled+E at a concentration of 25, 50, and 100 μg/ml). The newly synthesized milk proteins are shown to be sequestered within the membranes because in the absence of enzyme they are present in the membrane fraction, in the absence of detergent but presence of enzyme they are also present, whereas in the presence of enzyme and detergent they are degraded by the proteolytic enzymes. These and other experiments have also shown that α-LA and not the precursor is to be found within the oocyte membranes so that the oocyte is able to effect the cleavage of the signal peptide from α-LA precursor. These experiments therefore nicely complement those done on the translation of milk protein mRNA in cell free systems.

CHARACTERIZATION OF mRNA ASSOCIATED WITH FREE AND BOUND POLYRIBOSOMES

According to the signal hypothesis all species of mRNA in the cytoplasm should be able to associate with ribosomes to form free polyribosomes. Accordingly one should be

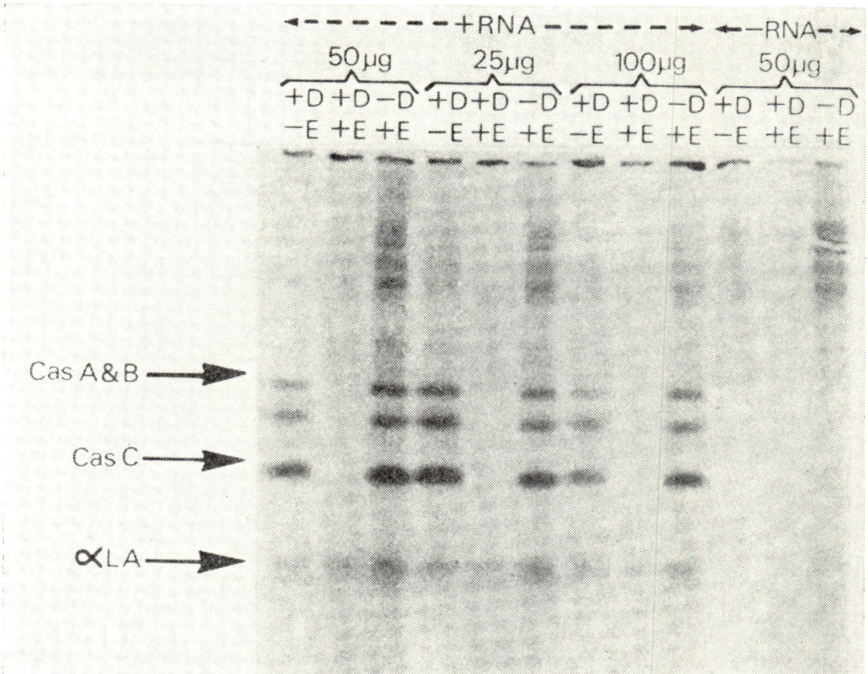

Fig. 8. The presence of guinea-pig milk protein within the light membrane fraction of *Xenopus* oocytes injected with guinea-pig mammry gland mRNA and incubated with [^{35}S] methionine. For explanation see text. From ref. 9.

able to detect the mRNA for milk proteins with the free polyribosomes of the lactating mammary gland. We[10] have isolated free and bound polyribosomes from lactating guinea-pig mammary gland and then isolated the poly (A) containing RNA from each fraction. When this was translated in the ascites tumour cell system we found that the efficiency of incorporation of [^{35}S]methionine into radioactive protein was very much less in the presence of mRNA from free polyribosomes compared with that from bound polyribosomes as shown in Table V. In terms of the percentage of the protein synthesized which reacted with antisera to milk proteins there was little difference. We then examined the nature of the milk proteins synthesized in the presence of the two different mRNA fractions. For this we used the wheat-germ system in order to avoid the complication of multiple products for the different proteins. As shown in Fig. 9 the milk proteins synthesized were

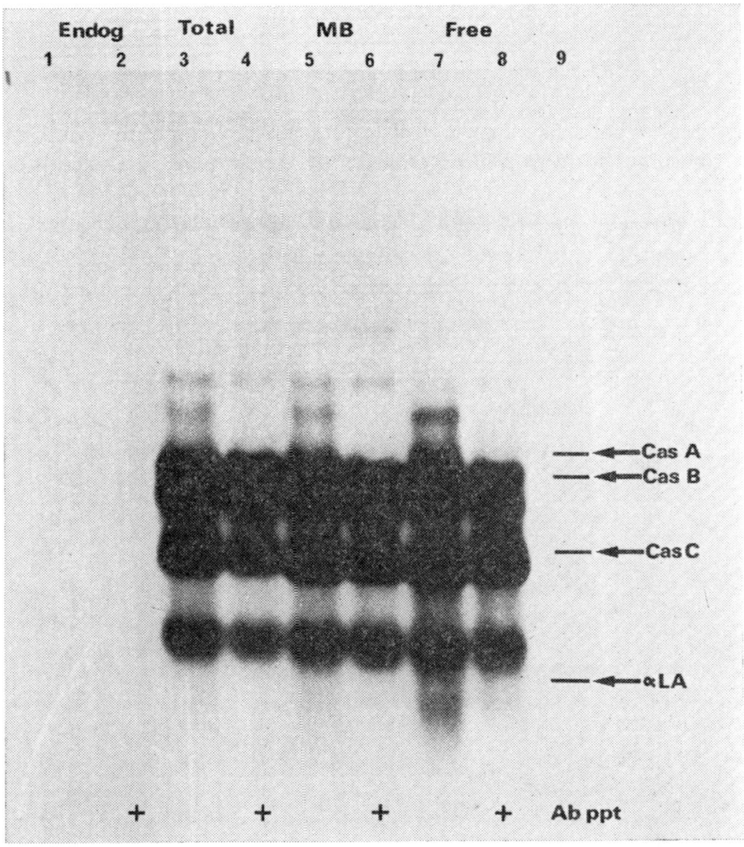

Fig. 9. Protein synthesis in a wheat-germ cell-free system directed by poly(A) mRNA derived from total polyribosomes from lactating mammary gland, membrane-bound polyribosomes (MB) and free polyribosomes (Free). Endog, in the absence of added mRNA. Incubation in the presence of [^{35}S]methionine. Ab ppt. indicates radioactive protein precipitated by the addition of a combined antisera for casein and α-LA.

TABLE V

DETERMINATION OF PERCENTAGE OF TRNASLATION PRODUCTS OF LACTATING MAMMARY GLAND mRNA ATTRIBUTABLE TO MILK PROTEINS*

The membrane-bound and free poly ribosomes were separated either over a sucrose cushion of 2.0 M or 2.3 M as described in ref. 10. The poly(A) containing mRNAwas isolated and translated in a cell-free system derived from Krebs II ascites tumour cells in the presence of a mixture of ^{3}H-labelled amino acids. Combined antisera to casein and α-LA was used to determine the proportion of protein synthesized which was milk protein.

Source of mRNA		*^{3}H cpm Total protein-Bg*	*^{3}H cpm in milk protein-Bg*	*% antibody precipitable*
2.0 M	Bound	183,660	159,600	84.7
	Free	127,010	106,590	91.1
2.3 M	Bound	60,980	52,810	86.6
	Free	23,930	22,840	95.4

*For explanation see text. From ref. 9.

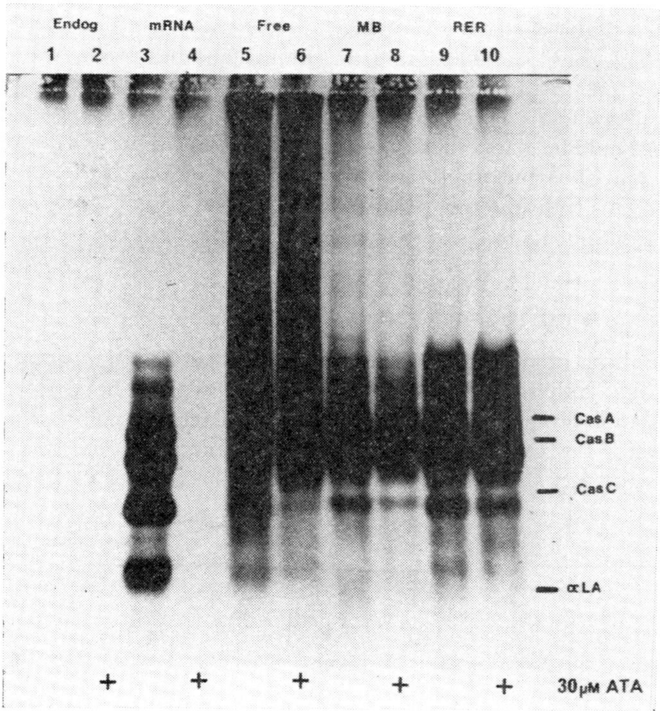

Fig. 10. Protein synthesized by free and membrane-bound polyribosomes when "run off" *in vitro* in the wheat-germ cell-free system in the presence of [^{35}S]methionine. The effect of the presence of an inhibitor of initiation, ATA, is shown. Endog, incubation in absence of added mRNA; mRNA, isolated mRNA from lactating mammary gland; Free, presence of free polyribosomes; MB, presence of membrane-bound polyribosomes; RER, presence of a crude microsome fraction.

virtually identical. We conclude therefore that it is possible to isolate from the free polyribosomes mRNA that directs the synthesis of α-LA and casein.

We then returned to the problem of the difference in the efficiency of translation of the two mRNA fractions. The isolated free-polyribosomes and detergent-treated membrane-bound polyribosomes were incubated in the wheat-getm system in the presence of ATA at a concentration that prevented initiation of protein synthesis. When the products of translation were examined the results obtained were as shown in Fig. 10. It will be seen that in both cases milk protein was produced. (In this particular experiment α-LA is not indicated as a product of the free polysome incubation but in other experiments this was synthesized as well as casein.) The difference between the polyribosomes is that the free polyribosomes unlike the bound polyribosomes have produced a wide range of larger non-milk proteins. This is, of course, the result to be expected since according to the signal hypothesis the free polyribosomes would be in the process of synthesizing many proteins in addition to milk proteins. It is noteworthy, however, that when the mRNA is isolated only the mRNA for milk proteins is translated. This implies either a selection mechanism in favour of certain proteins or is another example of a phenomenon previously noted that optimum conditions for the *in vitro* translation of mRNA may differ as between the different mRNA species[11]. In any event the low efficiency of free polyribosome mRNA translation (Fig. 9) is explained on the basis that this fraction contains non-milk protein mRNA which is not translated under the conditions used.

This experimental approach should also enable us to confirm another prediction of the signal hypothesis. The nascent proteins associated with polyribosomes as isolated are in varying stages of completion having been initiated *in vivo*. If their synthesis is completed in the wheat-germ system we should be able to demonstrate that the nascent proteins from the detergent-treated bound polyribosomes represent both precursor and authentic proteins whereas the nascent proteins from the free polyribosomes are exclusively precursor proteins. In this respect our experiments to date are encouraging but are not complete.

CONCLUSIONS FROM STUDIES ON SYNTHESIS OF MILK PROTEINS

Our results on the biosynthesis of guinea-pig milk protein are substantially in accord with the signal hypothesis for the synthesis of secretory proteins. So far we have not demonstrated that the primary translation products of mRNA for caseins possess a signal peptide and in this respect it is interesting that ovalbumin is synthesized without such a precursor.

Work is proceeding on a variety of subjects concerned with the synthesis of milk proteins (see review 12).

ACKNOWLEDGMENT

The assistance of Mr. David Parker is gratefully acknowledged as is the financial support of the Medical Research Council and the Wellcome Trust.

REFERENCES

1 H. R. B. PELHAM and R. J. JACKSON, *Eur. J. Biochem.*, 67 (1976) 247.
2 P. N. CAMPBELL and G. BLOBEL, *FEBS Lett.*, 72 (1976) 215.
3 C. MILSTEIN, G. G. BROWNLEE, T. M. HARRISON, and M. B. MATHEWS, *Nature New Biol.*, 239 (1972) 117.
4 S. YU and C. REDMAN, *Biochem. Biophys. Res. Commun.*, 76 (1977) 496; A. W. STRAUSS, A. M. DONOHUE, C. D. BENNETT, J. A. RODKEY, and A. W. ALBERTS, *Proc. Natl. Acad. Sci. U. S.*, 74 (1977) 1353.
5 G. BLOBEL and B. DOBBERSTEIN, *J. Cell Biol.*, 67 (1975) 835.
6 G. BLOBEL and D. D. SABATINI, in L. A. MANSON, *Biomembranes*, Plenum Press, New York, vol. 2, 1971, p. 193.
7 R. D. PALMITER, S. N. THIBODEAU, J. GAGNON, and K. A. WALSH, Abstracts of Proceedings of 11th FEBS Meeting, Copenhagen, No. A6-Z-L3-4, 1977.
8 R. K. CRAIG, P. A. BROWN, O. S. HARRISON, D. MCILREAVY, and P. N. CAMPBELL, *Biochem. J.*, 160 (1976) 57.
9 T. ZEHAVI-WILLNER and C. LANE, *Cell*, 11 (1977) 683.
10 O. S. HARRISON, R. K. CRAIG, and P. N. CAMPBELL, *Biocheim. Soc. Trans.*, 4 (1976) 340.
11 T. P. H. TSE and J. M. TAYLOR, *J. Biol. Chem.*, 252 (1977) 1272.
12 R. K. CRAIG and P. N. CAMPBELL, *Lactation*, Academic Press, New York, vol. IV, 1977, in press.

FERRITIN BIOSYNTHESIS AND ITS RESPONSE TO IRON

HAMISH N. MUNRO

Department of Nutrition and Food Science, Massachusetts Institute of Technology, Cambridge, Massachusetts (U.S.A.)

Although deposition of iron in tissues was long known to pathologists as hemosiderin, the major iron-storage protein, ferritin, was only isolated and described in 1937 by Laufberger. The capacity of organisms to synthesize ferritin appears to have developed early in evolution, first appearing in fungi and also widespread in plants as well as all forms of animal life so far examined. In the mammal, the tissues having the largest deposits of stored iron are liver, spleen, and bone marrow, but it can be found in all tissues including tumor cells, presumably as part of the equipment of cells necessary for utilizing iron. The recent recognition of ferritin in serum has made this a tool for studying iron stores in man, since the amount in serum reflects the magnitude of storage iron.

During the past decade, ferritin has been explored vigorously for several reasons. First, ferritin structure presents a challenge in which the variety of isoferritins and the number of their subunits are disputed. Second, the intracellular sites of ferritin protein synthesis and the response of the synthetic mechanism to iron stimulation provide some unusual features. Finally, the functions of ferritin in individual tissues combine the features of a depository for excess iron and a storage mechanism, but may have other functions. We have recently assembled a detailed review of these various aspects of ferritin.[1]

CURRENT CONCEPTS OF FERRITIN STRUCTURE

Many of the primary studies of ferritin structure—molecular size, subunit composition and catalytic groups—have been carried out on the ferritin of horse spleen. Horse spleen ferritin consists of an outer shell of 24 protein subunits with an aggregate molecular weight of about 450,000 daltons into which up to 4,500 atoms of iron can be packed as ferric oxyhydroxide. However, it has been demonstrated that other ferritins can show differences in molecular size, gel migration properties and amino acid composition even between ferritins from different tissues of the same animal. Studies of the properties of rat tissue ferritins have been particularly extensive. Preliminary experiments[2] showed that the gel migrations of ferritins from different rat tissues could differ, and that cardiac ferritin migrated as two major bands with different affinities for antibody to ferritin. Finer discrimination was achieved[3] by studying migration rates over a range of gel concentrations and expressing the data according to the Ferguson plot which provides information about the molecular sizes and charges of different ferritins. This demonstrated size and charge heterogeneity among ferritins prepared from liver, kidney, heart, and hepatoma of the rat. While molecular size was essentially similar (420,000 to 490,000

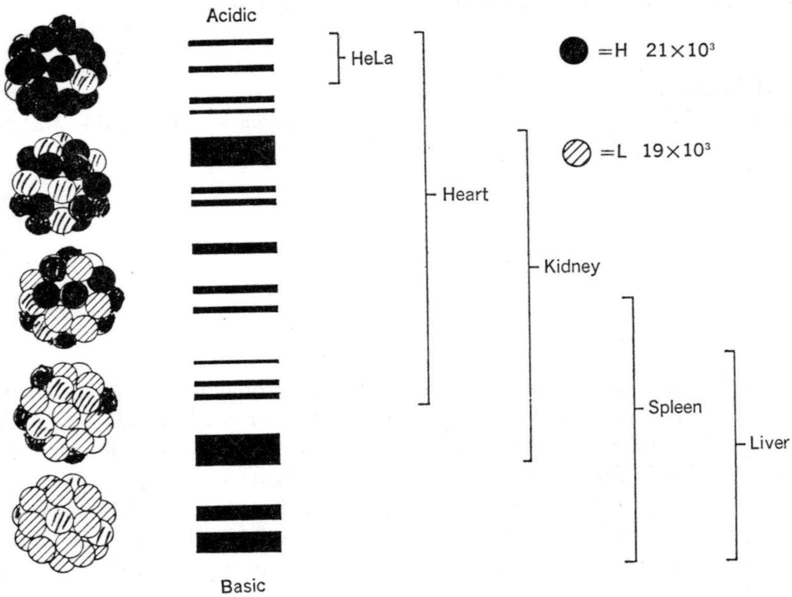

Fig. 1. Diagram illustrating the bands obtained on isoelectric focussing of ferritins extracted from human tissues. The p*I*'s of the bands vary from 4.6 (acidic end) to 5.7 (basic end). At the left, the proportions of large (H) and small (L) subunits corresponding to these bands are shown schematically. The diagram is modified from Drysdale *et al.*[5] by reducing the subunits from three to two (H and L), in accordance with the latest observations of this group. From ref. 1.

daltons) for most tissue ferritins, the ferritin in rat heart were distinctly larger (530,000 and 626,000 daltons), and the net charge on the larger rat heart ferritin was also much larger than that of other tissue ferritins. This structural heterogeneity among rat tissue isoferritins was confirmed by their distinctive individual amino acid analyses and peptide maps[4]. The evidence of heterogeneity of tissue ferritins in a single species has been amplified using gel isoelectric focusing to separate out human tissue ferritins according to p*I*. Drysdale *et al.*[5] have demonstrated that these consist of families of ferritins, some ferritin bands being common to several tissues (Fig. 1). These authors conclude that there are over 20 isoferritins ranging in isoelectric point from 4.8 to 5.8 in various human tissues. Worwood *et al.*[6] have shown with antibodies to spleen and to heart ferritins that the isofocussing bands of human ferritin at the basic, intermediate and acidic ends of the spectrum can be distinguished immunologically, implying that there are structural differences between them.

Originally, it was believed that the apoferritin shell consists of only one species of subunit, but evidence is accumulating to show that there may be more types of subunit even within the same shell. Thus, Adelman and Drysdale[7] have recently found that various horse and human tissue ferritins contain two subunits, one 19,000 and the other 21,000. They have determined the proportions of these subunits in different isoferritins resolved by isoelectric focussing and have found that the proportions of each subunit vary progressively from the basic end of the isoferritin series (p*I* 5.7) with 24 subunits of 19,000 daltons, to the acidic end of the spectrum (pI 4.6) with 24 subunits of 21,000 daltons (Fig. 1). Finally, the two ferritin subunits may differ in their content of a small number of sugar residues. In confirmation of Shinjyo *et al.*,[8] Cynkin and Knowlton[9] find that neutral sugars comprise 2.4% of the weight of liver and spleen apoferritins, but twice that amount in heart apoferritin and they believe that there are at least two types of carbohydrate chain present. Since heart ferritin contains predominantly the larger (21,000 daltons) subunit (Fig. 1), this finding suggests that the two subunits are distinctly different in sugar residue content.

These structural features of ferritin have considerable relevance to the intracellular site(s) of apoferritin biosynthesis and their response to iron administration.

INTRACELLULAR SITES OF SYNTHESIS OF FERRITIN

The mechanism of ferritin protein synthesis and its regulation by iron involves the question of where ferritin subunits are made. It has been generally accepted that proteins

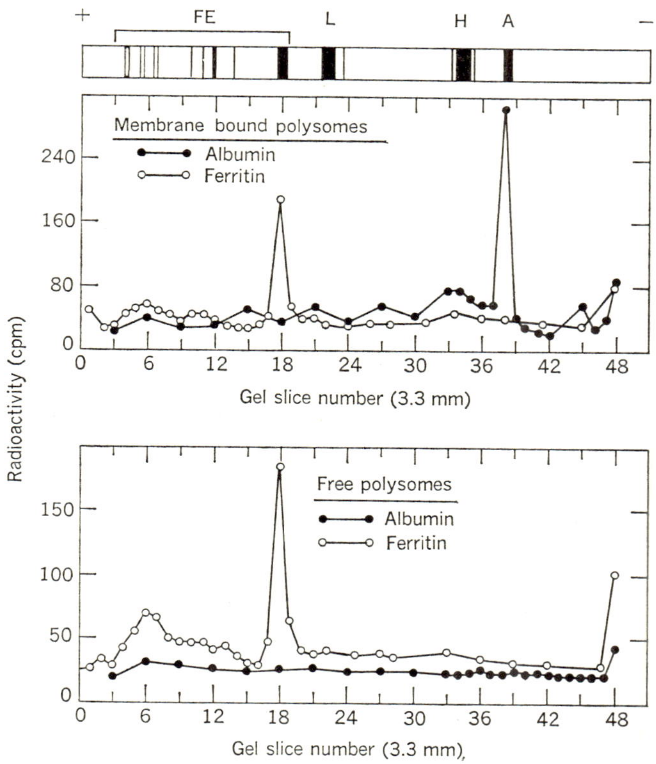

Fig. 2. Synthesis of ferritin and albumin by the mRNAs extracted from membrane-bound (top) and free (bottom) polysomes. After isolation, mRNA from each source was translated in a wheat germ S_{30} cell-free system. Following immunoprecipitation of the synthesized ferritin and albumin chains, immunoprecipitates were analysed on dodecyl sulfate-polyacrylamide slab gels. The gels were sliced and counted as shown (origin on the right). F, ferritin; A, albumin; L, L-chain; H, H-chain of antibody. From ref. 15.

secreted from cells are made on membrane-attached polyribosomes, whereas ribosomes free in the cytosol make retained proteins. This concept was first supported by the demonstration[10,11] that albumin is made on membrane-bound liver ribosomes, whereas ferritin is preferentially made on free liver ribosomes. However, this evidence regarding the site of ferritin synthesis was not clear-cut. Several authors[11-14] found a substantial number of nascent ferritin chains on membrane-bound liver ribosomes. Furthermore, evidence was obtained suggesting that induction of ferritin with iron is restricted to the free ribosome population, indicating a functional difference in the response of the two ribosomal populations.[15]

In recent studies[15] we extracted the mRNA's from the membrane-attached and the free ribosomes of rat liver and translated each mRNA sample in a cell-free wheat germ system containing ^{3}H-leucine. Labeled ferritin subunits formed were precipitated at the end of incubation with an antibody to ferritin and separated on a gradient polyacrylamide gel containing sodium dodecyl sulfate for radioactive counting (Fig. 2). In each case, a single major peak of radioactivity was found on the gel, corresponding to a molecular weight of about 20,000 daltons (the discrimination was inadequate to distinguish between 19,000 and 21,000 daltons). This confirms that mRNA's ferritin subunit synthesis are represented in the membrane-bound as well as the free polyribosmes. Figure 2 shows that serum albumin synthesis was restricted to the membrane-bound ribosomes. Administration of iron to the rats a few hours before killing increased the ferritin mRNA content in the free ribosome population three times, but left the membrane-bound ribosomes unchanged. This confirms the observation we made earlier.[14]

Some unanswered questions are raised by these observations. Are different ferritin subunits made by membrane-bound and free polyribosomes respectively? Are sugars added only to subunits made on the membrane-bound ribosomes?

RESPONSE OF APOFERRITIN SYNTHESIS TO IRON ADMINISTRATION

The acute response of ferritin protein synthesis to iron administration was investigated by Drysdale and Munro,[16] by giving rats a large dose of ferric ammonium citrate intraperitoneally and at various times during the next 24 hr administering ^{14}C-leucine followed by killed 2 hr later ("pulse dose"). Figure 3 shows that incorporation of this pulse dose of isotope into the mixed liver proteins was not affected by administered iron, but the activity of ferritin protein increased to a maximum level several-fold above basal 5 hr after iron administration. Thereafter, the amount of ferritin in the liver increased up to 12 hr. By separation of ferritins of different iron content on sucrose gradients, it was demonstrated that the initial product of biosynthesis is iron-poor apoferritin but later on more of the label passes into iron-rich ferritin.

Although this picture resembles the classical response observed in bacteria of a burst of new mRNA formation, nevertheless pre-treatment with adequate doses of actinomycin D failed to affect the induction of ferritin protein synthesis caused by iron administration.[17] Despite this evidence that new mRNA is not involved in the response to iron, a twofold increase in ferritin-synthesizing polyribosomes was observed in the liver cell cytoplasm of iron-treated rats.[18] It seemed unlikely that this could be accounted for by mRNA transported from a nuclear reserve, especially since pre-treatment with cordycepin, an inhibitor of poly-adenylic acid addition to mRNA prior to transport from nucleus to cytoplasm, failed to affect induction of liver ferritin by iron administration.[19] Thus there must be a

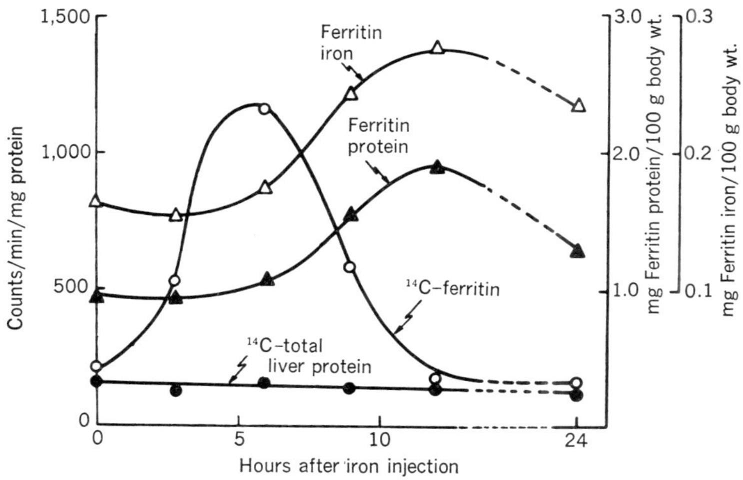

Fig. 3. Uptake of leucine-^{14}C into liver ferritin and into mixed liver proteins after a 2-hr pulse dose of leucine-^{14}C given to rats at various times after injection of iron. Each rat received 400 μg of iron/100 g of body wt., followed at 1, 3, 7, 10, and 22 hr 5 μCi of leucine-^{14}C/100 g of body wt. The animals were killed 2 hr after injection of leucine, and the specific activities of ferritin and of the mixed liver proteins were measured as cpm per mg of protein. The amounts of ferritin protein and ferritin iron per liver at the time of killing are also shown. From ref. 16. 1. Rats 150 g body weight fasting overnight. 2. Ferric ammonium citrate injected intraperitoneally, 0 hr. 3. ^{14}C-Leucine injected intraperitoneally: (a) at minus 2 hr killed at 0 hr (control no iron), (b) at 1 hr killed at 3 hr (standard time used), (c) at 3 hr killed at 5 hr, (d) at 7 hr killed at 5 hr, (e) at 10 hr killed at 12 hr, (f) at 22 hr killed at 24 hr.

cytoplasmic source for the additional ferritin-synthesizing polyribosomes. On extracting the liver cytosol, a high content of free mRNA for ferritin was in fact obtained.[19] When the rats were given parenteral iron salts 5 hr before extracting free mRNA from the cytosol, the store of unused (free) ferritin mRNA diminished sharply, coincident with the increase in the number of poly-ribosomes making ferritin peptides.[19]

To explain the rapid activation of this reserve of ferritin mRNA after giving iron salts, it has been postulated (Fig. 4) that a subunit of ferritin is attached to the initiation site of the ferritin mRNA in the tissues of untreated animals, thus preventing the mRNA from binding to the ribosome. On entry of iron into the cell, the equilibrium is shifted towards assembly of completed ferritin shells, and in consequence these inhibitory subunits are mobilized so that more ferritin mRNA becomes available to initiate new chains on ribosomes. An additional cytoplasmic control mechanism is suggested by the studies of Drysdale and Shafritz,[20] who added iron to a cell-free system synthesizing ferritin subunits and observed increased incorporation of labeled free amino acids into apoferritin. This response appeared to be due to acceleration of the transfer of subunits to the apoferritin shell. The reserve of free ferritin mRNA in the cytosol may therefore provide a rapid mechanism for protein synthesis, probably limited to a few proteins performing similar emergency functions.

Finally, the adaptive mechanism proposed by us refers only to ferritin mRNA present in free polyribosomes in the liver. The function of the subunits made on membrane-bound

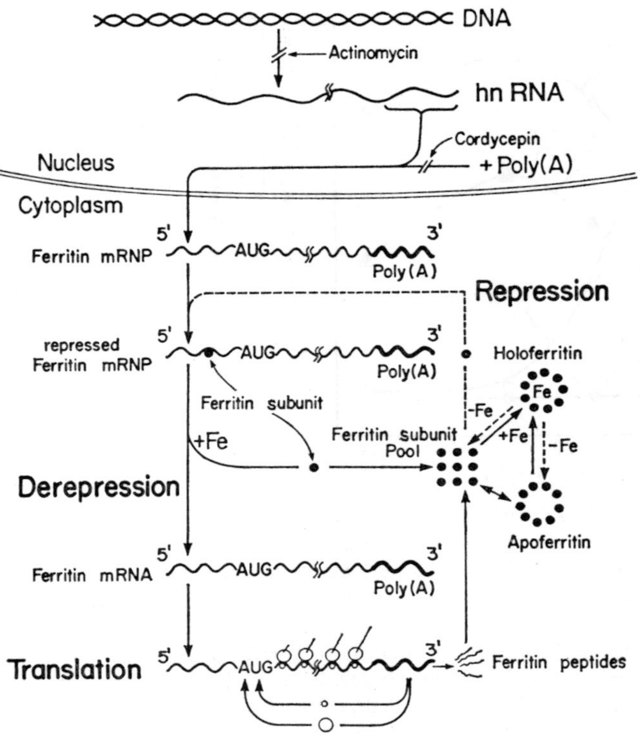

Fig. 4. Proposed model from the translational control mechanism by which iron specifically regulates the synthesis of ferritin. From ref. 19.

polyribosomes remains obscure; they may be secreted into a different cell compartment such as pinocytotic vesicles that become secondary lysosomes.

Additionally, we measured liver ferritin degradation rate in untreated rats following ^{14}C-leucine injection (ref. 16), or ^{14}C-guanido-arginine,[21] the latter being used to prevent reutilization of label. Figure 5 shows that in the case of the control group, loss of label from ferritin protein was at the same rate as from mixed liver protein, the ratio remaining constant over the 72 hr period. Following a single injection of iron, there was initially a higher uptake of ^{14}C into ferritin protein, but subsequent loss of label was faster than that of general liver protein. Loss of ^{14}C-label was accelerated by bleeding the animals, and was inhibited by repeated injections of iron throughout the experimental period, indicating that the supply of iron to the liver regulates rates of both synthesis and degradation.

ROLE OF FERRITIN IN CELL METABOLISM

Ferritin accepts iron in the ferrous form and stores it as ferric iron, a process in which catalytic sites within the apoferritin shell act as oxidizing foci. Similarly, intracellular release of iron occurs from intact ferritin molecules through reduction of the iron. Many reducing or chelating agents small enough to negotiate the channels in the ferritin shell can

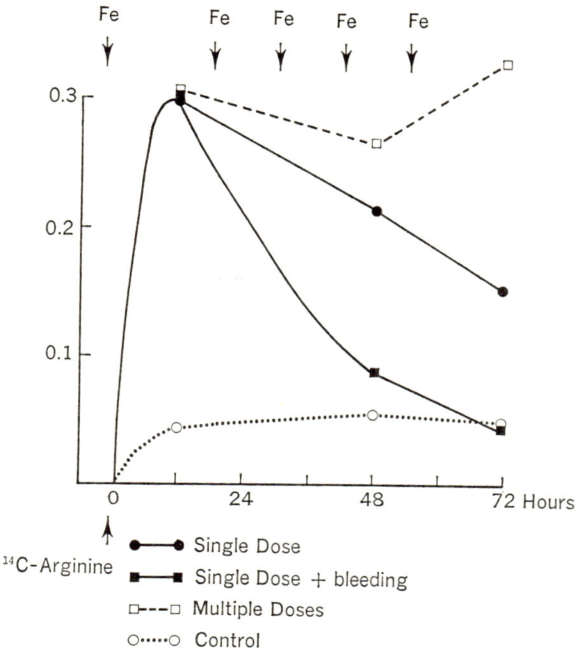

Fig. 5. Effect of varying the iron content of the liver on the rate of loss of ^{14}C-arginine from rat liver ferritin. The percent of ^{14}C-arginine in ferritin as compared with general protein is plotted against time after injection of the isotope. All groups except controls were injected with 400 μg iron/100 g body wt. at zero time; one group received multiple doses. From ref. 21.

cause iron release from ferritin *in vitro*. In the intact cell the most likely candidates are dihydroflavins such as $FMNH_2$. This function of ferritin in iron uptake and release can be integrated with other aspects of iron metabolism in the cell. Figure 6 is an attempt to provide a composite picture of the entry of iron sources into various cells and the fate of the iron once it enters the cell. Most cells are presumed to have specific receptors for transferrin Fe^{3+} which enters the cell sap by endocytosis and releases its iron to an intracellular pool, while the apotransferrin returns to the plasma. Hepatocytes have specific receptors for any hemoglobin-haptoglobin or heme-hemopexin complexes present in plasma, and for serum ferritin. The hepatocyte can also take up iron salts and complexes injected into the animal. All these iron-containing sources enter the hepatocyte and become encapsulated in pinocytic vesicles which then acquire lysosomal enzymes to become phagosomes (secondary lysosomes). Within the phagosomes, the iron is released, and some may be trapped by ferritin entering the phagosome from the cell sap or made on membrane-bound polyribosomes attached to the vesicles. Unlike the hepatocyte, the Kupffer cell and other reticulo-endothelial cells do not accept free hemoglobin and heme nor serum ferritin, but take up intact red cells to be rapidly digested in the phagosomes and their iron released. Iron also enters the secondary lysosome system through turnover of ferritin from the cytoplasm. Masses of cytoplasm, including organelles and cell sap with ferritin, become engulfed in autophagic vacuoles which then receive lysosomal enzymes. Much of the ferritin iron is probably released again to the iron pool in the cell sap. In some cells,

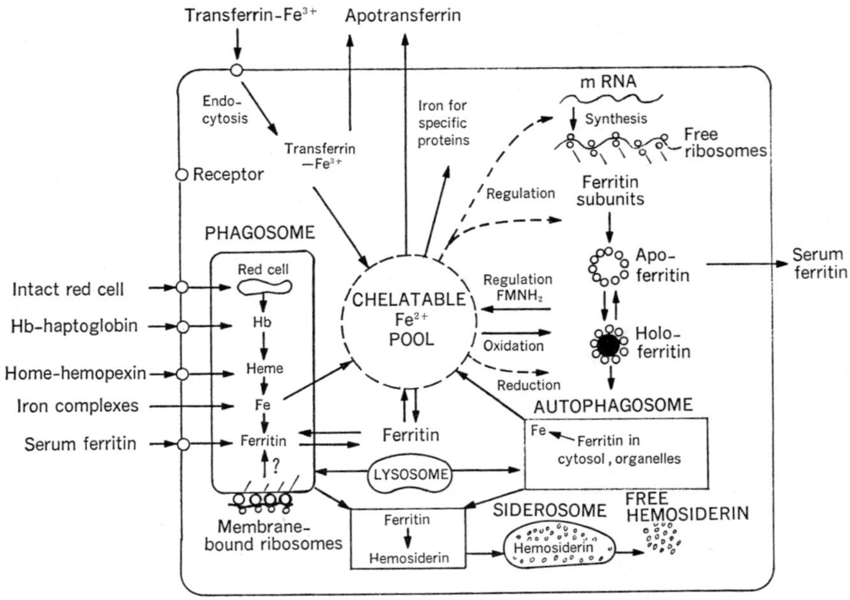

Fig. 6. Schematic representation of iron uptake and utilization by cells of various types. See text for description. From ref. 1.

such as reticuloendothelial cells, some of the ferritin goes on to hemosiderin and is permanently retained in the cell within solid particles.

There is now good evidence[22] of a pool of chelatable iron in cell sap, which is the source of iron for synthesis of specific cell products such as heme. This pool probably receives iron from all sources and is in equilibrium with the Fe^{3+} in ferritin. Changes in the size of this pool appears to regulate synthesis of ferritin protein through changes in availability of mRNA for ferritin. Finally, ferritin is secreted by reticuloendothelial cells into the serum in proportion to the amount of iron stored in these cells.

This picture probably applies to all cells, including tumor cells. Variations from one cell type to another depends on the types of receptors for iron-containing compounds in the blood (*e.g.*, receptors for hemoglobin-haptoglobin on hepatocytes, and for aging erythrocytes on reticuloendothelial cells), the capacity of the secondary lysosomes to form hemosiderin, and the functional needs of the cell for iron (*e.g.*, the maturing erythrocyte removes iron from the pool for hemoglobin, while the mucosal cell of the small intestine passes it unidirectionally to the plasma). The evidence for this integrated picture of intracellular iron metabolism is discussed elsewhere.[1]

REFERENCES

1 H. N. Munro and M. C. Linder, *Physiol. Rev.*, 58 (1978) 317.
2 M. Linder-Horowitz, R. T. Ruettinger, and H. N. Munro, *Biochim. Biophys. Acta*, 200 (1969) 442.
3 L. Vulimiri, M. C. Linder, H. N. Munro, and N. Catsimpoolas, *Biochim. Biophys. Acta*, 491 (1977) 67.

4 M. C. Linder, J. R. Moor, H. N. Munro, and H. P. Morris, *Biochim. Biophys. Acta*, 386 (1975) 409.
5 J. W. Drysdale, P. Arosio, T. Adelman, J. T. Hazard, and D. Brooke, in R. R. Crichton, *Proteins of Iron Storage and Transport in Biochemistry and Medicine*, North-Holland, Amsterdam, 1975, p. 359.
6 M. Worwood, M. Wagstaff, B. M. Jones, S. Dawkins, and A. Jacobs, in E. B. Brown, P. Aisen, J. Fielding, and R. R. Crichton, *Proteins of Iron Metabolism*, Grune and Stratton, New York, 1977, p. 79.
7 T. G. Adelman and J. W. Drysdale, in E. B. Brown, P. Aisen, J. Fielding, and R. R. Crichton, *Proteins of Iron Metabolism*, Grune and Stratton, New York, 1977, p. 49.
8 S. Shinjyo, H. Abe, and M. Masuda, *Biochim. Biophys. Acta*, 411 (1975) 165.
9 M. A. Cynkin and M. Knowlton, in E. B. Brown, P. Aisen, J. Fielding, and R. R. Crichton, *Proteins of Iron Metabolism*, Grune and Stratton, New York, 1977, p. 115.
10 S. J. Hicks, J. W. Drysdale, and H. N. Munro, *Science* 164 (1969) 584.
11 C. M. Redman, *J. Biol. Chem.*, 244 (1969) 4308.
12 D. G. Puro and G. W. Richter, *Proc. Soc. Exp. Biol. Med.*, 138 (1971) 399.
13 S. S. C. Lee and G. W. Richter, *J. Biol. Chem.*, 252 (1977) 2054.
14 A. Konijn, B. S. Baliga, and H. N. Munro, *FEBS Lett.*, 37 (1973) 249.
15 J. Zähringer, B. S. Baliga, R. L. Drake, and H. N. Munro, *Biochim. Biophys. Acta*, 474 (1977) 234.
16 J. W. Drysdale and H. N. Munro, *J. Biol. Chem.*, 241 (1966) 3630.
17 J. W. Drysdale and H. N. Munro, *Biochim. Biophys. Acta*, 103 (1965) 185.
18 J. Zähringer, A. M. Konijn, B. S. Baliga, and H. N. Munro, *Biochim. Biophys. Res. Commun.*, 65 (1975) 583.
19 J. Zähringer, B. S. Baliga, and H. N. Munro, *Proc. Natl. Acad. Sci. U.S.*, 73 (1976) 857.
20 J. W. Drysdale and D. A. Shafritz, *Biochim. Biophys. Acta*, 383 (1975) 97.
21 H. N. Munro and J. W. Drysdale, *Fed. Proc.*, 29 (1970) 1469.
22 G. P. White, R. Bailey-Wood, and A. Jacobs, *Clin. Sci. Mol. Med.*, 50 (1976) 145.

USE OF LIVER CELLS IN PRIMARY CULTURE FOR BIOCHEMICAL STUDIES OF LIVER FUNCTION

AKIRA ICHIHARA, KEIJI TANAKA, YUMIKO TOMITA, AND MITSURU SATO

Institute for Enzyme Research, School of Medicine, Tokushima University, Tokushima (Japan)

For biochemical studies of divergent and complexed liver functions a simple system is required, but this system must retain the normal organized cellular structure of liver. The systems most commonly used for this purpose are perfused liver, liver slices and isolated liver cells. However, perfusion techniques are laborious and costly, and although slices are simpler, the results obtained are sometimes quite variable, possibly due to damage of the cells. Therefore, isolated liver cells seem the most promising system, and there have been many attempts to isolate functionally normal liver cells.[1,2] However, classical procedure of mechanical dispersion of liver cells causes severe damage of the cells with much leakage of intracellular materials and the cells are usually not viable. There have also been many attempts to use established liver cell lines, but these cells retain very few of the specific functions of liver, although some cell lines express limited functions, such as inducibility of tyrosine transaminase by hormones or synthesis of albumin.[3] It should be mentioned that these established cell lines have mostly been isolated from slow-growing hepatomas, and even when they are derived from normal liver they become transformed and their chromosomal numbers are grossly deviated. Therefore, these cells are not suitable for studies of "normal liver functions."

Howard *et al.* first used collagenase to disperse liver cells from slices in 1967, and subsequently Berry and Friend modified this method to perfuse whole liver with collagenase and hyaluronidase and in this way obtained about 10 times more cells than by enzymatic dispersion of liver slices. Since then their method has been widely used and many metabolic studies on liver function have been carried out using freshly isolated liver cells.[2]

However, although these cells retain various liver functions, their functions are definitely impaired, possibly due to damage of the cell membrane. For example, Kletzien *et al.* showed that freshly isolated cells have low activity for transport of amino acids, but that when they were cultured for a few hours this activity increased and insulin enhanced the recovery.[4] We also found that protein synthesis in freshly isolated cells is very low and scarcely any protein is secreted, but after 24 hr culture synthesis of proteins increased severalfold and the proteins were secreted actively to the medium.[5] The increase of protein synthesis continues for several days and the polysomes in freshly isolated cells are almost completely disaggregated, but they also recover partially after a few days culture. Bissell *et al.*[6] also showed the enhancement of protein synthesis and the recovery of ATP content in cultured liver cells.[6] Therefore, it is more desirable to use liver cells cultured at least 24 hr.

Freshly isolated cells are round morphologically, but within a few hours in culture they become attached firmly to the dish and become flat. They also aggregate forming clusters and their ultrastructure is very similar to that of cells from intact liver.[7,8] Laishes and Williams[9] showed that insulin enhanced the attachment and dexamethasone increased the life span of these cells. We have adopted the procedure of culturing cells in Williams medium E with 10% fetal bovine serum in Falcon plastic dishes under 5% CO_2 and 95% air, and we also observed the effectiveness of insulin and dexamethasone on viability and attachment of the cultured cells and hence the recovery of various functions, such as inductions of tyrosine transaminase and ornithine decarboxylase and synthesis and secretion of various serum proteins; these proteins have been identified as albumin, fibrinogen, transferrin, and lipoproteins by electrophoresis and immunochemical techniques.[5] Although serum greatly enhances cell viability and attachment, some workers have used serum-free medium and coated the petri dishes with collagen to promote cell attachment.[10-12] We found that addition of dexamethasone to serum-free medium causes comparable cell attachment to that in medium containing serum.[5]

It is interesting that these cells in primary culture do not proliferate and that their viability decreases gradually within a week[6,9,12,13]; only cells isolated 20 hr after partial hepatectomy showed significant DNA synthesis.[14] However, in some cultures after one week a different type of cells is found among the parenchymal cells.[5,12,13]. These large polymorphous cells with clear cytoplasm are called clear cells. It is unknown whether clear cells are derived from parenchymal cells or from latent immature cells. The clear cells appear earlier after 2–3 days in cultures obtained by dissociating liver cells by perfusion with trypsin than in cultures of cells dissociated by collagenase. The properties of these clear cells are still unknown, but they seem to be an immature type of liver cells and possibly they may propagate to undifferentiated established cell lines. Leffert *et al.* reported that not only cells isolated from fetal rat liver but also these isolated from adult rat liver could proliferate in culture.[15,16] The reason for this difference in results is unknown; Leffert's cells may have been immature hepatocytes, because they secreted α-fetoprotein.[15]

These studies suggest that liver cells in primary culture are useful for studies on liver functions, such as regulation of gluconeogenesis,[17] glycogenesis,[8] lipogenesis,[18,19] urea formation,[10,20] the syntheses of various serum proteins,[5,6,12,15] and the effects of various hormones on these activities. However, not all differentiated markers were retained by these cells in primary culture; the various kinases of glycolysis, cytochrome P-450 and carbamyl phosphate synthetase all decreased during culture.[6,10,12,13,17] However, decrease of cytochrome P-450 was prevented by addition of various hormones to the culture medium.[21] Further studies may indicate methods for retaining other labile functions of the cells *in vitro*.

ACKNOWLEDGMENT

This work was supported by a grant from the Ministry of Education, Science and Culture (No. 287035).

REFERENCES

1 G. Schreiber and M. Schreiber, *Sub-Cell. Biochem.*, 2 (1973) 321.
2 P. O. Seglen, *Methods Cell Biol.*, 13 (1976) 29.
3 A. Ichihara, in W. E. Criss, T. Ono, and J. R. Sabine, *Control Mechanisms in Cancer*, Raven Press, New York, 1976, p. 317.
4 R. F. Kletzien, M. W. Pariza, J. E. Becker, V. R. Potter, and F. R. Butcher, *J. Biol. Chem.*, 251 (1977) 3014.
5 K. Tanaka, M. Sato, Y. Tomita, and A. Ichihara, *J. Biochem.*, 84 (1978) 937.
6 D. M. Bissell and P. S. Guzelian, in L. E. Gerschenson and E. B. Thompson, *Gene Expression and Carcinogenesis in Cultured Liver*, Academic Press, New York, 1975, p. 119.
7 J.-C. Wanson, P. Drochmans, R. Mosselmans, and M.-F. Ronveaux, *J. Cell Biol.*, 74 (1977) 858.
8 D. Bernaert, J.-C. Wanson, P. Drochmans, and A. Popowski, *J. Cell Biol.*, 74 (1977) 878.
9 B. A. Laishes and G. M. Williams, *In Vitro*, 12 (1976) 521, 821.
10 R. C. Lin and P. J. Snodgrass, *Biochem. Biophys. Res. Cummun.*, 64 (1975) 725.
11 G. Michalopoulos and H. C. Pitot, *Exp. Cell Res.*, 94 (1975) 70.
12 M. W. Pariza, J. D., Yager, Jr. S. Goldfarb, J. A. Gurr, S. Yanagi, S. H. Grossman, J. E. Becker, T. A. Barber, and V. R. Potter, in L. E. Gerschenson and E. B. Thompson, *Gene Expression and Carcinogenesis in Cultured Liver*, Academic Press, New York, 1975, p. 137.
13 U. Junge, S. Nagamori, G. Brunner, and H. D. Söling, in J. M. Tager, H. D. Söling, and J. R. Williamson, *Use of Isolated Liver Cells and Kidney Tubulus in Metabolic Studies*, North-Holland, Amsterdam, 1976, p. 201.
14 H. Hirshinger, J. R. Gautchi, and R. Schindler, *Exp. Cell Res.*, 100 (1976) 356.
15 S. Sell, H. Skelly, H. L. Leffert, U. Muller-Eberhard, and S. Kida, *Ann. N. Y. Acad. Sci.*, 259 (1975) 45.
16 H. L. Leffert, T. Moran, R. Boorstein, and K. S. Koch, *Nature*, 267 (1977) 58.
17 P. R. Walker and J. Grindle, *J. Cell. Physiol.*, 91 (1977) 181.
18 P. A. Watkins, D. M. Tarlow, and M. D. Lane, *Proc. Natl. Acad. Sci. U.S.*, 74 (1977) 1497.
19 R. C. Feldhoff, J. M. Taylor, and L. S. Jefferson, *J. Biol. Chem.*, 252 (1977) 3611.
20 P. O. Seglen, *Biochim. Biophys. Acta*, 496 (1977) 182.
21 G. M. Decad, D. P. H. Hsieh, and J. L. Byard, *Biochem. Biophys. Res. Commun.*, 78 (1977) 279.

REFERENCES

AMPLIFICATION OF DIHYDROFOLATE REDUCTASE GENES IN METHOTREXATE-RESISTANT CULTURED MOUSE CELLS

ROBERT T. SCHIMKE,*[1] FREDERICK W. ALT,*[1] RODNEY E. KELLEMS,*[1] RANDAL KAUFMAN,*[1] AND JOSEPH R. BERTINO*[2]

*Department of Biological Sciences, Stanford University, Stanford, California**[1] *and Departments of Pharmacology and Medicine, Yale University, New Haven, Connecticut**[2] (*U.S.A.*)

Our laboratory has been investigating the mechanism whereby cultured cells acquire resistance to the 4-amino analogs of folic acid, a phenomenon often associated both in cultured cells and in human neoplasms[1] with elevated levels of DHFR activity. Resistant cell variants containing up to a 200-fold increase in DHFR activity can be obtained by growth of cells in progressively increasing concentrations of MTX.[2-4] Previous reports from this laboratory employing cell variants derived from a mouse sarcoma (S-180) have demonstrated that the increase in DHFR results solely from an increased rate of enzyme synthesis,[5] and that there is a proportionality between the rate of enzyme synthesis and the content of specific mRNA as assayed in a rabbit reticulocyte translation system.[6] Littlefield and his colleagues, employing a cell line derived from baby hamster kidney cells, have come to similar conclusions.[7,8]

We summarize here studies employing cDNA complementary to the DHFR mRNA to quantitate the number of mRNA sequences and the number of gene copies. These experiments were done with the mouse sarcoma-derived AT-3000 cell line (high resistance), which reverts to sensitivity upon growth in MTX-free medium, as wellas with a mouse lymphoma-derived resistant cell line, L 1210, where the property of high resistance and high DHFR levels is retained in the absence of MTX. In both the stable and unstable cell lines we find a direct correlation between the content of enzyme and the relative amount of DHFR mRNA, comparing sensitive and resistant cell lines. More importantly, we also find that this correlation extends to the number of gene copies. Thus we conclude that the level of DHFR is directly proportional to the number of gene copies, *i.e.*, amplification, and that in some cell lines the genes are subject to rapid loss, whereas in other cell lines, they are fixed in the genome.

The cells and culture methods have been described previously.[5,6] The figure legends provide certain details of experimental procedures, and extensive descriptions of methods and corroborating data are published elsewhere.[9]

SYNTHESIS OF DIHYDROFOLATE REDUCTASE

Figure 1 compares the pattern of pulse-labeled soluble protein in S3 (sensitive) and AT-3000 (resistant) cells in which there is approximately a 200-fold difference in DHFR

Abbreviations: DHFR, dihydrofolate reductase; MTX, methotrexate; cDNA, DNA complementary to specific mRNA.

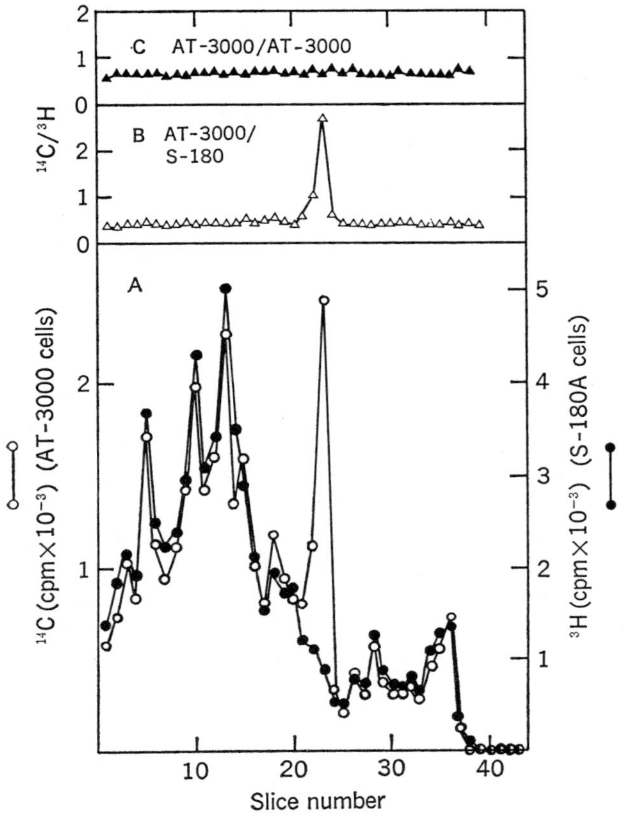

Fig. 1. Analysis of pulse-labeled soluble proteins from sensitive and resistant cells. A, logarithmically growing cultures of S-180 and AT-3000 cells were pulse-labeled with [^{3}H]leucine (6 μCi/ml) and [^{14}C]leucine (2.5 μCi/ml), respectively. Cells were mixed and processed, and 100-μl aliquots of the cellular extract were precipitated with 10% trichloroacetic acid. The precipitates were dissolved and electrophoresed on sodium dodecyl sulfate-polyacrylamide gels. Radioactivity in gels was determined separately for ^{3}H (●) or ^{14}C (○). B, each *point* gives the ratio of ^{14}C to ^{3}H for the corresponding *point* on the gel shown in Fig. 2A. C, duplicate cultures of AT-3000 cells were pulselabeled with either [^{3}H]leucine (6 μCi/ml) or [^{14}C]leucine (2.5 μCi/ml). The cells were mixed and processed, and aliquots of the extract were electrophoresed as described above. Each point gives the ratio of ^{14}C to ^{3}H in that gel slice. Details are given in ref. 5.

enzyme activity.[5] As displayed by electrophoresis on sodium dodecyl sulfate-acrylamide gels, there is no difference in the patterns of labeled proteins except for the prominent peak of ^{14}C label (resistant cells) which in other experiments we have shown comigrates with DHFR. We conclude that the only detectable difference in the pattern of synthesis of proteins between the two cell lines can be ascribed to increased synthesis of the enzyme.

We have observed a variety of parameters which alter DHFR levels, including different clones of the AT-3000 line, duration of cell growth in the absence of MTX, as well

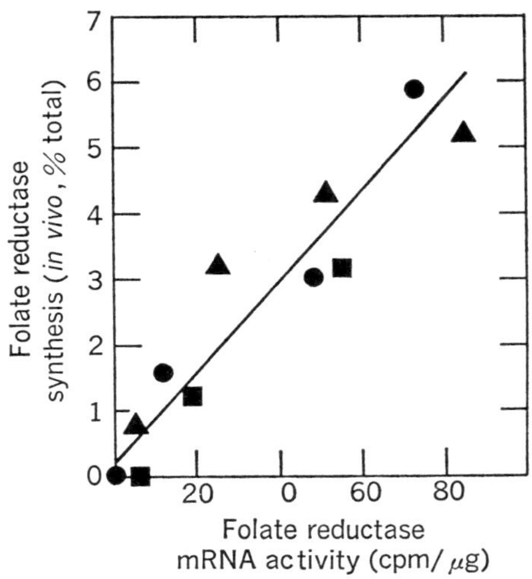

Fig. 2. The relative rate of folate reductase synthesis in cells as a function of folate reductase mRNA activity. The data from several independent experiments are gathered in this figure to illustrate the relationship between folate reductase mRNA activity and *in vivo* folate reductase synthesis. Details concerning the measurement of folate reductase synthesis and mRNA activity are given in ref. 6. ● AT-3000 cells ±MTX; ■ R-1 cells±MTX; ▲ AT-3000 cells, growth phase.

as the growth phase of the culture.[5] When cytoplasmic RNA is extracted from such cells and quantitated for ability to code for DHFR synthesis in a rabbit reticulocyte lysate, we find a good correlation between the proportional rate of enzyme synthesis (percent of radioactivity incorporated into immunoprecipitable dihydrofolate reductase relative to incorporation into total soluble protein), and the amount of translatable mRNA (Fig. 2). Thus, we conclude, by this relatively crude assay, that cells synthesize more enzyme because they contain more specific mRNA activity.

QUANTITATION OF DHFR mRNA AND GENE NUMBER

In order to obtain more accurate quantitation of the relative number of specific mRNA sequences, as well as to determine the number of gene copies, we have purified cDNA to DHFR mRNA. The DHFR mRNA contains poly (A) sequences, but its size distribution relative to total poly (A) RNA is not sufficiently distinct to allow for meaningful purifications by size fractionation. Therefore we have obtained DHFR cDNA by a combination of the two techniques. We undertook an initial enrichment of the mRNA by means of immunoprecipitation of the specific polysomes[10] which resulted in an mRNA preparation approximately 25–30% pure. We have then synthesized cDNA with this material.

We have also made use of the fact that there is more DHFR mRNA in resistant cells (Fig. 2), and that it would appear that only DHFR synthesis is vastly increased in resistant cells (Fig. 1) to remove the contaminating cDNA species by hybridization of the cDNA generated from the immunoprecipitated poly (A) RNA to a 40-fold (mass) excess of poly (A) RNA from sensitive cells. By hybridizing this cDNA to a limited excess of mRNA from sensitive cells and subsequently selecting the cDNA that did not hybridize by chromatography on hydroxylapatite, we remove from the cDNA preparation those cDNA sequences which are of similar abundance in mRNA from both sensitive and resistant cells. Secondly, we have hybridized the resulting cDNA preparation to poly (A) RNA from the resistant cells, and selected those cDNA sequences whose rate of hybridization is very rapid, *i.e.*, those mRNA sequences present in high abundance in the resistant cells. Details of the purification and evidence supporting the conclusion that the cDNA obtained is specific for DHFR mRNA are provided elsewhere.[9]

Figure 3A shows the hybridization kinetics of cDNA with poly (A) RNA from sensi-

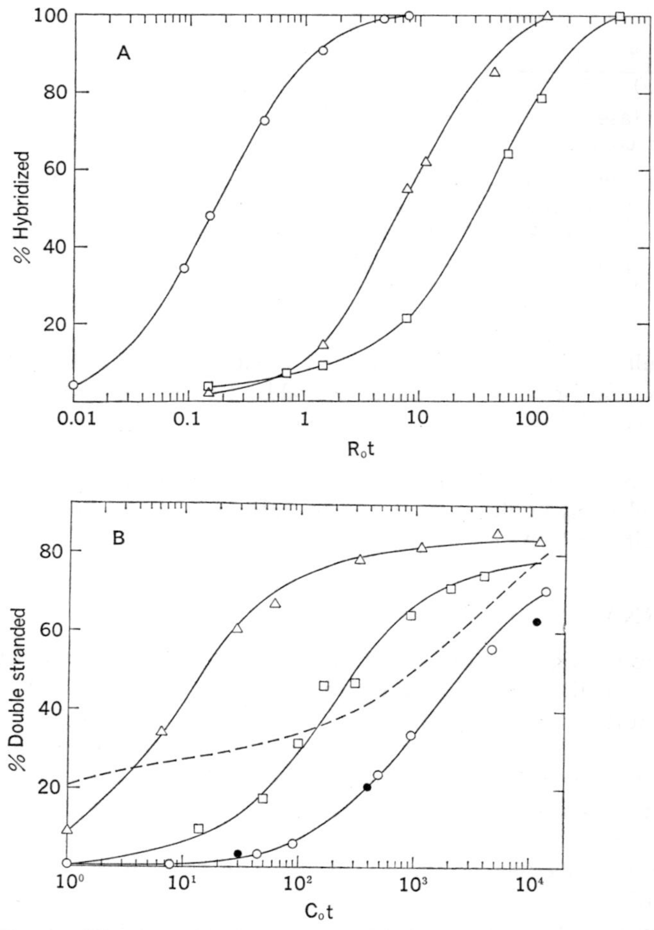

Fig. 3. Kinetics of hybridization of DHFR cDNA probe to poly(A) RNA and DNA from MTX-sensitive and -resistant mouse S-180 cells. The three cell lines are described in the text. A, cDNA: poly(A) RNA hybridizations; □ sensitive; △ revertant 400; ○ resistant. B, cDNA: DNA hybridization, ○ sensitive; □ revertant 400; △ resistant; ● sensitive with added poly(A) RNA from resistant cells (see text); ----- *C₀t* curve of total DNA.

tive, resistant (200-fold increase in enzyme relative to sensitive cells) and resistant S-180 cells grown in the absence of MTX for 400 cell doublings, designated as R-400 (10-fold increase in enzyme over sensitive cells). Three points are of note: (1) The hybridization approaches 100%; (2) the kinetics of the reactions are essentially defined by a single pseudo-first order reaction characteristic of the interaction of a single reacting species of cDNA with a single reacting species of RNA reacting with RNA present in equal concentrations); (3) the different RNA preparations contain different abundances of the RNA species reacting with the cDNA, and the $R_0t_{1/2}$ values of the reactions are consistent with the differences in DHFR levels (and the rate of enzyme synthesis) in the different

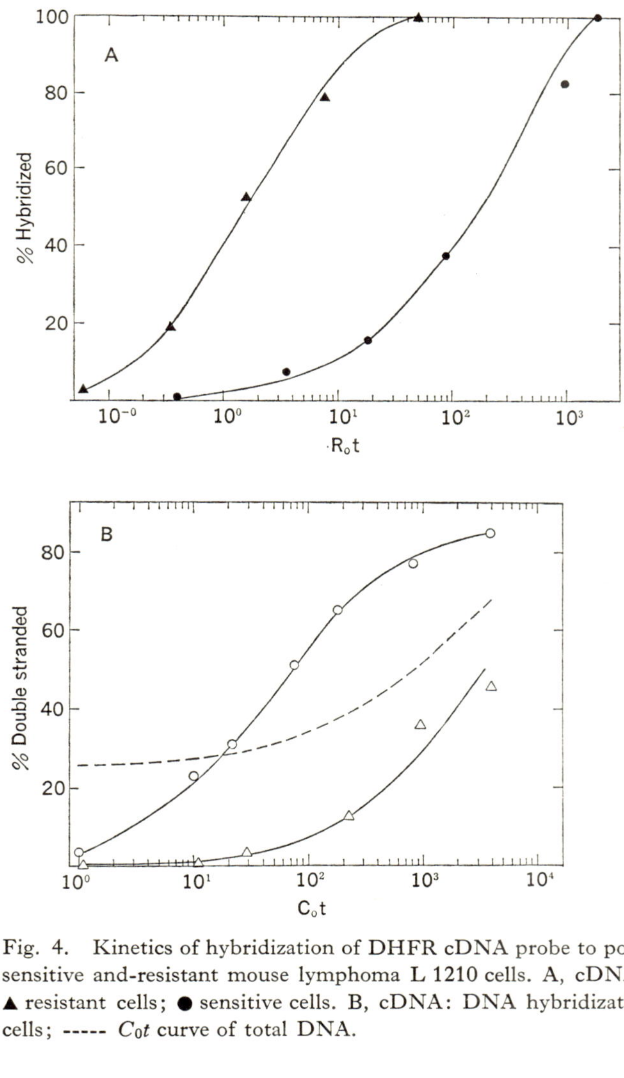

Fig. 4. Kinetics of hybridization of DHFR cDNA probe to poly(A) RNA and DNA from MTX-sensitive and-resistant mouse lymphoma L 1210 cells. A, cDNA: poly (A) RNA hybridizations; ▲ resistant cells; ● sensitive cells. B, cDNA: DNA hybridizations; ○ resistant cells; △ sensitive cells; ----- C_0t curve of total DNA.

cells. We therefore conclude that there is a direct correlation between the rate of enzyme synthesis and the abundance of mRNA complementary to the cDNA.

Figure 3B shows hybridization of the cDNA to DNA from the sensitive, resistant and revertant cell lines of S-180, as well as the C_0t curve for total cell DNA (dotted lines). The hybridizations approximate 80–90% completion with kinetics characteristic of a unique second-order reaction. Most important is the finding that there is an acceleration in the rate of hybridization when DNA from resistant and revertant cells is used and that the degree of acceleration is consistent with the amount of DHFR enzyme and mRNA content in these cell lines. We therefore conclude that there are different numbers of DHFR genes and, furthermore, the number is directly proportional to the rate of enzyme synthesis. An important control is shown by the closed circles in Fig. 3B, in which an amount of poly (A) RNA from resistant cells equivalent to that derived from the amount of cells used to obtain the DNA for each C_0t point was added to the DNA from sensitive cells prior to base hydrolysis (to remove RNA). This result shows that all of the RNA was destroyed. Hence the acceleration of the cDNA:DNA hybridization cannot be ascribed to contaminating RNA in the DNA preparations from the resistant cells.

Figures 4A and 4B show comparable hybridization analyses with the mouse lymphoma-derived sensitive and resistant L1210 cell lines, in which the resistance and high enzyme level is stable in the absence of MTX in the growth medium. The relative content of mRNA and genes between sensitive and resistant cell lines is consistent with the approximately 50- to 75-fold difference in DHFR activity in these lines. Thus, we find a direct relationship between the number of genes and the rates of specific protein synthesis in the L1210 lines as well as the S-180 lines.

The property of high enzyme content and rate of DHFR synthesis is not stable in the

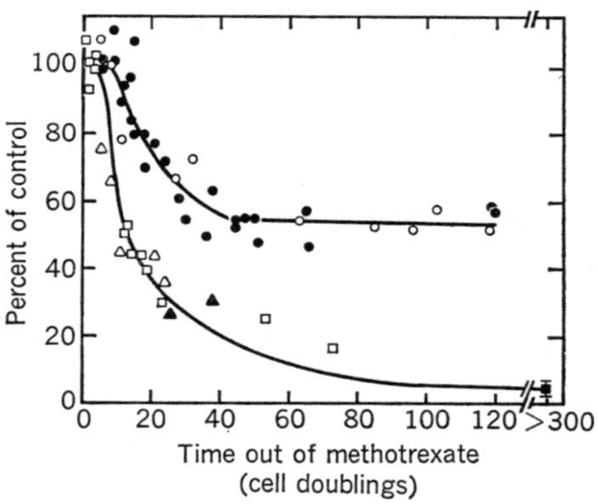

Fig. 5. Effect of MTX on folate reductase synthesis. Resistant cells maintained in a medium containing 50 μM MTX were split in duplicate into flasks containing medium with and without 50 μM MTX. At various cell doublings thereafter, midlog phase cells were pulse-labeled with [^{3}H]leucine and the relative rate of isotope incorporation into immunoprecipitable DHFR (open symbols) or enzyme activity (closed symbols) was measured. Each point represents the relative value for cells grown in the absence of MTX expressed as a percent of the corresponding value for control cells grown in the presence of MTX. □ data from ref. 5; △ data from these same cells frozen in liquid nitrogen for 2 years prior to this experiment; ○ cells maintained continuously for 2 years in 50 μM MTX prior to the experiment.

S-180 cells we have been studying. Furthermore, we have found that the rate of reversion varies, depending on the particular resistant cells we have employed. This is shown in Fig. 5 which shows the relative rate of DHFR synthesis in cells after removal of MTX from the growth medium. All of the cells studied in this figure were obtained from a single clone of the parental AT-3000 cell line. For cells maintained for a relatively short time in a medium containing 50 μM MTX prior to MTX withdrawal, whether those cells were studied 30 months ago (squares) or 4 months ago (triangles), there is a rapid decrease in the rate of enzyme synthesis, as well as a related decrease in mRNA content and gene number (data not shown). For the same cell clone that had been maintained over 2 years continuously in 50 μM MTX, removal of MTX from the medium results in a slower loss of enzyme synthesis capacity, and after some 40 cell doublings, high enzyme synthesis is now a stable property of the cells. Therefore something has happened to the cells during the 2-year period of constant growth in MTX that has now led to fixation of the amplified genes in the genome of these cells.

The observation that under appropriate selection conditions the rate of synthesis of a specific protein, *i.e.*, DHFR can be altered by changes in the number of specific genes in cultured mammalian cells, to the best of our knowledge has not been clearly documented previously. We know very little about the mechanism(s) of the process whereby this occurs, and our initial observations open up a number of experimental approaches to the problem. Modulation of the number of specific gene copies has been documented in various organisms, including the classical study of Sturtevant in 1925 involving the Bar locus in *Drosophila*, as well as more recently in various prokaryotic systems,[11-13] Amplification of the ribosomal genes in *Xenopus* during oocyte maturation is a classical example in higher organisms.[14] That an increase in the number of specific genes can occur in such a wide spectrum of biological material suggests that it can occur in all organisms.

It is perhaps instructive to compare the alteration in gene number in other cases with our studies in cultured mammalian cells. Classically in *E. coli* the duplication of genes has been observed when cells have been placed under selection such that those cells with an increased number of gene copies (and gene expression) will have a growth advantage, *e.g.*, *E. coli* with a defective aminoacyl tRNA synthetase selected for more rapid growth in limiting amino acid concentration.[12] Anderson *et al.*[13] have suggested recently that in *Salmonella typhimurium* there is a random duplication of genes, and hence the selection process will obtain those individual cells that are duplicated for the specific gene at any given time. The development of resistance in *Proteus mirabilis* to chloramphenicol is analogous to MTX resistance in cultured cells, and results from an increased capacity for synthesis of chloramphenicol acetyltransferase and an increase in the number of genes specifying chloramphenicol resistance as well as other antibiotic resistances.[15]

Similarly the presence of MTX in the growth medium subjects mammalian cells to selection for growth. Inhibition of DHFR inhibits *de novo* purine, thymidine, and glycine synthesis, and hence selects for cells capable of increased enzyme synthesis. Selection of resistant cell lines requires a slow incremental increase in MTX concentration in the medium. Subjecting cells to a high drug concentration has uniformly failed to result in obtaining resistant cells. We would suggest that the progressive amplification of genes is a relatively rare event. Our preliminary estimates, as well as those of Hakala and Ishihara[16] are that approximately 1 in 10^6 or 10^7 cells survive each incremental increase in MTX concentration and cells must undergo a number of amplifications to attain high enzyme levels and high resistance. That the phenomenon of increased gene copies may not be unique to DHFR is suggested by recent studies of Stark and his colleagues who have observed the emergence of resistance in cultured hamster cells to PALA, a specific inhibitor of aspartyl transcarbamylase. They have found that there is more enzyme activity in resistant cells.[17] I nboth cases the inhibitors are highly specific for enzymes required for cell growth. It will be interesting to determine if the same phenomenon (increased gene copies) can be observed with a variety of specific enzyme inhibitors, or whether the phenomenon is limited to certain genes. It should be noted that the inhibitor must be highly specific, since if it inhibits several enzymes, the chances of two genes being amplified in the same cell at any specific time would be highly unlikely.

In the cases of increased gene numbers studied in *Drosophila* and prokaryotes the phenomenon appears to be one of tandem duplication (refs. 11–13), and in the *Drosophila* case, Sturtevant originally proposed that it occurred by unequal crossing over during DNA replication.[18] Although we do not know if the genes in our cultured cells are tandemly duplicated, the karyology studies of Biedler and her colleagues are most interesting. They have reported both in hamster cells,[19] as well as in the L1210 (ref. 20) cell line we have studied, that there is a well-defined alteration in a specific chromosome in MTX-resistant cells, but not in the sensitive cells. *In situ* hybridizations of the DHFR cDNA to mitotic chromosomes are currently in progress in our laboratory with both the S-180 and L1210 cells to determine if the chromosomal abnormality observed by Biedler's group corresponds to the DHFR genes, or whether the genes are dispersed at different sites within the chromosomes. If the genes appear to be localized to a specific chromosomal segment, it will be most interesting to determine by restriction fragment analysis and sequence studies of recombinant DNA clones whether the genes and their adjacent sequences are similar or not. If the former is observed, it would suggest that the amplification process occurs at specific DNA sequences. Such sequences would then have analogy with insertion sequences as observed in prokaryote cells[21] and suggest a possible role in genome structure (and flexibility) in higher eukaryotes.

We have employed the term "amplification" to describe an increased number of gene copies in a context different from that employed to describe the process where there is amplification of ribosomal genes in *Xenopus*. In our case there appears to be a selection pressure for obtaining those cells randomly in a state of specific gene duplication. We differentiate this process from that which is specifically regulated as part of a developmental sequence. It is of interest to note that the rDNA amplification in *Xenopus* occurs by amplification of a subset of rDNA sequences in a given oocyte by a so-called rolling circle process which results in the generation of extra-chromosomal rDNA segments.[22] Gene amplification during a developmental sequence has not been observed in cases where large amounts of differentiated cell products are synthesized, *e.g.*, globin,[23] ovalbumin,[24] silk fibroin,[25] implying that regulation of these genes occurs by modulation of expression of a limited number of gene copies. However, it would appear that the rate of DHFR synthesis in the cultured cells we have studied is proportional to the number of specific genes, implying that little modulation of the activity of each gene has occurred.

The finding that certain cell lines "revert" to MTX sensitivity with differing rates, and to differing degrees, is both interesting and puzzling. Reversion (gene loss) is a well-known phenomenon in instances of tandem duplication in prokaryotes, and a reversal of such a duplication process can be envisaged readily as a mechanism for gene loss in our cells. One can consider two general processes which would lead to "fixation" of genes in the genome. One is a secondary alteration in cells resulting in lack of an enzymatic process that "excises" genes. Perhaps more likely is an alteration in the sequence structure of the multiplied genes, either by translocation, or loss of specific flanking sequences (insertion or recombinational sequences[21]) that prevents subsequent excision. The analogy between the generation of increased gene copies and their fixation in the genome in our cultured cells and the process of gene duplication, fixation, and random mutation-selection in evolution[26] is striking and bears further study.

Our results add further evidence to support the emerging concept that the genome in higher organisms is not constant, but can undergo a variety of changes, including duplications, as well as the clearly documented instances of translocation of the variable and league in fragmentation of macro nuclear genomes in protozoa,[28] ascaris[29] and the loss of entire chromosomes in insect somatic cells.[30] It is equally interesting to note that in the case of insects and protozoa where the genome disruption occurs, as well as in the vast majority of higher organisms, the germ cell line is sequestered (differentiated) early in the process of cell division and differentiation. Hence those cells carrying the full complement of the genome and involved in sexual conjugation need not be subject to potential possible deletions, inversions, translocations, *etc*. While the striking alteration in the genomic structure of a limited number of species need not be characteristic of all differentiating organisms, less obvious alterations may underlie a number of controls of differentiation.

REFERENCES

1 J. R. Bertino, D. M. Donohue, B. Simmons, B. W. Gabrio, R. Silber, and F. M. Huennekens, *J. Clin. Invest.*, 42 (1963) 466.

2 M. T. Hakala, S. E. Zakrgewski, and C. Nichol, *J. Biol. Chem.*, 236 (1961) 952.

3 G. A. Fisher, *Biochem. Pharmacol.*, 7 (1961) 75.

4 K. Friedkin, E. S. Crawford, S. R. Humphreys, and A. Goldin, *Cancer Res.*, 22 (1962) 600.

5 F. W. Alt, R. E. Kellems, and R. T. Schimke, *J. Biol. Chem.*, 251 (1976) 3063.

6 R. E. Kellems, F. W. Alt, and R. T. Schimke, *J. Biol. Chem.*, 251 (1976) 6987.

7 U. J. Hanggi and J. W. Littlefield, *J. Biol. Chem.*, 251 (1976) 3075.

8 S. Chang and J. W. Littlefield, *Cell*, 7 (1976) 391.

9 F. W. Alt, R. E. Kellems, J. R. Bertino, and R. T. Schimke, submitted to *J. Biol. Chem.* (1977).

10 D. J. Shapiro, J. M. Taylor, G. S. McKnight, R. Palacios, C. Gonzalez, M. L. Kiely, and R. T. Schimke, *J. Biol. Chem.*, 249 (1974) 3665.

11 S. W. Emmons, V. MacCosham, and R. L. Baldwin, *J. Mol. Biol.*, 91 (1975) 133.

12 W. R. Folk and P. Berg, *J. Mol. Biol.*, 58 (1971) 595.

13 R. P. Anderson, C. G. Miller, and J. R. Roth, *J. Mol. Biol.*, 105 (1976) 201.

14 D. D. Brown and I. B. Dawid, *Science*, 160 (1968) 272.

15 D. Perlman, T. M. Twose, M. J. Holland, and R. H. Rownd, *J. Bacteriol.*, 123 (1975) 1035.

16 M. T. Hakala and T. Ishihara, *Cancer Res.*, 22 (1962) 987.

17 T. D. Kempe, E. A. Swyryd, M. Bruist, and G. R. Stark, *Cell*, 9 (1976) 541.

18 A. H. Sturtevant, *Genetics*, 10 (1925) 117.

19 J. L. Biedler and B. A. Spengler, *Science*, 191 (1976) 185.

20 J. L. Biedler, A. M. Albrecht, and D. J. Hutchison, *Cancer Res.*, 25 (1965) 246.

21 S. N. Cohen, *Nature*, 263 (1976) 731.

22 D. Hourcade, D. Dressler, and J. Wolfson, *Cold Spring Harbor Symp. Quant. Biol.*, 38 (1973) 537.

23 S. Packman, H. Aviv, J. Ross, and P. Leder, *Biochem. Biophys. Res. Commun.*, 49 (1972) 813.

24 D. Sullivan, R. Palacios, J. Stavnezer, J. M. Taylor, A. J. Faras, M. L. Kiely, N. M. Summers, J. M. Bishop, and R. T. Schimke, *J. Biol. Chem.*, 248 (1973) 7530.
25 Y. Suzuki, L. P. Gage, and D. D. Brown, *J. Mol. Biol.*, 70 (1972) 637.
26 S. Ohno, *Evolution by Gene Duplication*, Springer-Verlag, Berlin, New York, 1970.
27 N. Hozumi and S. Tonegawa, *Proc. Natl. Acad. Sci. U.S.*, 73 (1976) 3628.
28 D. M. Prescott, K. G. Murti, and C. J. Bostock, *Nature*, 242 (1973) 576, 597.
29 H. Tobler, K. D. Smith, and H. Ursprung, *Dev. Biol.*, 27 (1972) 190.
30 I. Geyer-Duszynska, *J. Exp. Zool.*, 141 (1959) 391.

ROLE OF DIPEPTIDASES AND DIPEPTIDE ABSORPTION IN INTESTINAL DIGESTION OF PROTEINS*

V. GANAPATHY AND A. N. RADHAKRISHNAN
School of Life Sciences, University of Hyderabad, Hyderabad (India)

Digestion of dietary proteins takes place in the small intestine of animals by a variety of proteolytic enzymes present in the gastrointestinal tract. Pepsin in the stomach, perhaps, plays only a limited role in protein digestion. Pancreatic enzymes notably trypsin, chymotrypsin, and carboxypeptidases and the mucosal enzyme leucineaminopeptidase generally attack large proteins although some of these enzymes attack smaller peptides also. However, till recently there had been a tacit assumption that by the concerted or sequential action of the enzymes in the gastrointestinal tract, the dietary proteins are broken down all the way to amino acids which are then actively absorbed. It was also the belief that since only amino acids and no peptides are present in the portal blood soon after a protein meal, absorption must have taken place in the form of amino acids. Evidence has been accumulating to suggest that small peptides are actually taken up by the enterocyte and that peptides might be intermediates in the digestion and absorption of proteins.

Several earlier observations in support of this concept were entirely ignored.

a) Messerli and others almost 60 years ago observed that enzymatic hydrolysates of proteins were absorbed faster than an equivalent mixture of individual amino acids.[1]

b) In 1954, Fisher noted that the time taken for complete hydrolysis of proteins by pancreatic proteases *in vitro* was so slow compared to the observed rate of absorption of proteins *in vivo* that complete hydrolysis of proteins to amino acids seemed unlikely.[2] More recently, a similar conclusion was drawn by Nixon and Mawer[3] who showed that certain amino acids were released too slowly from proteins to be absorbed in the free form.

c) In the 1950's, homopeptides of glycine were shown to be taken up and found inside the enterocyte,[4-7] but the work was ignored since glycyl-glycine, glycyl-glycyl-glycine, *etc.* were considered to be unusual and perhaps unnatural peptides.

There has been in recent years a renewed interest in peptide absorption as perhaps a major aspect of protein absorption. There exists a separate uptake system for peptides in the intestine of many mammalian species (for reviews, see refs. 8, 9). The presence of separate uptake systems for peptides in bacteria is a well-established fact,[10,11] and more recently it has been shown that uptake of peptides occur in higher plants also during germination.[12] A decisive proof for the distinct nature of peptide transport in man came from studies in hartnup disease and in cystinuria.[13-16] In hartnup disease, the neutral amino acid transport

* The work reported here was carried out at the Wellcome Research Unit, Christian Medical College Hospital, Vellore-632004, Tamil Nadu, India.

TABLE I

SUBSTRATE SPECIFICITY OF THE "MASTER" DIPEPTIDASE

All the peptides contained amino acids of the L-configuration. The peptides that were inactive as substrates are underlined.

C-terminal	*Gly*	*Ala*	*Ile, Leu Val*	*Ser, Thr*	*Phe, Tyr Trp, His*	*Met*	*Asp, Glu*	*Lys, Arg*
N-terminal			Gly-Ile		Gly-Trp			
Gly	Gly-Gly	Gly-Ala	Gly-Leu	Gly-Thr	Gly-Phe	Gly-Met	Gly-Glu	Gly-Lys
			Gly-Val		Gly-His			
Ala	Ala-Gly	Ala-Ala	Ala-Leu	Ala-Ser	Ala-Phe	Ala-Met	Ala-Asp	Ala-Arg
			Ala-Val					Ala-Lys
Ile, Leu	Leu-Gly	Leu-Ala	Leu-Leu					
Val			Val-Leu	Leu-Ser	Leu-Phe	Leu-Met		
Ser, Thr	Ser-Gly	Ser-Ala	Ser-Leu	Ser-Ser	Ser-Phe	Thr-Met		
His			His-Leu					
Phe, Tyr			Phe-Leu					
Trp	Phe-Gly	Phe-Ala	Tyr-Leu		Phe-Phe	Phe-Met	Tyr-Glu	Tyr-Lys
			Trp-Leu					
Met	Met-Gly	Met-Ala	Met-Leu	Met-Ser	Met-Phe			
			Met-Val	Met-Thr	Met-Tyr	Met-Met	Met-Glu	
	Glu-Glu						Glu-Glu	Glu-Lys
Asp, Glu	Asp-Gly	Glu-Ala	Glu-Val		Glu-Tyr		Glu-Asp	Asp-Lys
								Lys-Lys
Lys	Lys-Gly	Lys-Ala	Lys-Leu		Lys-Phe		Lys-Asp	
Arg	Arg-Gly	Arg-Ala					Arg-Asp	Arg-Arg
								Arg-Lys

From Das and Radhakrishnan.[18]

system is impaired and pellagra-like symptoms develop due to a deficiency in tryptophan absorption. These patients, however, absorb tryptophan very efficiently when it is presented as a peptide. Similarly, in cystinuria, the patients efficiently absorb cystine and basic amino acids when present as peptides while the absorption of these amino acids when present as free amino acids is impaired.

INTESTINAL DIPEPTIDASES

The major problem in demonstrating peptide absorption is that intact peptides are seldom seen in the enterocyte and in the portal blood. This is because of the presence of powerful peptidases in the intestine. Our efforts have, hence, been directed mostly towards a detailed study of peptidases—their nature, cellular localization, substrate specificity and the possible number of peptidases. Another aspect of our work has been to study the role of peptidases in the transport of peptides.

If we consider the number of theoretically possible dipeptides with 20 and more amino acids, it will be well over 400, and for tripeptides it will be over 8,000. Thus the crucial question is whether there are a limited number of peptidases with a broad specificity or whether there is a whole fleet of peptidases, each with limited specificity.

Dipeptide hydrolysing activity is present both in the cytosol and the brush border fractions of the enterocyte. However, the bulk of the activity (about 90%) is in the cytosol fraction. Our work suggests that there are only a limited number of dipeptidases in the cytosol, with characteristic specificity. The following enzymes have been adequately characterized: a) The "master" dipeptidase which hydrolyses over 80% of the possible dipeptides; b) glycyl-glycine hydrolase; c) glycyl-histidine hydrolase; d) glycyl-proline hydrolase (imido dipeptidase); e) prolyl-glycine hydrolase (imino dipeptidase). In the case of c) to e), glycine may be replaced by several other amino acids. It is possible that some of the dipeptides with acidic amino acids are hydrolysed by a separate enzyme, as suggested by the work of Andria *et al.*[17] Even though dipeptide hydrolysing activity is present in the brush border fraction of the enterocyte, so far no "true" dipeptidase has been isolated.

Table I shows the substrate specificity of our "master" dipeptidase, isolated from the cytosol fraction of monkey intestinal mucosa.[18] It has a very broad spectrum of substrate specificity and it is one of the most active enzymes in the body with a molecular activity 1.4×10^6 mol of glycyl-leucine hydrolysed/mol of dimer enzyme/min. The enzyme contains no sugar residues. It has two identical subunits of molecular weight 54,000.

INTESTINAL DIPEPTIDE TRANSPORT

We next studied several aspects of dipeptide transport in monkey and in man. Using monkey intestinal strips (20–30 mg) and with radioactive glycyl-leucine, we demonstrated that there is a broad spectrum dipeptide uptake system.[19] We came to this conclusion in view of the inhibition of the uptake of glycyl-leucine by a variety of dipeptides (Table II). Using judiciously selected dipeptides, the inhibition was shown to be competitive. In a limited study, this type of inhibition was also noted in human biopsy specimens. Although we found that the tripeptides glycyl-glycyl-leucine, glycyl-leucyl-glycine and glycyl-glycyl-glycine inhibited glycyl-leucine uptake, it was not possible to conclude that there was a common transport system for dipeptides and tripeptides. The inhibition may well

TABLE II

SPECIFICITY OF THE MONKEY INTESTINAL GLYCYL-L-[^{14}C]LEUCIN UPTAKE SYSTEM

In these experiments, the concentration of ^{14}C-labelled glycyl-L-leucine was 0.5 mM and the concentration of the unlabelled peptides was 10 mM in all cases. All the peptides, except glycyl-D-leucine, contained amino acids of the L-configuration. Z, N-benzyloxycarbonyl; Gly-γ-Abu, glycyl-γ-aminobutyric acid.

Peptide	*Inhibition (%)*	*Peptide*	*Inhibition (%)*
Gly-Gly	20	Gly-Asp	50
Gly-Ala	50	Gly-Glu	42
Gly-Val	65	Gly-Asn	63
Gly-Ile	78	Ala-Asp	62
Gly-Leu	86	Met-Glu	64
Gly-Ser	70	Asp-Gly	40
Gly-Phe	73	Glu-Ala	54
Gly-Trp	67	Glu-Val	58
Gly-His	63	Glu-Glu	54
Gly-Met	86	Gln-Gln	76
Ala-Gly	70	Tyr-Lys	77
Ala-Ala	73	Lys-Phe	67
Ala-Leu	92	Lys-Lys	62
Ala-Ser	74	Gly-D-Leu	10
Ala-Phe	86	Z-Gly-Leu	30
Ala-Met	86	Gly-β-Ala	20
Leu-Gly	87	Gly-γ-Abu	32
Ser-Leu	85	Gly-Gly-Leu	58
Met-Leu	91	Gly-Leu-Gly	58
Gly-Pro	69	Gly-Gly-Gly	20
Pro-Gly	51		

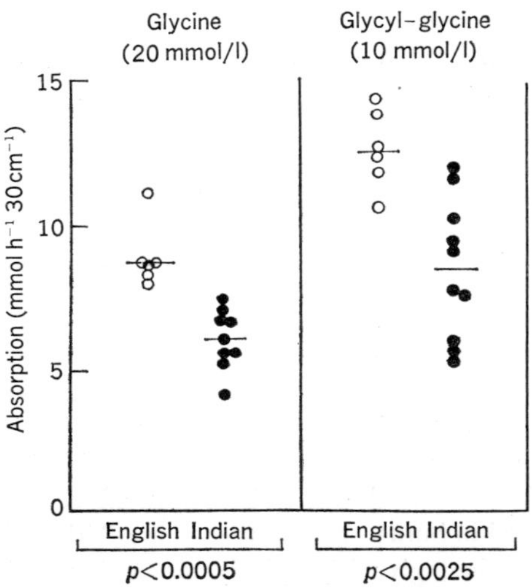

Fig. 1. Absorption of glycine (20 mM) and glycyl-glycine (10 mM) in normal English and Indian people. Horizontal lines represent means.

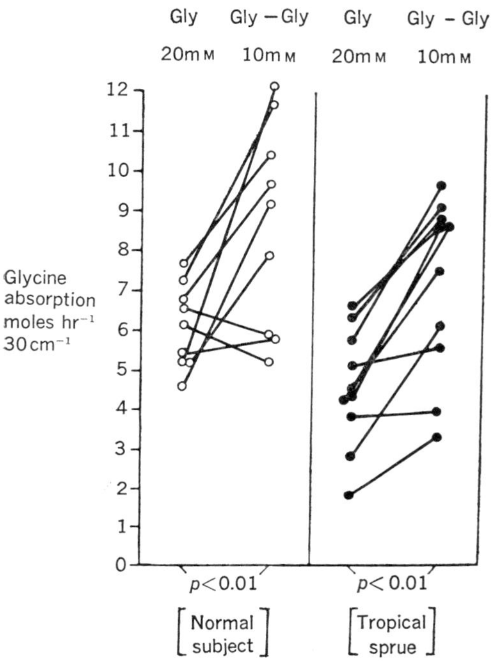

Fig. 2. Absorption of glycine (20 mM) and glycyl-glycine (10 mM) in control subjects and tropical sprue patients.

be due to the formation of dipeptides by the intestinal aminotripeptidase action and these dipeptides might be expected to cause the inhibition. Recently, using the non-hydrolysable tripeptide glycyl-sarcosyl-sarcosine, Addison *et al.*[20] have shown that the dipeptide transport system may also be shared by tripeptides.

Studies in the human with perfusion of glycine and glycyl-glycine showed that there was an impaired absorption of amino acid and dipeptide in normal Indian subjects compared to the British.[21] However, the kinetic advantage of dipeptide uptake over that of free amino acids was maintained (Fig. 1). Using the same technique, we studied the intestinal absorption of glycine, leucine, glycyl-glycine and glycyl-leucine in tropical sprue patients. Both the amino acid and dipeptide transport systems were impaired in these patients.[22] Nevertheless, the kinetic advantage was retained (Fig. 2).

AMINO ACID INTERACTION WITH DIPEPTIDE TRANSPORT AND DIPEPTIDE HYDROLYSIS

Further intensive studies with the monkey uptake system revealed that amino acids at higher concentrations inhibited dipeptide uptake. This finding came as a surprise since an interaction between amino acids and dipeptides during transport was not known. But many workers had earlier shown that amino acids can interfere with the hydrolysis of peptides at the enzyme level.[23,24] It can, therefore, be argued that the inhibition of dipeptide uptake by amino acids observed in our studies is due to inhibition of hydrolysis of the peptide inside the cell resulting in a reduction of peptide transport by decreasing the con-

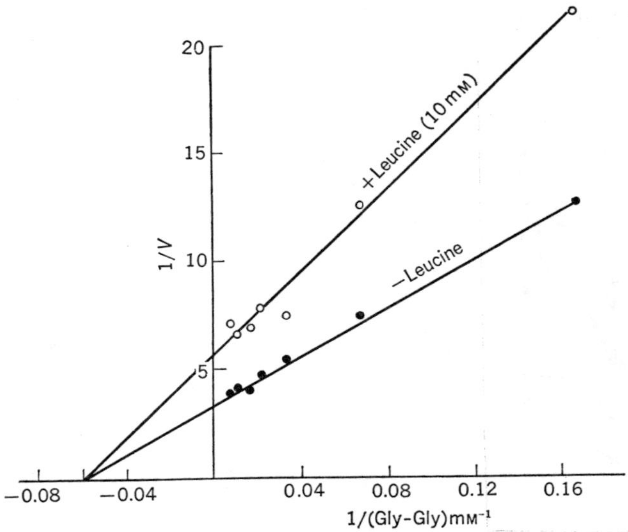

Fig. 3. Lineweaver-Burk plot showing non-competitive inhibition of glycyl-glycine hydrolysis by leucine (brush border enzyme from monkey intestine). V: μmol of glycyl-glycine hydrolysed (30 min)$^{-1}$ (30 μg protein)$^{-1}$.

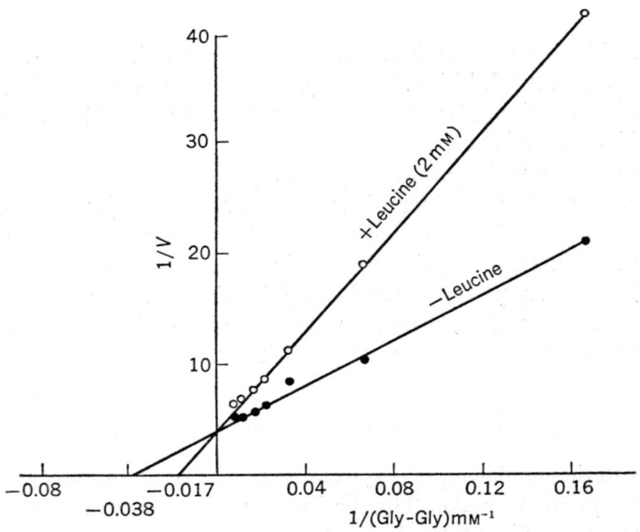

Fig. 4. Lineweaver-burk plot showing competitive inhibition of glycyl-glycine hydrolysis by leucine (cytosol enzyme from monkey intestine). V: μmole of glycyl-glycine hydrolysed (30 min)$^{-1}$ (3 μg protein)$^{-1}$.

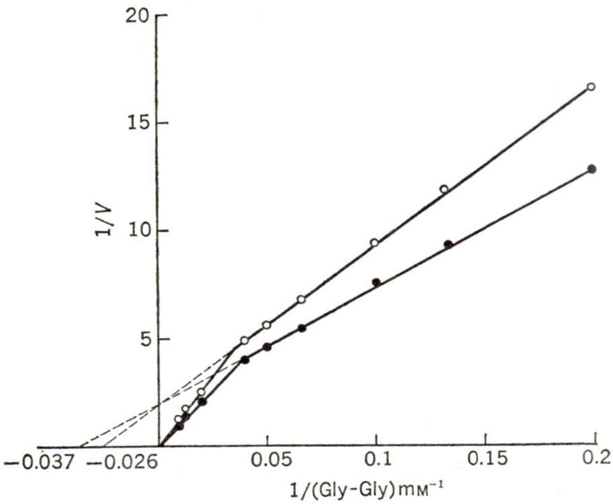

Fig. 5. Lineweaver-Burk plot showing competitive inhibition of uptake of glycyl[^{14}C]-glycine by leucine, using monkey intestinal strips. Inhibitor concentration, 50 mM. V: $10^{-3}\times$ counts min^{-1} (mg tissue)$^{-1}$.

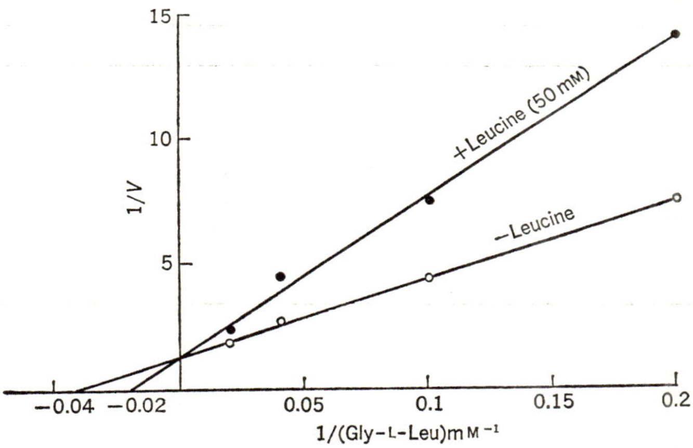

Fig. 6. Lineweaver-Burk plot showing competitive inhibition of uptake of glycyl[^{14}C]-leucine by leucine, using monkey intestinal strips. Inhibitor concentration, 50 mM. V: $10^{-3}\times$ counts min^{-1} (mg tissue)$^{-1}$.

centration gradient. Hence, we did a very careful and systematic study of the interaction of amino acids on the dipeptide hydrolysis by cytosol and brush border fractions and on the dipeptide transport. These results will now be discussed.

Leucine is one of the amino acids which inhibit glycyl-glycine hydrolysis. The kinetics of the inhibition by leucine of glycyl-glycine hydrolysis by cytosol and brush border fractions of the monkey small intestine were studied after separating the two fractions to a reasonable extent. While the brush border glycyl-glycine hydrolysing activity is inhibited non-competitively, the cytosol glycyl-glycine hydrolase is inhibited competitively (Figs. 3 and 4). But the uptake of both glycyl-glycine (Fig. 5) and glycyl-leucine (Fig. 6) was inhibited by leucine and the nature of inhibition was found to be competitive. Dissimilarity in the kinetics of inhibition excludes the possibility of the involvement of brush border enzyme in the transport of peptides. Even though the inhibition of cytosol enzyme and the inhibition of peptide uptake are kinetically similar, it is rather unlikely that these are related since an additional parameter, the brush border barrier, is also involved. Thus, these studies show that leucine interacts with the dipeptide uptake at the level of transport step and not at the hydrolysis step.

We then studied the effect of a number of amino acids on glycyl-leucine hydrolysis (both brush border and cytosol) and on glycyl-leucine transport to look for any possible relationship between the hydrolysis and the transport. Table III shows the effect of amino acids on glycyl-leucine hydrolase of monkey intestine, and Table IV shows the effect of amino acids on glycyl-leucine uptake by monkey intestinal strips. It was found that there was no correlation between the inhibition by amino acids of the two processes, transport

TABLE III

EFFECT OF AMINO ACIDS ON GLYCYL-LEUCIN HYDROLASE OF MONKEY INTESTINE

Gly, Ala, Pro, and Glu had no effect; Gly-Leu, 8 mM; Dopa, 20 mM.

L-Amino acid (40 *mM*)	*Inhibition (%)*		*L-Amino acid* (40 *mM*)	*Inhibition (%)*	
	Cytosol	*Brush border*		*Cytosol*	*Brush border*
Cys	100	100	Asp	45	39
His	95	74	Lys	34	0
Met	73	31	Val	31	16
Leu	64	36	Dopa	26	38
Nor-Leu	63	25	Thr	21	43
Trp	63	25	Hyp	12	0
Phe	62	47	Arg	10	23
Ile	59	22	Ser	8	19

TABLE IV

EFFECT OF AMINO ACIDS ON GLYCYL-[^{14}C]LEUCIN UPTAKE BY MONKEY INTESTINAL STRIPS

Gly-Leu, 2 mM.

L-Amino acid (50 *mM*)	*Inhibition* (%)	*L-Amino acid* (50 *mM*)	*Inhibition* (%)
Phe	62	Trp	31
Ala	59	Arg	30
Met	58	Pro	30
Leu	56	Ser	28
Cys	53	Hyp	27
Lys	49	Gly	27
Thr	47	Asn	24
Val	43	Glu	7
His	42	Asp	5
Gln	42		

and hydrolysis. This study provides an additional evidence for the direct interaction of amino acids and the dipeptides during their uptake.

Amino acid inhibition of glycyl-glycine uptake was also observed in perfusion studies in man. The uptake of glycyl-glycine was unaffected by the presence of glycine but was inhibited by about 30% in the presence of a mixture of leucine and glycine, thus suggesting inhibition *in vivo* of glycyl-glycine uptake by leucine.

HARMALINE AND DIPEPTIDE TRANSPORT

We did a limited study on the effect of harmaline, an hallucinogenic alkaloid, on the transport of dipeptides in the monkey small intestine. Harmaline is a well-known inhibitor of Na^+-K^+ adenosine triphosphatase system. It has already been shown to inhibit the transport of glucose and amino acids in guinea pig intestine.[25] Since the transport of dipeptides is also partially dependent on the presence of sodium, we expected harmaline might inhibit dipeptide transport. We found that preincubation of the tissue with harmaline at least for 10 min was necessary to obtain maximal inhibition and the study of the effect of harmaline concentration on the extent of inhibition revealed that 4 mM harmaline was optimal. Under these optimal conditions, harmaline inhibited glycyl-leucine transport to about 50%. However, Robinson *et al.*, who have carried out detailed studies on the

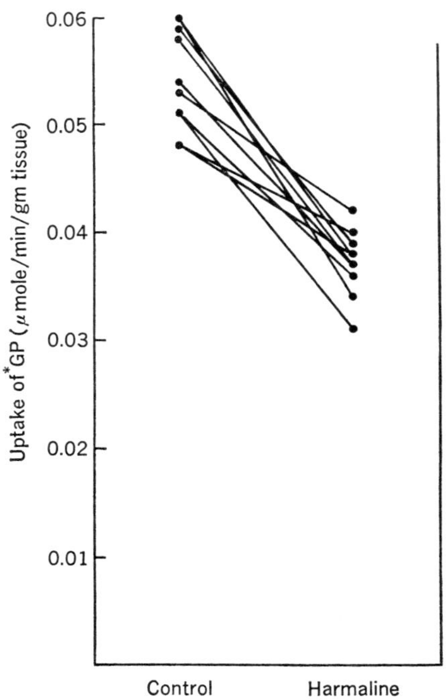

Fig. 7. Uptake of glycyl[^{14}C]-proline by monkey intestinal strips in presence and absence of harmaline (4 mM).

effect of harmaline on the transport of amino acids, found that harmaline inhibited phenylalanine transport to about 90%.[26] They have also established that the harmaline effect is incubation-time dependent. Thus, the difference in the results can be reasonably explained by the longer incubation time 60 min used by Robinson *et al.* compared to the 2 min incubation time used in our experiments.

In order to make certain that the harmaline inhibition of peptide uptake does not operate at the uptake of amino acids resulting from surface hydrolysis, we selected the peptide glycyl-proline against which there is no hydrolysing activity in the brush border preparations although as we mentioned earlier there is an active glycyl-proline hydrolase associated with the cytosol. Harmaline inhibits glycyl-proline uptake by about 30% (Fig. 7).

The effect of harmaline on the uptake of glycyl-leucine and glycyl-proline was studied in the presence and absence of sodium ions. The results show that absence of sodium reduces glycyl-leucine uptake by 57% and glycyl-proline uptake by 35%. Harmaline inhibits glycyl-leucine uptake by 60% and glycyl-proline uptake by 36% when sodium containing buffer is used. But the uptake of these two dipeptides are not affected by harmaline when sodium-free buffer is used. Thus, harmaline is inhibitory only when sodium ions are present in the medium. However, the sodium-independent uptake of glycyl-leucine and glycyl-proline is inhibited by other dipeptides. Alanyl-phenylalanine inhibits glycyl-leucine uptake by 62% and glycyl-leucine inhibits glycyl-proline uptake by 49%, even when sodium-free buffer is used.

A GENERAL SCHEME FOR PROTEIN DIGESTION AND ABSORPTION

The available information from our work as well as from others on protein digestion

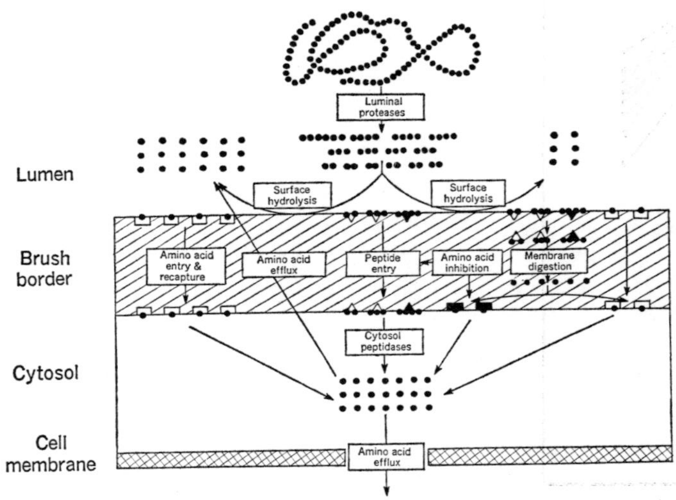

Fig. 8. A general scheme of protein digestion and absorption. ● amino acids; ●● ●●● ●●●● di-, tri-, and tetra-peptide; □ carrier proteins for amino acids (general entry); ■ carrier proteins for amino acids (special entry); △ common carrier for di- and tri-peptide; ▲ other special peptide carriers.

can be diagrammatically represented as in Fig. 8. We believe that the following mechanisms may operate in the terminal stages of protein digestion.

1) Proteins are hydrolysed in the lumen by the concerted action of pepsin, proteolytic enzymes present in the pancreatic juice and the mucosal surface proteases to a mixture of free amino acids and small peptides (dipeptides to hexapeptides), among which we believe the peptides predominate.

2) The free amino acids are taken up by the well established group-specific amino acid transport systems which can also operate in the recapture of amino acids effluxing from inside the cell.

3) Peptides are absorbed by three mechanisms.

a) Peptides crossing the brush border membrane intact, enter the cell where they are hydrolysed to amino acids by the powerful cytosol peptidases.

b) Peptides are converted to amino acids by surface hydrolysis (membrane digestion) and the amino acids then make use of group-specific amino acid transport systems to enter the cell. This component of peptide absorption would then behave just like the group-specific amino acid transport systems in all respects.

c) Surface hydrolysis (membrane digestion) yields amino acids but which are not in free equilibrium with the luminal amino acids. They are hence not available for the group-specific amino acid transport systems but are transported by a special transport system not yet rigorously established. This component of peptide transport would be susceptible to general amino acid inhibition without showing any group specificity, and kinetically it would be indistinguishable from the intact peptide entry system.

Under physiological conditions, all these mechanisms may operate, and this would explain the rapid absorption of proteins observed *in vivo*.

ACKNOWLEDGMENTS

We are deeply indebted to our colleague Dr. Manjusri Das who has collaborated in this work, and to Dr. M. D. Hellier for his contributions and stimulating discussions during his sabbatical year in Vellore. We would like to thank Prof. S. J. Baker, who was head of our unit during the project, for his help and encouragement. Our thanks are due to Dr. Annie Gammon and Dr. V. I. Mathan for their collaboration and to Mr. P. Dakshinamurthy for his help in the preparation of the manuscript. We also gratefully acknowledge financial assistance from the Wellcome Trust, London and C.S.I.R. (India).

REFERENCES

1 H. Messerli, *Biochem. Z.*, 54 (1913) 446.
2 R. B. Fisher, *Protein Metabolism*, Methuen, London, 1954.
3 S. E. Nixon and G. E. Mawer, *Br. J. Nutr.*, 24 (1970) 227.
4 W. T. Agar, F. J. R. Hird, and G. S. Sidhu, *J. Physiol.*, 121 (1953) 255.
5 D. S. Wiggans and J. M. Johnston, *Biochim. Biophys. Acta*, 32 (1959) 69.
6 H. Newey and D. H. Smyth, *J. Physiol.*, 145 (1959) 48.
7 H. Newey and D. H. Smyth, *J. Physiol.*, 164 (1962) 527.
8 D. M. Matthews, *Physiol. Rev.*, 55 (1975) 537.
9 M. Das and A. N. Radhakrishnan, *World Rev. Nutr. Diet.*, 24 (1976) 58.
10 J. W. Payne, in D. M. Matthews and J. W. Payne, *Peptide Transport in Protein Nutrition*, North-Holland, Amsterdam, 1975, p. 283.

11 J. W. Payne, in A. H. Rose and D. W. Tempest, *Advances in Microbial Physiology*, Academic Press, London, vol. 13, 1976, p. 55.
12 T. Sopanen, D. Burston, and D. M. Matthews, *FEBS Lett.*, 79 (1977) 4.
13 A. M. Asatoor, B. Cheng, K. D. G. Edwards, A. F. Lant, D. M. Matthews, M. D. Milne, F. Navab, and A. J. Richards, *Gut*, 11 (1970) 380.
14 J. V. Leonard, T. C. Marrs, J. M. Addison, D. Burston, K. M. Clegg, J. K. Lloyd, D. M. Matthews, and J. W. Seakins, *Pediat. Res.*, 10 (1976) 246.
15 M. D. Hellier, D. Perrett, and C. D. Holdsworth, *Br. Med. J.*, 4 (1970) 782.
16 M. D. Hellier, C. D. Holdsworth, D. Perrett, and C. Thirumalai, *Clin. Sci.*, 43 (1972) 659.
17 G. Andria, A. Marzi, and S. Auricchio, *Biochim. Biophys. Acta*, 419 (1976) 42.
18 M. Das and A. N. Radhakrishnan, *Biochem. J.*, 135 (1973) 609.
19 M. Das and A. N. Radhakrishnan, *Biochem. J.*, 146 (1975) 133.
20 J. W. Addison, D. Burston, J. A. Dalrymple, D. M. Matthews, J. W. Payne, M. H. Sleisenger, and S. Wilkinson, *Clin. Sci. Mol. Med.*, 49 (1975) 313.
21 M. D. Hellier, A. N. Radhakrishnan, V. Ganapathy, A. Gammon, and S. J. Baker, *Br. Med. J.*, 24 (1976) 186.
22 M. D. Hellier, A. N. Radhakrishnan, V. Ganapathy, V. I. Mathan, and S. J. Baker, *Gut*, 17 (1976) 511.
23 C. I. Cheesman and D. H. Smyth, *J. Physiol.*, 218 (1971) 39.
24 C. I. Cheesman and D. H. Smyth, *Proc. Roy. Soc. Lond. B*, 190 (1975) 149.
25 F. V. Sepulveda and J. W. L. Robinson, *Biochim. Biophys. Acta*, 373 (1974) 527.
26 F. V. Sepulveda and J. W. L. Robinson, *Naunyn-Schmiedeberg's Arch. Pharmacol.*, 291 (1975) 201.

INTESTINAL ABSORPTION OF ENZYME PROTEINS

TAKASHI MURACHI
Department of Clinical Science, Faculty of Medicine, Kyoto University, Kyoto (Japan)

The small intestine of certain *neonatal* mammalian species can absorb large quantities of macromolecules as a transient phenomenon for acquiring passive immunity. It is said that macromolecular absorption ceases when the epithelial cell membrane matures.[1]

However, in the early 1960s some enzyme preparations began to be used as anti-edema or anti-inflammation drugs given through the mouth.[2] One of these enzyme drugs was bromelain, a proteolytic enzyme from pineapple tissue, with which we were working at that time with a basic interest in enzymology.[3] We decided, therefore, to investigate whether bromelain molecule or other enzyme proteins could be absorbed *as such* through the adult intestine.

We first employed an *in vitro* system called the "everted sac method," which was usually used for studying absorption of small molecular weight substances such as glucose, amino acids, and certain antibiotics.[4] Quite unexpectedly, we obtained definite positive results showing small but significant transfer of proteolytic enzymes from the mucosal to the serosal side of the rabbit small intestine.[5] Positive results were also obtained in perfusion experiments.[6] Questions then arose regarding the structural and functional integrity of the intestinal preparations used for these *in vitro* studies and also regarding the use of proteolytic enzymes as the test protein since these enzymes could have digested the intestinal tissue and made it leaky.

After a number of trials, we found that an *in situ* system of experiment was far more successful in maintaining viability of the intestine as compared with *in vitro* systems.[7] We then avoided the use of proteolytic enzymes and, instead, used microbial lipase and hen egg-white lysozyme as the test proteins. Again we obtained the results showing positive absorption. As a result of a further series of *in situ* experiments with native and modified lysozyme, we have come to conclude that the absorption of enzyme proteins through the adult mammalian intestine is a physiological phenomenon.[8]

THE *in vitro* EXPERIMENTS

The first and the simplest system we adopted was the "everted sac method." A segment of rabbit intestine was everted to make it "inside-out," and the sample protein to be tested was added to the outside fluid, *i.e.*, to the mucosal side. The fluid in the sac lumen was tested from time to time to see whether the sample protein added could traverse to the serosal side.

Figure 1 shows the transfer of hen egg-white lysozyme across the adult rabbit jeju-

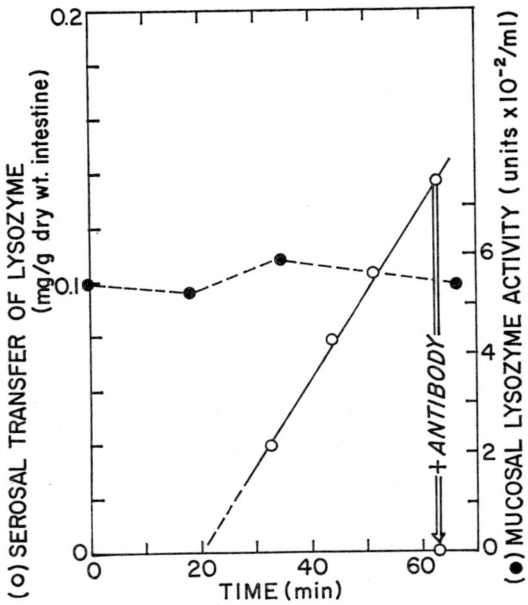

Fig. 1. Transfer of lysozyme across rabbit intestine, from the mucosal to the serosal side of an everted sac.[9] The lysozyme activity was assayed by measuring the rate of lysis of cell suspension of *Micrococcus lysodeikticus*. The weight of tissue was determined after drying under an infrared lamp for 20 hr.

num. Open circles represent such transfer, while solid circles respect the lysozyme activity in the outside fluid, *i.e.*, the mucosal side. The lysozyme activity transferred into the serosal fluid was completely inhibited by anti-hen egg-white lysozyme antibody, indicating that we were dealing with exogenous lysozyme absorbed rather than endogenous lysozyme that happened to be emerged.[9] Figure 2 is an example showing that the transfer of lysozyme is insensitive to a metabolic inhibitor. The transfer was not influenced also by 12 mM monoiodoacetic acid and by 3.4 mM DL-*p*-fluorophenylalanine added to the mucosal fluid.

We then continued with the more complicated *in vitro* perfusion experiments. A rabbit intestinal segment was cannulated at both the mesenteric arterial and venous vessels. Enzyme sample was added into the intestinal lumen, and the appearance of enzyme activity in the outflowing perfusate from venous cannula was monitored.

Figure 3 shows the time course of the absorption of stem bromelain. Open circles indicate the appearance of bromelain activities in venous perfusate in definite quantities. Similar results were obtained with α-chymotrypsin and amylase. The amount of test emzymes absorbed for 60 min was calculated to be a few percent of the amount added to the lumen.

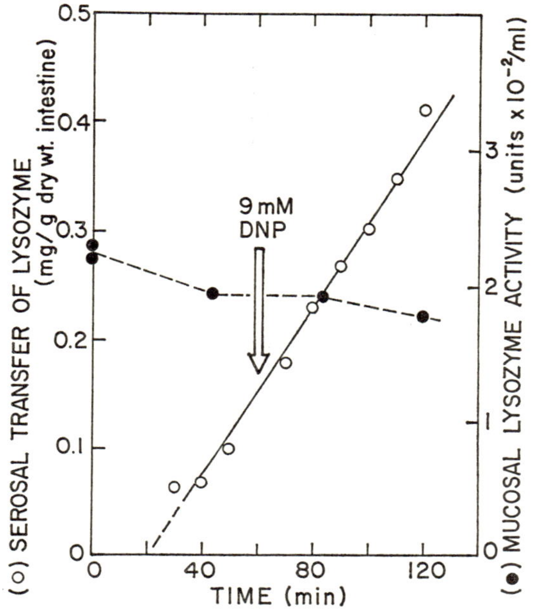

Fig. 2. Effect of 2,4-dinitrophenol (DNP) on the transfer of lysozyme across rabbit intestine. DNP was added to the mucosal fluid at the time indicated by the arrow in the figure.

THE *in situ* EXPERIMENTS

While the *in vitro* experiments were in progress in our laboratory, evidence was also accumulating to suggest that adult animals can absorb large molecules in antigenic and biologically active quantities. The lines of such evidence were based on either *in vitro* or *in vivo* observations.[10-14] We wanted to investigate further using an *in situ* system. We thought that an *in situ* system could offer quantitation as accurate as an *in vitro* experiment, while at the same time the *in situ* experiment guarantees the continuous and ample supply of nutrients, particularly oxygen in blood, that are essential for maintaining the integrity of the intestinal tissue under study. For example, the histology of a piece of intestinal mucosa after a perfusion experiment for 120 min shows such extensive damage to the mucosal tissue that one hesitates to claim that one is doing a physiologic experiment. We studied extensively ways of evaluating the integrity, or viability, of the intestine and came to the conclusion that the most sensitive index was the release of various enzymes of epithelial cells into the lumen.

Figure 4 shows the comparison between *in vitro* and *in situ* experiments in release of three different kinds of enzymes from or together with the epithelium into the lumen. For *in vitro* experiment we used the everted sac, and the results are shown with open symbols. The solid circles represent an *in situ* experiment as shown below in Fig. 5. It is obvious that an *in situ* system is much better in maintaining the structural integrity of the intestine than an *in vitro* system.[7]

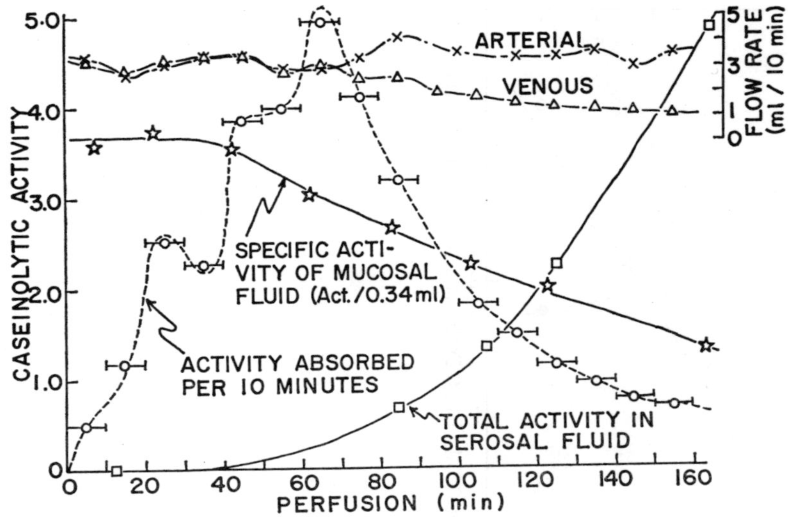

Fig. 3. Absorption of stem bromelain through rabbit intestine *in vitro*.[6] A 10-cm segment of the jejunum was perfused with Krebs-Ringer bicarbonate solution containing 0.1% glucose (KRBG) through mesenteric arterial (×) and venous (△) cannulae at flow rates shown in the figure. The solution of stem bromelain (0.05 %) was added into the intestinal lumen at time 0 min, while the segment was placed in 50 ml of the serosal KRBG fluid which was maintained at 37°. Caseinolytic activities at pH 7.2 in the presence of 5 mM cysteine were determined with aliquots of the venous perfusate (○), the mucosal fluid (☆), and the serosal fluid (□).

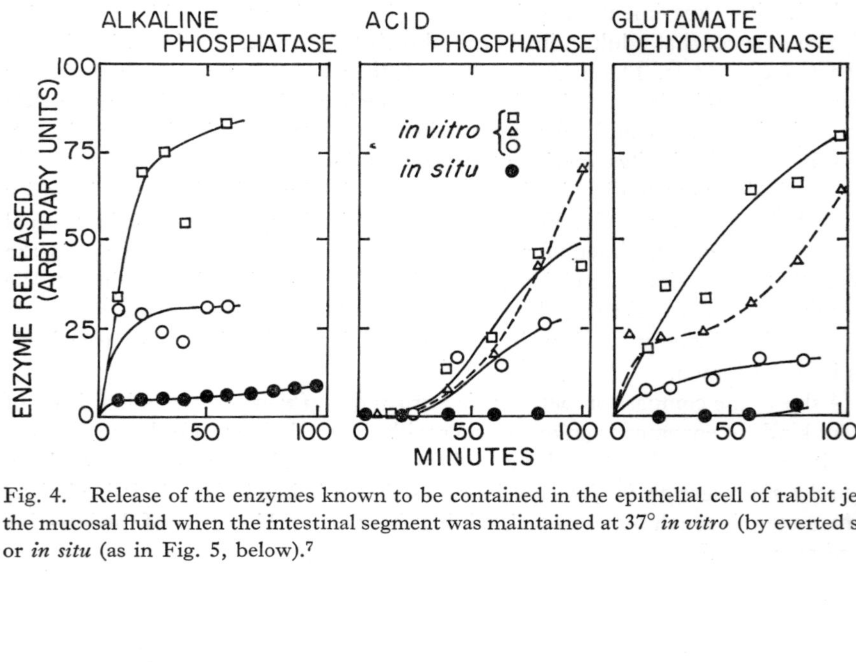

Fig. 4. Release of the enzymes known to be contained in the epithelial cell of rabbit jejunum into the mucosal fluid when the intestinal segment was maintained at 37° *in vitro* (by everted sac method) or *in situ* (as in Fig. 5, below).[7]

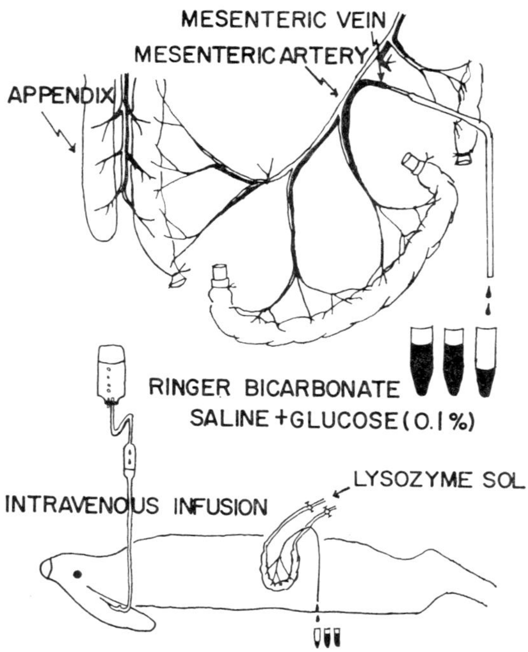

Fig. 5. Schematic diagram of *in situ* experiment. The upper part shows anatomical position of the intestinal segment used. The lower part is a diagrammatic illustration of the experiment during the collection of blood samples.[7]

A rabbit jejunum segment approximately 10 cm in length was connected with glass tubing at both ends. The mesenteric vein was cannulated while the supplying artery was left open. The intestinal loop was replaced in the abdominal cavity, as shown in the lower half of Fig. 5. The test enzyme was then added through glass tubing into the loop lumen, and the venous blood was collected in portions for analysis. The animal was given heparin before the surgery and it survived usually for 2 hr.

Lipase GA-56 from a strain of pseudomonad was used as a test enzyme. This lipase has a molecular weight of approximately 30,000; it is an acidic protein and stable against heating at 60° for 15 min which almost abolishes the activity of the intrinsic lipase found in rabbit plasma. Thus, the heat treatment could be used to distinguish the exogenous lipase from the endogenous.

The results are shown in Fig. 6. The abscissa is the time in min after the moment the test enzyme at a concentration of 0.05% was added to the loop lumen. The rate of blood flow coming out through the venous cannula is shown as the shaded area. The horizontal bars show the amount of the enzyme found in each fraction collected. It can be seen that the rate of absorption increased during the initial 30 min and then leveled off or decreased. The total amount of the enzyme absorbed is plotted with open circles. From the slope of this plot, one can estimate the average rate of absorption.[8,15]

No doubt lipase GA-56 was absorbed through the rabbit jejunum. However, the ques-

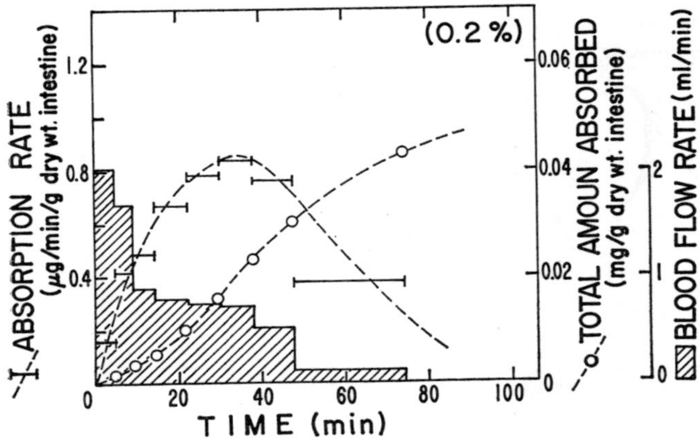

Fig. 6. Intestinal absorption of lipase GA-56 into the blood vessel by rabbit *in situ*.[8,15] The lipase activity was determined at pH 7.0 and at 37° using albumin-fattogen emulsion as substrate. Intrinsic lipase activity of rabbit plasma was inactivated by heat treatment at 60° for 15 min.

tion then arose as to whether the catalytic activity found in the plasma meant the presence of macromolecular enzyme or the appearance of smaller pieces like active fragments. The latter possibility was ruled out by analyzing the gel filtration profile of the rabbit plasma on a Sephadex G-50 column after the absorption experiment. The lipase activity emerged only in high-molecular weight fractions.

EFFECT OF MOLECULAR SIZE AND CONCENTRATION OF TEST PROTEINS

Similar *in situ* experiments were carried out with hen egg-white lysozyme as the test protein. Figure 7 shows the results obtained with 0.2% lysozyme in the lumen. The sharp decrease in the absorption rate after 50 min must have been caused by poor supply of blood in the later part of this experiment. However, in the initial 30 min, the absorption profile is essentially the same as in the case of lipase.[8,15]

We then found that when the concentration of the test enzyme in the loop lumen was lowered from 0.2% to 0.01%, the rate of absorption decreased considerably. This means that the absorption rate is dependent on the concentration of the enzyme protein that interacts with the surface of the mucosal epithelium. The dose response was extensively studied, and the results obtained are compared for lipase and lysozyme as shown in Fig. 8.[8,15]

Lipase GA-56, as mentioned earlier, is an acidic protein having a molecular weight of approximately 30,000. Lysozyme, on the other hand, is a basic protein, and its molecular weight, 14,307, is less than half of that of lipase GA-56. Keeping these features of the two enzymes in mind, one must be surprised to see that the larger molecule is absorbed several times faster than the smaller molecule. This is to say that the rate of absorption is independent of the size of the macromolecule to be absorbed. The rate must be regulated by some other factor or factors.

The second special feature in Fig. 8 is that in the cases of both lipase and lysozyme,

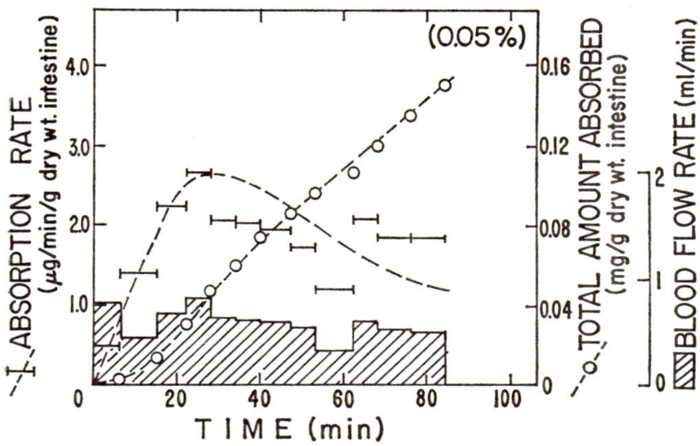

Fig. 7. Intestinal absorption of lysozyme into the blood vessel by rabbit *in situ*.[8,15] Intrinsic lysozyme activity of rabbit plasma was inhibited by the addition of enough amount of anti-hen egg-white lysozyme IgG to the sample plasma.

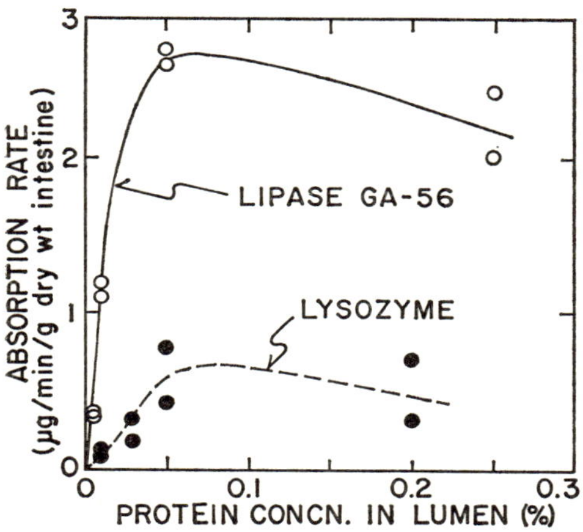

Fig. 8. Dependence of the rate of absorption on the concentration of protein in the intestinal lumen of rabbits *in situ*.[8,15] The rate of absorption is an averaged rate for the initial 30 min.

the rate of absorption increases as the protein concentration in the lumen increases up to 0.05%, but beyond this, the absorption rate does not increase or even decreases slightly. Therefore, the overall pattern looks like a saturation curve, which is often the case in dose response to drugs.

MECHANISM OF ABSORPTION

The data summarized in Fig. 8 clearly eliminate the possibility of mechanical leakage and the possibility of passive diffusion. What are the possibilities remaining for the transport mechanism we have found so far? The saturation curves in Fig. 8 are compatible with the active transport mechanism. However, as shown in Fig. 2, the *in vitro* transfer was found to be insensitive to 2,4-dinitrophenol. We have also found that the absorption phenomenon was almost insensitive to 0.1 mM ouabain, added to the medium in an *in situ* experiment. Therefore, any mechanism that requires energy as a driving force seems to be less plausible.

In order to look more deeply into the mechanism of such absorption, we have recently been studying the effect of chemical modification of lysozyme on the rate of absorption from the intestine. The chemical modifications employed are listed in Table I. The acylation includes acetylation with acetic anhydride and isobutyrylation with isobutyric anhydride. For attachment of glucose, N-acetyl-glucosamine, and cellobiose, lysozyme was coupled with 2-imino-2-methoxyethyl-1-thioglycoside.[16] Fortunately, these modified lysozymes were found to cross-react with anti-hen egg-white lysozyme antibody, inhibiting their enzymatic activities.

With these derivatives of lysozyme synthesized, we carried out the *in situ* experiment and found that the absorption profile was quite similar to what we had seen with unmodified lysozyme or lipase.

However, when the rates of absorption for the initial 30 min were compared, definite differences were found to exist among these derivatives of lysozyme. As shown in Fig. 9, acetylated lysozyme was absorbed approximately three times as fast as the unmodified lysozyme, while isobutyrylated enzyme did not enhance absorption. Among three sugar-bound lysozyme species, only glucose-bound derivative distinctly accelerate the absorption.[17] Obviously, the rate of absorption is strongly influenced by the chemical nature of the protein molecule, but we have not obtained enough data to explain the mechanism by which such selectivity is executed.

We have demonstrated that the absorption of enzyme proteins through rabbit intestine is a physiological phenomenon. It never represents an artifact. Our experiments have indicated, for the first time, that the rate of absorption is regulated by the chemical nature of the protein molecule that has come in contact with the surface of the intestinal epithelium rather than by the molecular size or the electric charge of the macromolecule. This may imply that one could chemically modify an enzyme protein which one wants to

TABLE I

LYSOZYME DERIVATIVES SYNTHESIZED

*Modification**1	*Enzymatic activity* (%)	*Amino group**2 (*number/molecule*)
Unmodified	100	7.3
Acetylated	23	3.1
Isobutyrylated	56	5.9
IE-S-Glc	85	3.4
IE-S-GlcNAc	76	3.4
IE-S-cellobioside	88	4.2

*1 Lysozyme coupled with 2-imino-2-methoxyethyl-1-thioglycoside is abbreviated as IE-S-Glc, *etc.*[16]

*2 Determined by the method using 2,4,6-trinitrobenzene sulfonic acid. Lysozyme has seven primary amino groups.

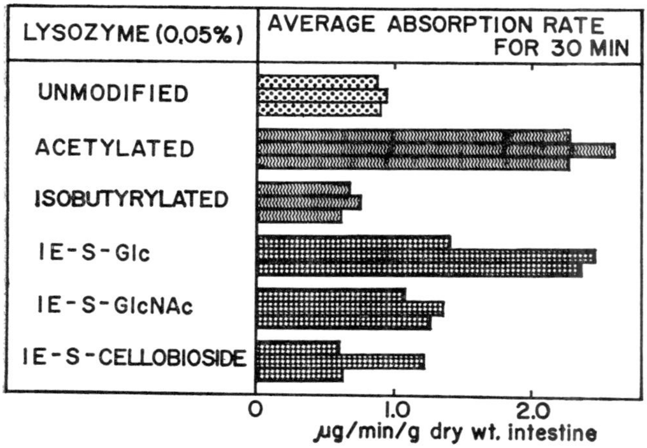

Fig. 9. Intestinal absorption of lysozyme derivatives into the blood vessels by rabbit *in situ*.[17] For abbreviations, see Table I.

use as a drug given through the mouth, for example, so that it can be absorbed more readily or more slowly depending upon the purpose and condition of administration of that drug.

In this connection, however, we wish to emphasize that our positive results in the absorption experiments have nothing to do directly with the pharmacological mechanism of the actions of enzymes used as drugs which are administered orally. We also wish to emphasize the possibility of immunological hazard as a result of absorption of non-self proteins through the intestine, although to our present knowledge such clinical cases have not been reported.

ACKNOWLEDGMENT

This work was supported in part by a grant from the Ministry of Education, Science and Culture of Japan, and by a grant from the Naito Foundation, Tokyo, Japan.

REFERENCES

1 G. Wiseman, *Absorption from the Intestine*, Academic Press, New York, 1964.
2 *New and Non-official Drugs*, Council on Drugs, American Medical Association, Chicago, Ill., 1964.
3 T. Murachi, in L. Lorand, *Methods in Enzymology*, Academic Press, New York, vol. 45, 1976, p. 475.
4 R. K. Crane and T. H. Wilson, *J. Appl. Physiol.*, 12 (1958) 145.
5 T. Murachi, *Saishin Igaku*, 20 (1965) 2971 (in Japanese).
6 S. Kimura, M. Oida, and T. Murachi, Abstr., 7th International Congress of Biochemistry, Tokyo, 1967, p. 919.
7 S. Kimura, M. Totani, and T. Murachi, *Japan. J. Exp. Med.*, 43 (1973) 163.
8 T. Murachi, Abstr. 10th International Congress of Biochemistry, Hamburg, 1976, p. 588.
9 S. Kimura, *J. Nagoya City Univ. Med. Assoc.*, 20 (1970) 701 (in Japanese).
10 D. E. Bockman and W. B. Winborn, *Anat. Rec.*, 155 (1966) 603.

11 N. Ogawa, H. Tajima, T. Kinoshita, and K. Tajima, *Seikagaku*, 42 (1970) 718 (in Japanese).
12 W. A. Walker, R. Cornell, and L. M. Davenport, *J. Cell Biol.*, 54 (1972) 195.
13 K. Katayama and T. Fujita, *Biochim. Biophys. Acta*, 288 (1972) 181.
14 A. L. Warshaw, W. A. Walker, and K. J. Isselbacher, *Gastroenterology*, 66 (1974) 987.
15 T. Murachi, *Seibutsu Butsuri Kagaku*, 19 (1975) 307 (in Japanese).
16 Y. C. Lee, C. P. Stowell, and M. J. Krantz, *Biochemistry*, 15 (1976) 3956.
17 Y. Sakaguchi and T. Murachi, *Seikagaku*, 49 (1977) 833 (abstr. in Japanese).

FATTY ACID SYNTHETASE OF YEAST AND 6-METHYLSALICYLATE SYNTHETASE OF *PENICILLIUM PATULUM*—TWO MULTIENZYME COMPLEXES

F. LYNEN,*[1] H. ENGESER,*[1] J. FRIEDRICH,*[1] W. SCHINDLBECK,*[1]
R. SEYFFERT,*[1] F. WIELAND*[1], AND E. SIESS*[2]
Max-Planck-Institut für Biochemie, Martinsried[1] *and Institut für Diabetesforschung, München*[2] *(F.R.G.)*

The biosynthesis of fatty acids from acetyl CoA is achieved by the action of acetyl CoA carboxylase and the multienzyme complex fatty acid synthetase. We have studied the latter enzyme of yeast. From ruptured yeast cells we isolated a protein fraction which synthesizes a mixture of palmityl and stearyl CoA according to the following equation (n=7 or 8):

$$\text{Acetyl CoA} + n \text{ malonyl CoA} + 2n \text{ NADPH} + 2n \text{ H}^+ \rightarrow$$
$$\text{CH}_3(\text{CH}_2\text{CH}_2)_n \text{ CO-CoA} + n \text{ CO}_2 + n \text{ CoA} + 2n \text{ NADP}^+ + n\text{H}_2\text{O}$$

The purified fatty acid synthetase proved to be homogeneous by electrophoresis and ultracentrifugation and could be crystallized from ammonium sulfate solution.[1] Its molecular weight was estimated to be 2.3 million.

The transformation of malonyl CoA into fatty acids is achieved through intermediates which are covalently bound to two types of sulfhydryl groups of the multienzyme complex which we denoted as "central" ($-S_cH$) and "peripheral" ($-S_pH$) and which belong either to 4′-phosphopantetheine, the functional group of the ACP component, or to cysteine in the active center of the condensing enzyme.

The synthetic process, as summarized in Fig. 1 is initiated by the transfer of an acetyl residue from acetyl CoA to the "peripheral" SH-group *via* the "central" SH-group. After the following transfer of a malonyl residue from malonyl CoA to the "central" SH-group, condensation occurs between the two enzyme-bound acyl groups, resulting in the formation of acetoacetate with the concomitant liberation of CO_2. The stepwise conversion of the β-keto acid into the saturated acid is accomplished with acids bound to the "central" SH-group. At the stage of the saturated acid, the butyryl group finally is transferred to the "peripheral" SH-group, thus liberating the "central" group for introduction of the next malonyl residue. The reaction sequence is then repeated until long-chain saturated fatty acids with 16 or 18 carbon atoms are formed, which in the terminal step are transferred from the "central" SH-group to coenzyme A with the formation of palmityl or stearyl CoA and the regenerated enzyme.

The multienzyme complex may be visualized as a strict compartmentation of a metabolic multistep reaction sequence in the smallest possible space. According to this concept the multienzyme complexes represent intracellular factories in which the building blocks

Abbreviations: ACP, acyl carrier protein; DMMA, dimethylmaleic anhydride; 6-MSA, 6-methylsalicylic acid; TAE, triacetic acid ethyl ester; AAC, acetoacetyl-N-acetyl cysteamine.

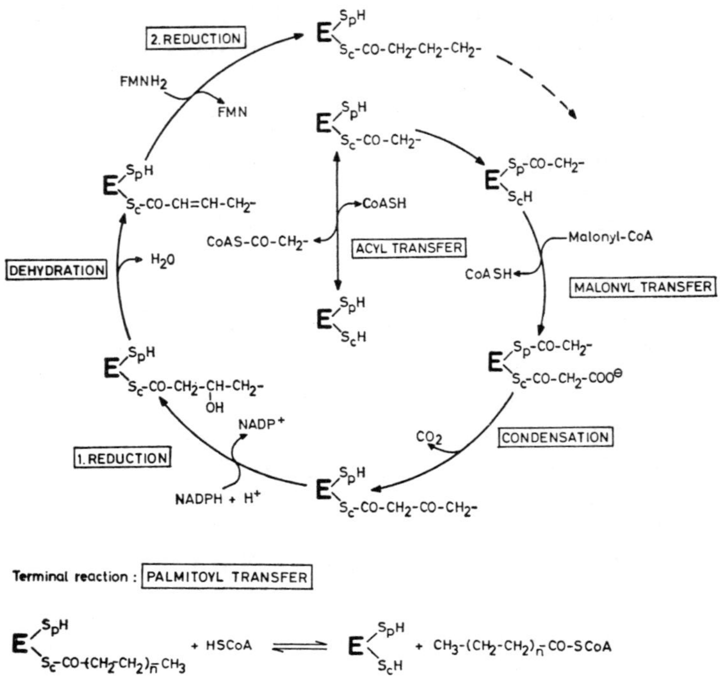

Fig. 1. Reaction scheme of fatty acid biosynthesis.

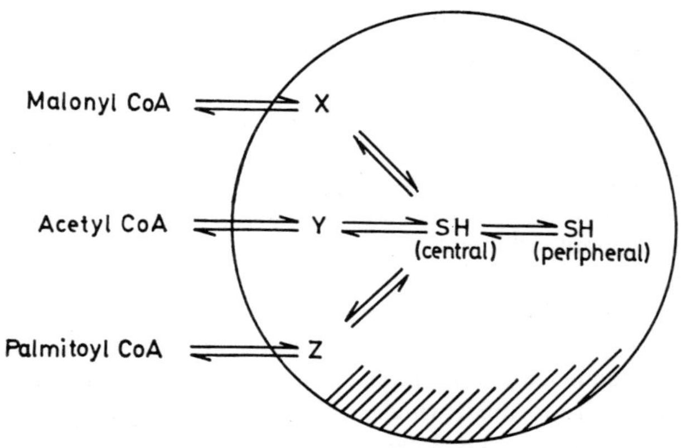

Fig. 2. Schematic representation of the functions of acyl transferases in fatty acid synthetase. $SH_{central}$, ACP component; $SH_{peripheral}$, functional group of the condensing enzyme; X, Y, and Z, active sites of acyl transferases.

are assembled piece by piece and only the finished product is released from the complex. With this picture in mind it is tempting to draw an analogy between the yeast fatty acid synthetase and the mitochondrion. The function of the mitochondrial membrane, serving as a selective barrier which guarantees the availability of certain metabolites and the exclusion of others in the fatty acid synthetase, is taken over by the acyl transferase enzyme components which deliver acetyl and malonyl fragments to the complex and release the long-chain fatty acids from it. In fatty acid synthesis the transferases play the critical role in compartmentalization. It was found that the active sites of all transferases labeled X, Y, and Z in Fig. 2, are represented by the OH-groups of serine residues. However, even more interestingly, it was found by genetic analysis in Schweizer's laboratory,[2] and also by binding studies as well as by protein chemical analysis of the binding sites performed by Engeser[3] in our laboratory, that one and the same transferase component enzyme is responsible for the transfer of malonate and that of palmitate. As a result the incorporation of malonate into fatty acids is blocked as long as the long-chain fatty acids are not released from the complex. That may be of great regulatory significance.

In order to explain the double specificity of this acyl transferase we may assume that there exist three binding sites in the active center of this enzymic domain. The first interacts with the thiolester grouping, which would be present in all acyl thiolester intermediates of the synthetic process. The additional binding sites leading to the specificity of the enzyme are assumed to be represented by a positively charged group of the enzyme which can interact with the negatively charged carboxylate anion of malonyl thiolesters and an hydrophobic area of the enzyme more distant from the first binding site which comes into play if the number of carbon atoms in the acyl residue exceeds 13. As Sumper and Oesterhelt[4] in our laboratory have calculated from their experiments the binding energy for this site increases by 0.9 kcal for each $-CH_2-$ group in the acyl residue exceeding 13.

THE ARCHITECTURE OF FATTY ACID SYNTHETASE

With respect to the architecture of the multienzyme complex, Knobling *et al.*[2] in 1973 showed with genetic methods that all partial activities are coded for by only two gene loci, designated as fas 1 and fas 2, each coding for one single multifunctional polypeptide chain. By genetic analysis the distribution of most of the partial reactions on the gene products of fas 1, named polypeptide chain β, and fas 2, named chain α, could be found (Fig. 3). The gene product for fas 2, α, carries the condensing enzyme activity, the first reductase as well as the integrated acyl carrier protein. On β are located malonyl/palmitoyl transferase, acetyl transferase, dehydratase, and the second reductase. By SDS-gel-electrophoresis the two subunits were analytically separated and their molecular weights were estimated to be about 185,000 and 180,000 (Table I). For the experiments to be discussed in the following,

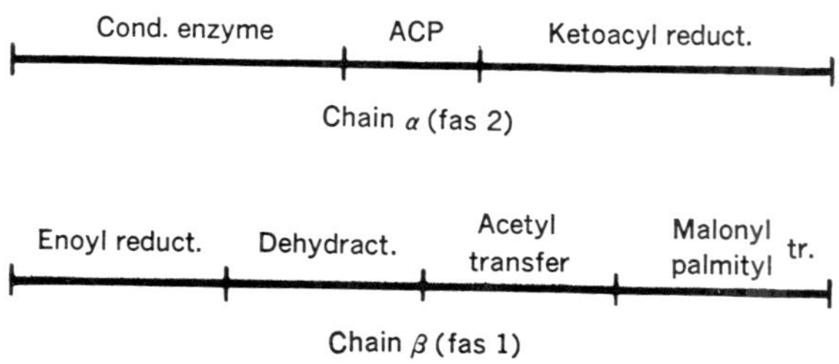

Fig. 3. Localization of the component enzymes on the polypeptides α and β.

TABLE I

COMPOSITION OF YEAST FATTY ACID SYNTHETASE

	Mol. wt.
Native enzyme ($\alpha_6\beta_6$)	2.3×10^6
Chain α	185,000
Chain β	180,000

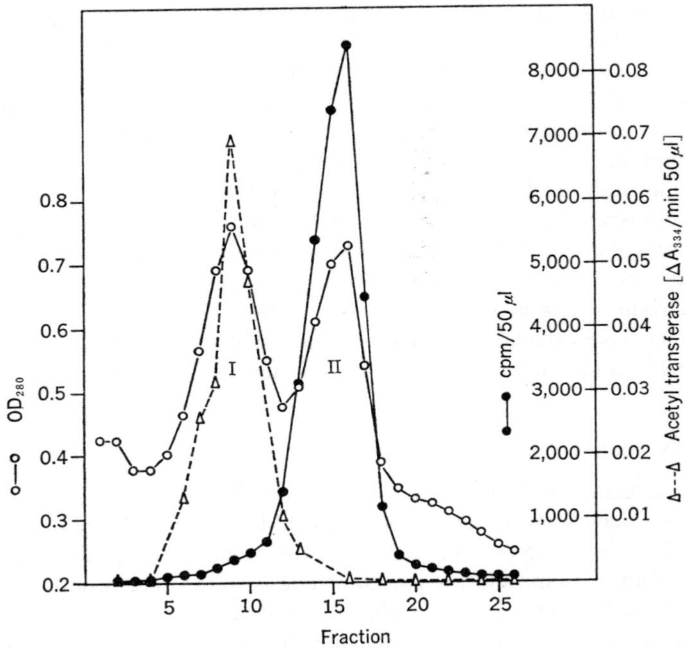

Fig. 4. Separation of chain α and β after treatment of fatty acid synthetase with DMMA. Centrifugation for 42 hr at $230{,}000\times g$ in a linear density gradient (10–20 % sucrose) 5–6 mg purified and ^{14}C-iodoacetamide treated enzyme per ml of 0.3 M potassium phosphate, pH 7.5, containing 10 mM 2-mercapto-ethanol were brought to 10 mM DMMA and incubated for 30 min at 0°. The sample was then chromatographed over a Sephadex G-50 column in 20 mM Tris-HCl, pH 7.5, 1 mM dithiothreitol and loaded on sucrose density gradients containing the same buffer.

it should be mentioned that Kresze *et al.*[6] were able to confirm by protein chemical methods that the condensing enzyme activity is located on chain α. It was known from previous studies of Oesterhelt and Hagen in our laboratory that iodoacetamide is a specific reagent for the "peripheral" SH-group, which represents the active site of the condensing enzyme. Fatty acid synthetase was specifically labeled with ^{14}C-iodoacetamide and analyzed by SDS-gel-electrophoresis. Radioactivity was found only in the α chain.

Fatty acid synthetase can be reversibly dissociated by the freezing and thawing procedure of Sumper.[7] In this procedure the solution of the multienzyme complex in the presence of 1 M lithium chloride is repeatedly frozen and thawed. This leads to the loss of enzymic activity concomitant to the disaggregation of the complex to the separated polypeptide chains. But our attempts to separate the two subunits prepared in this way were without success.

The separation became only possible when Wieland[8] tried to modify the complex chemically, hoping to change the chemical properties of one chain more than those of the other one. Acylation of the ε-amino-group of lysine by treatment with cyclic dicarbonic anhydrides like citraconic anhydride and DMMA under mild conditions led to a total loss of the overall activity. On disk-gel-electrophoresis a resolution into two proteins could be observed.

The preparative isolation of the two subunits became possible on Martin and Ames sucrose density gradients. Centrifugation for 45 hr at $230{,}000 \times g$ led to the appearance of two protein peaks (Fig. 4), of which the slower sedimenting protein contained all radioactivity and therefore represented α. The faster one showed high activity in acetyl transferase which was not observed in α but was present in β (see Fig. 3).

Table II summarizes the distribution of the partial enzymic activities in both fractions: Acetyl transferase, dehydratase, malonyl transferase, and enoyl reductase were found in peak I protein (β), whereas the condensing enzyme is located in peak II protein (α) as shown by its radioactivity, due to the labeling with the ^{14}C-carboxamidomethyl group.

Using DMMA in order to dissociate the complex is advantageous, because the ε-amino-lysyl-dimethylmaleic amide formed is much easier to hydrolyse under mild acidic conditions than the products of other cyclic dicarbonic anhydrides. Its half life at pH 3.5 and 20° was found to be about 2 min. Therefore it could be expected that the dissociation of the complex by treatment with DMMA could be reversed. The reconstitution was finally achieved by removal of dimethylmaleic acid by incubation at pH 4.6 in the presence of ammonium sulfate at 0° (10 hr). Though the reactivated protein exhibits only about 50% of the original activity, it sedimented like untreated fatty acid synthetase in the analytical ultracentrifuge. In addition the protein behaves like the untreated complex in the Maurer disk-gel electrophoresis system. From this we may conclude that, at least under appropriate conditions, the complex state of the enzyme is favored over the subunit state and over possible intermediate subcomplexes which we were not able to find with this method.

The isolated α and β polypeptides were used by Wieland to immunize rabbits and in this way he obtained specific antibodies, which, in collaboration with Dr. Elmar Siess, he used to obtain some insight into the architecture of the multienzyme complex. Native fatty acid synthetase was incubated with non-precipitating amounts of each immunoglobulin fraction. Such incubations were centrifuged in sucrose density gradients with the results

TABLE II

DISTRIBUTION OF THE COMPONENT ENZYME ACTIVITIES ON THE TWO PROTEIN FRACTIONS FROM FIG. 4.

Peak I protein	*Peak II protein*	*Activity*
+	−	Acetyl transfer
+	−	Malonyl transfer
−	−	β-Ketoacylreduction
−	+	Condensation (radioactivity)
+	−	Dehydratation
+	−	Enoylreduction

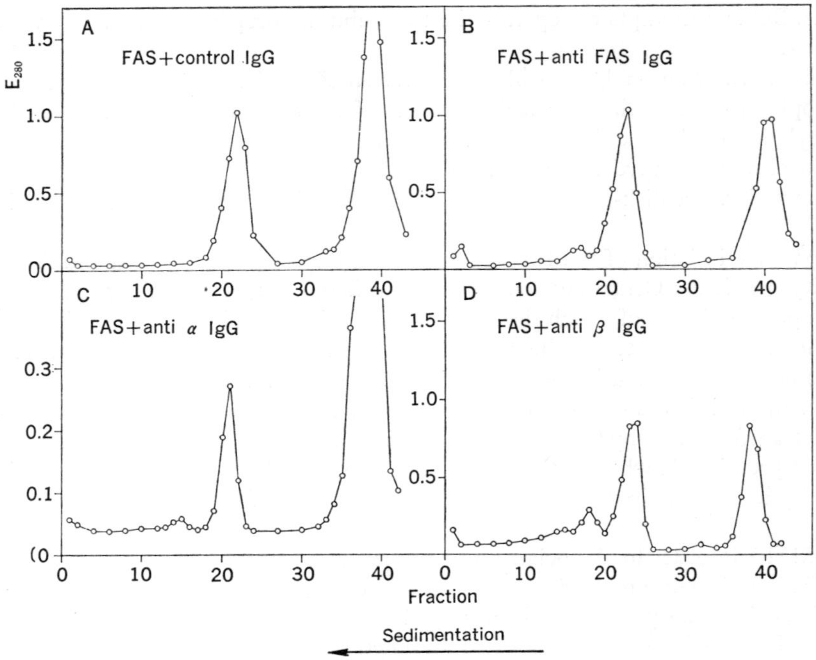

Fig. 5. Sucrose density gradient centrifugation of fatty acid synthetase (FAS) in presence of non-precipitating amounts of antibodies.

shown in Fig. 5. Fatty acid synthetase treated with control immunoglobulin from non-immunized rabbits shows only one peak corresponding to native fatty acid synthetase. Incubation with anti-α immunoglobulin led to the appearance of small amounts of a faster sedimenting protein peak before fatty acid synthetase and so did also the incubation with anti-β immunoglobulin and fatty acid synthetase immunoglobulin. This faster sedimenting material was expected to be immunoglobulin crosslinked fatty acid synthetase dimers or oligomers.

Figure 6a, an electronmicrograph of untreated fatty acid synthetase, shows a random distribution of the individual complex molecules over the whole area. In Fig. 6b, protein from the faster sedimenting peak of the specific immunoglobulin fatty acid synthetase interaction is shown. As expected they are no longer randomly distributed but fatty acid synthetase molecules are predominantly arranged in dimeric and oligomeric groups. Anti-α immunoglobulin crosslinked and anti-β immunoglobulin corsslinked material now was investigated at higher magnification, and Fig. 6c gives a representative survey of anti-β crosslinked fatty acid synthetase. For interpretation it must be added that only those structures were taken into account which possessed a visible immunoglobulin as a link between the synthetase molecules. Many other dimeric and oligomeric structures without visible antibody were present but were not evaluated. We don't know why antibody bridges were not always visible and why in some of the dimers the molecules were closely attached. It may be that parts of the antibodies are able to penetrate into the hollow body of the enzyme and bind internally. In our pictures of evaluated structures we are able to localize a preferable region for anti-β antibody binding on fatty acid synthetase. This region

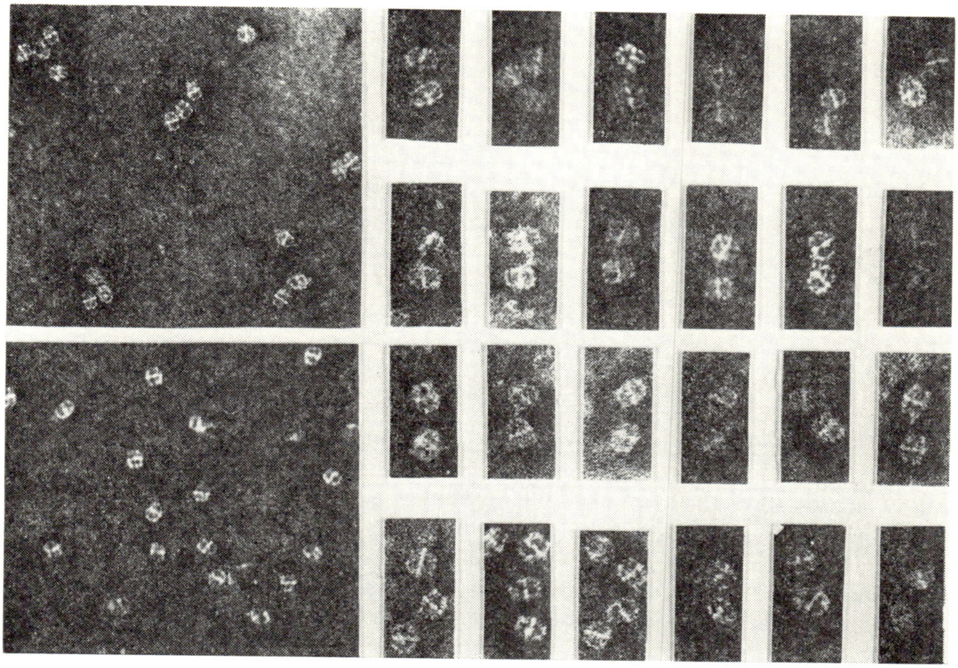

Fig. 6. Electronmicrographs of fatty acid synthetase (FAS). Alone (b) or after interaction with anti-FAS antibodies (a), anti-β antibodies (d), and anti-β antibodies (c).

is spanned in the central part between equator and poles of the enzyme structure. Figure 6d gives a survey of typical anti-α antibody crosslinked complexes. The region of complexation by anti-α immunoglobulin seems to be concentrated at the equator of the enzyme structure.

This information was used to extend a three-dimensional model for the yeast fatty acid synthetase complex in our laboratory in the past year. A comparison of the molecular weights of the subunits with the molecular weight of the complex as already mentioned suggests that each subunit is present six times in the complex (see Table I). Further evidence for this stoichiometry results from the presence of 5.5 to 6 FMN molecules[1] and between 5 and 6 phosphopantetheine molecules[9] per one molecule of fatty acid synthetase complex. Small angle X-ray scattering analysis of the complex made with Pilz and Kratky,[10] as well as the results of Hoppe and his colleagues,[11] supported the assumption that the enzyme is a hollow body, separated into two halves by a center wall, having a 3/2 symmetry.

To combine these data with the analytical results mentioned above, we assumed in Fig. 7 that the complex is built from six protomers, each consisting of one α and one β subunit, which are connected in the form of the letter V. Combination of these six protomers in such a manner that all of the polypeptides of one type are arranged in hexagonal order forming a single plane. The binding of these polypeptide chains is achieved by the interaction of identical binding sites, *i.e.*, in our model the gray sites bind to the gray sites

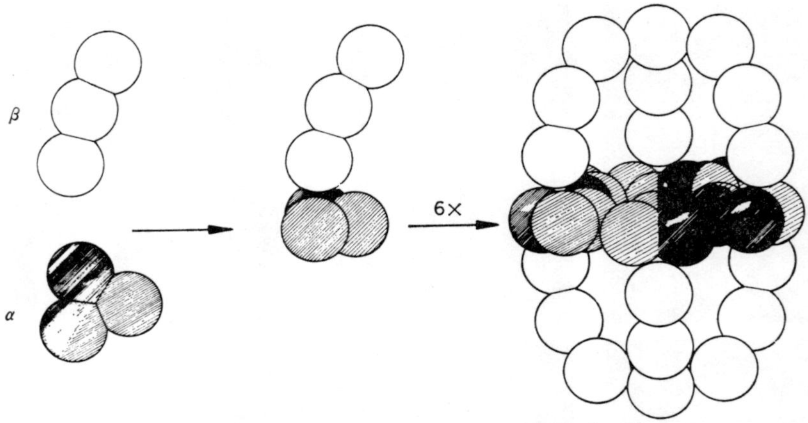

Fig. 7. Three-dimensional model of yeast fatty acid synthetase.

and the black sites to the black sites. The result is a hexagonal basic disk resembling the central wall of the complex, from which three polypeptide chains of the other type protrude upward and three subunits protrude downwards. Those chains protruding upwards are displaced by 60 degrees from those protruding downwards. This model has a shape similar to the shape of the complex seen in electronmicrophotographs (see Fig. 6a) and is compatible with the proposed symmetry. Twisting three times around the long axis and twice around the short axis results in a identical, hollow rotation ellipsoid.

From our electronmicroscopic studies with specific antibodies, we would like to propose that the central wall consists of six α-subunits, separating the complex into two halves, each of which is built from three β-subunits.

6-METHYLSALICYLATE SYNTHETASE

Let us now turn to a discussion of recent results with the 6-methylsalicylate synthetase of *Penicillium patulum*. We were interested in this multienzyme complex because it uses the same substrates as fatty acid synthetase, namely: Acetyl CoA as primer, malonyl CoA, and NADPH. But instead of straight chain fatty acids, it synthesizes the benzene derivative 6-MSA according to the following equation:

$$\text{Acetyl CoA} + 3\ \text{malonyl CoA} + \text{NADPH} + \text{H}^+ \longrightarrow$$

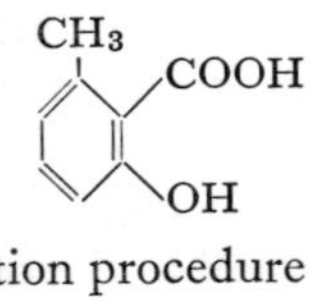

$$+ 4\ \text{CoA} + 3\ \text{CO}_2 + \text{NADP}^+ + \text{H}_2\text{O}$$

Friedrich[12] in our laboratory recently developed a new purification procedure which leads to a homogeneous protein. This is summarized in Table III.

The enzyme catalyzes the synthesis of 6-MSA in the following way (Fig. 8). It contains two types of SH-groups, analogous to fatty acid synthetase, which we again called "central" and "peripheral" and which belong to 4′-phosphopantetheine[13] bound at a serine residue of the multienzyme complex and to a cysteine residue in the active center of the condensing enzyme component. The synthesis of 6-MSA proceeds in a manner rather analogous to fatty acid synthesis: First transfer of acetyl and malonyl residues to the active SH-groups, then condensation of sulfur-bound acetate and malonate to form

TABLE III

PURIFICATION OF 6-MSA SYNTHETASE FROM *Penicillium patulum*

Step	*Volume (ml)*	*Total activity (mU)*	*Protein (mg)*	*Specific activity (mU/mg)*	*Recovery (%)*
1. Centrifuged extract	3,000	54,400	38,900	1.4	100
2. Polyethylene-glycol-6,000-precipitation (3–10% w/v)	410	42,950	6,400	6.7	79
3. Polyethylene-glycol-6,000-precipitation (4–9% w/v)	75	66,110	2,900	22.7	121
4. 22–37% ammonium-sulfate fractionation	52	56,060	1,940	28.8	103
5. Hydroxyapatite concentrated eluate	24	35,880	356	101	66
6. Centrifugation in a discontinuous sucrose gradient	10	28,730	177	162	53

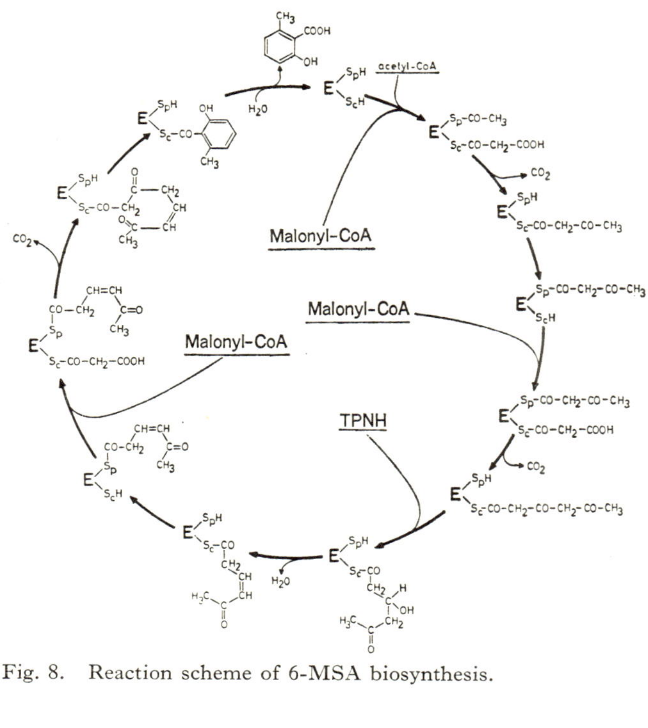

Fig. 8. Reaction scheme of 6-MSA biosynthesis.

acetoacetate. Whereas in fatty acid synthesis acetoacetate is reduced, in 6-MSA synthesis it condenses once more with malonate to form triacetic acid before reduction occurs. After dehydration, which probably leads to the formation of 5-keto-*cis*-3-hexenoic acid, the condensation with the third malonyl-unit follows and the product then cyclizes by an aldol condensation to form 6-MSA bound to the enzyme. In the final step the product is released from the enzyme complex by hydrolysis.

TABLE IV

COMPARISON OF 6-MSA SYNTHETASE AND FATTY ACID SYNTHETASE

6-MSA synthetase	*Fatty acid synthetase*
1. Acetyl transfer	1. Acetyl transfer
2. Malonyl transfer	2. Malonyl transfer
3. Condensation $C_2 \rightarrow C_4 \rightarrow C_6$	3. Condensation $C_2 \rightarrow C_4$
4. β-Keto acyl reduction	4. β-Keto acyl reduction
5. Dehydration [β, γ → *cis*]?	5. Dehydration [α, β → *trans*]
	6. Enoyl acyl reduction
3.′ Condensation $C_6 \rightarrow C_8$	⋮
6. Condensation (aldol type) ⟶aromatic ring	Repetition of 2 to 6
7. Hydrolysis	7. Palmitoyl transfer to CoA-SH (stearoyl transfer)

Table IV (in the left column) summarizes the reactions just mentioned and compares them with the partial reactions of fatty acid synthesis (in the right column).

In order to demonstrate many of the reactions listed here we applied two methods:

1) The enzyme complex was used in stoichiometric amounts and the transfer of the acyl groups from ^{14}C-acetyl- or ^{14}C-malonyl-CoA to the carrier sites of the complex was measured directly. In this way Schindlbeck[14] could demonstrate that acetate and malonate were not only bound to SH-groups on the enzyme but also to OH-groups. We assume that the latter groups represent the active sites of acetyl and malonyl transferase respectively and belong to peptide bound serine residues as in the case of fatty acid synthetase. Friedrich[12] continued these studies and obtained experimental evidence showing that in 6-MSA synthetase the acyl transferases for acetate and malonate are identical, or in other words, the same catalytic domain transfers acetate and malonate.
2) The second method took advantage of the fact that some of the enzymic functions of 6-MSA synthetase, like those of fatty acid synthetase, can also act on substrate models. For comparative studies Seyffert[15] used either TAE (I) or S-AAC (II) as substrate models.

$$CH_3-\overset{\overset{\displaystyle O}{\|}}{C}-CH_2-\overset{\overset{\displaystyle O}{\|}}{C}-CH_2-\overset{\overset{\displaystyle O}{\|}}{C}-OC_2H_5$$

I (TAE)

$$CH_3-\overset{\overset{\displaystyle O}{\|}}{C}-CH_2-\overset{\overset{\displaystyle O}{\|}}{C}-SCH_2CH_2NH-COCH_3$$

II (AAC)

In the experiment shown in Fig. 9, various protein fractions obtained by sucrose gradient centrifugation during our enzyme purification procedure were assayed with both substrate models: AAC and TAE. It was found that the heaviest protein fraction, representing fatty acid synthetase, very actively catalyzes the reduction of AAC, whereas the middle fraction, representing 6-MSA synthetase, is inactive in that respect. On the other hand this fraction can catalyze the reduction of TAE. Fatty acid synthetase can also reduce

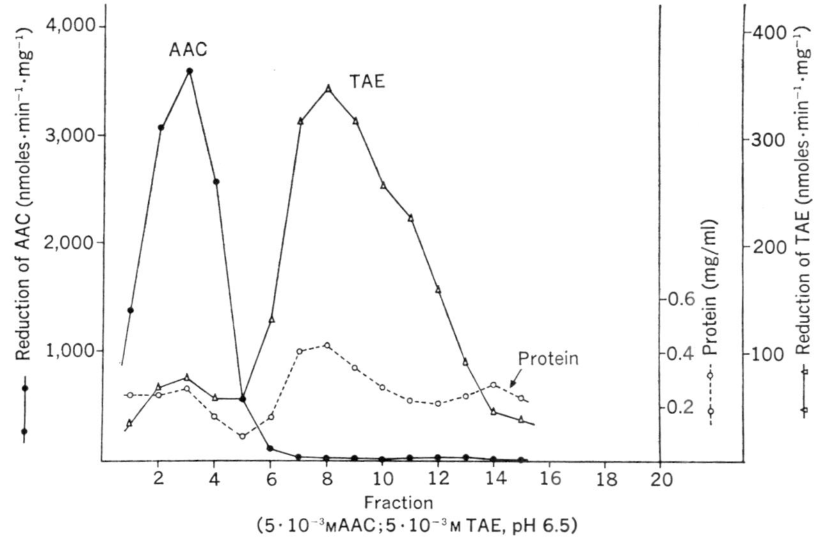

Fig. 9. Reduction of AAC and TAE by various protein fractions obtained by sucrose gradient centrifugation.

TAE but only at a slow rate. The observations of Seyffert in our laboratory indicate that the specificity of the reducing enzyme, to some extent, determines which product is formed by the particular multienzyme complex. In both processes, fatty acid synthesis and 6-MSA synthesis, the condensation of acetate and malonate leads to the formation of acetoacetate bound to the ACP component of the particular multienzyme complex. Due to the specificity of the reducing enzyme component of fatty acid synthetase, the acetoacetate is rapidly reduced to β-hydroxy-butyrate which then is further transformed into butyrate and, thus, channeled into the synthesis of fatty acids. In 6-MSA synthetase, however, acetoacetate is not reduced. On the contrary, it enters another condensation with malonate to form triacetic acid. Only then reduction occurs, leaving the keto group in position 5 untouched. It seems to be essential that this group, after dehydration and elongation of the carbon chain by condensation with another malonate residue, eventually enters an aldol condensation and thus leads to the formation of the benzene ring.

It is interesting to note that the ability to reduce triacetic acid was found to be present also in fatty acid synthetase to a small extent. If we now assume that by mutation of the reductase protein component this low activity towards triacetic acid became strongly potentiated and at the same time activity towards acetoacetate was lost, we would come to the conclusion that 6-MSA synthetase might have been evolved from a precursor fatty acid synthetase in the course of evolution.

Friedrich[12] was able to support this hypothesis by immunological studies. He prepared specific antibodies against the purified 6-MSA synthetase and tested them with the Ouchterlony double diffusion technique against 6-MSA synthetase, purified fatty acid synthetase from *P. patulum* and purified fatty acid synthetase from yeast. As Fig. 10 illustrates, we observed a cross reaction with fatty acid synthetase from *Penicillium* but

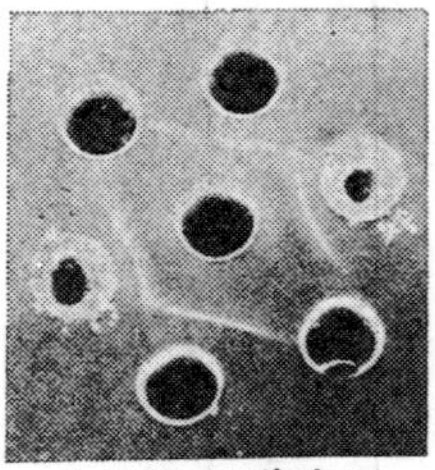

Fig. 10. Immunological comparison of 6-MSA synthetase, fatty acid synthetase (FAS) of *P. patulum* and FAS of yeast by the Ouchterlony technique. Anti 6-MSA synthetase immunoglobulin was pipetted into the center well, the various enzymes in the outer wells as indicated in the figure.

TABLE V
COMPOSITION OF 6-MSA SYNTHETASE

	Mol. wt.
Native enzyme	760,000
Subunits	176,000

not with the one from brewer's yeast. This observation is in good accord with our hypothesis that fatty acid synthetase and 6-MSA synthetase have a common ancestor.

With respect to the quaternary structure, both synthetases differ from each other. Fatty acid synthetase from *P. patulum*, like the one from yeast, has a molecular weight of 2.3×10^6 daltons and probable is built up from two polypeptides α and β, each present six times. The molecular weight of the purified 6-MSA synthetase was found to be only 760,000 daltons[12] correcting the value of 1.1 million given by Dimroth[16] and to be composed of four subunits having a molecular weight of 176,000 daltons (Table V). According to the results of SDS-gel-electrophoresis, these subunits appear to be identical. This would be in contrast to the situation with fatty acid synthetase. If further experiments should support this observation, we have to conclude that all the component enzyme activities of 6-MSA synthetase are present in only one multifunctional polypeptide chain which occurs four times in the purified enzyme. In agreement with this assumption, in binding experiments to the serine of acetyl/malonyl transferase, Friedrich already found 3.1–3.8 acetyl or malonyl residues bound per mol of enzyme.[12]

The dissociation of the tetrameric enzyme can be achieved by incubation with 2 M LiCl at 0° for 4 hr.[12] Under this conditions total activity disappears completely, the partial activities for the formation of triacetic acid, the reduction step and the acyl transferase reaction, respectively, disappear only partially, or not at all. Reconstitution of the total enzymic activity can be achieved by removal of the high LiCl-concentration and incubation at 25° in presence of dithiothreitol. Under optimal conditions 70% of the original enzyme activity can be recovered.

In conclusion, our main results may be briefly summarized:

1) Fatty acid synthetase and 6-MSA synthetase are multienzyme complexes built from multifunctional polypeptide chains present in the complexes several times.
2) According to the results of immunological studies, both enzymes appear to have

had a common ancestor and the mutation in the course of evolution has principally affected the specificity of the reducing enzyme component.

3) A structure model of fatty acid synthetase was suggested which is in good accord with the electronmicroscopic picture of the multienzyme complex.

REFERENCES

1 D. Oesterhelt, H. Bauer, and F. Lynen, *Proc. Natl. Acad. Sci. U.S.*, 63 (1969) 1377.
2 A. Knobling, D. Schiffmann, H.-D. Sickinger, and E. Schweizer, *Eur. J. Biochem.*, 56 (1975) 359.
3 H. Engeser, Ph. D. Thesis, University of Munich, München, 1978.
4 M. Sumper, D. Oesterhelt, C. Riepertinger, and F. Lynen, *Eur. J. Biochem.*, 10 (1969) 377.
5 E. Schweizer, B. Kniep, H. Castorph, and U. Holzner, *Eur. J. Biochem.*, 39 (1973) 353.
6 G. B. Kresze, D. Oesterhelt, F. Lynen, H. Castorph, and E. Schweizer, *Biochem. Biophys. Res. Commun.*, 69 (1976) 893.
7 M. Sumper, C. Riepertinger, and F. Lynen, *FEBS Lett.*, 5 (1969) 45.
8 F. Wieland, Ph. D. Thesis, University of Munich, München, 1978.
9 W. Winnewisser, Ph. D. Thesis, University of Munich, München, 1979.
10 I. Pilz, M. Herbst, O. Kratky, D. Oesterhelt, and F. Lynen, *Eur. J. Biochem.*, 13 (1970) 55.
11 W. Hoppe, J. H. Schramm, M. Sturm, N. Hunsmann, and J. Gassmann, *Z. Naturforsch.*, 31a (1976) 1380.
12 J. Friedrich, Ph. D. Thesis, University of Munich, München, 1977.
13 G. Greull, Ph. D. Thesis, University of Munich, München, 1973.
14 W. Schindlbeck, Ph. D. Thesis, University of Munich, München, 1974.
15 R. Seyffert, W. Schindlbeck, and F. Lynen, Abstr. 10th Meet. Fed. Eur. Biochem. Soc., 675, Société de Chimie Biologique, Paris, 1975.
16 P. Dimroth, H. Walter, and F. Lynen, *Eur. J. Biochem.*, 13 (1970) 98.

MOLECULAR MECHANISMS FOR BIOLOGICAL REGULATION OF LIPOGENESIS

SHOSAKU NUMA, TATSUYUKI KAMIRYO, MASAYOSHI MISHINA, SHIN-ICHI TASHIRO, SHIGETADA NAKANISHI, SABURO HORIKAWA, TADASHI TANABE, SATOSHI YAMASHITA, KOHEI HOSAKA, ULRICH SCHIELE, AND YOSHINOBU MIKI

Department of Medical Chemistry, Faculty of Medicine, Kyoto University, Kyoto (Japan)

Lipid is an essential component of all living cells, playing an important role not only as the most concentrated store of energy but as a constituent of all biological membranes. Therefore, it is essential for the living organism to regulate the process of lipid biosynthesis. The present paper is focused upon our recent studies on the molecular mechanism underlying the regulation of synthesis of acetyl coenzyme A carboxylase [acetyl-CoA: carbon-dioxide ligase (ADP-forming), EC 6.4.1.2], a key enzyme for the control of fatty acid synthesis, as well as on the enzymic mechanism effecting the asymmetric fatty acid distribution in naturally occurring glycerolipids.

REGULATION OF ACETYL-CoA CARBOXYLASE SYNTHESIS

Acetyl-CoA carboxylase, which mediates the initial step of *de novo* synthesis of long-chain fatty acids, plays a critical role in the regulation of this biosynthetic process.[1] During the past several years, studies have been made to elucidate the mechanism by which the acetyl-CoA carboxylase content of the liver is regulated under different metabolic conditions, including dietary alteration, diabetes, and obesity, in which the rate of fatty acid synthesis varies markedly. It is now well established that the variations in the enzyme content are due principally to corresponding changes in the rate of synthesis of the enzyme, while the degradation of the enzyme plays no significant role except in a non-steady state like starvation.[1-3] Our efforts have therefore been concentrated on the molecular mechanism involved in the regulation of synthesis of acetyl-CoA carboxylase, specifically on two questions, *i.e.*, at which step of protein synthesis the rate of synthesis of acetyl-CoA carboxylase is regulated and which metabolite is responsible for the regulation of synthesis of this enzyme.

To approach the first question, we estimated the contents of specific polysomes involved in the synthesis of acetyl-CoA carboxylase in the livers of animals under various metabolic conditions. Acetyl-CoA carboxylase-synthesizing polysomes were quantitated by two independent methods. First, the binding of ^{125}I-labelled specific antibody to isolated liver polysomes was measured according to the procedure developed by Schimke's group.[4] The radioactivity bound was determined after separation of polysomes by sucrose density gradient centrifugation. In the experiment shown in Fig. 1, we compared the extents of binding of ^{125}I-labelled antiacetyl-CoA carboxylase to polysomes isolated from livers of normally fed, fasted, and fat-free refed rats. The results showed that, after subtraction of the background radioactivity, the amount of bound radioactivity was approxi-

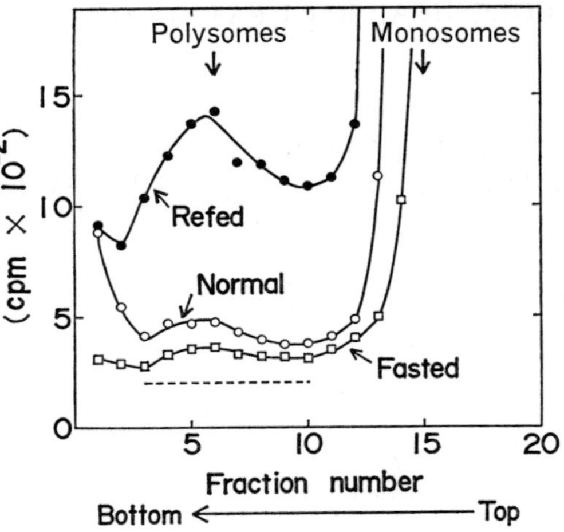

Fig. 1. Binding of ^{125}I-labelled antiacetyl-CoA carboxylase to liver polysomes derived from rats fed a balanced diet ("normal"), rats starved for 48 hr ("fasted"), and rats starved for 48 hr and subsequently refed a fat-free diet for 72 hr ("refed"). Polysomes (15 A_{254} units), were incubated at 0° for 60 min with 18.5 μg of ^{125}I-labelled antiacetyl-CoA carboxylase and then centrifuged at 41,000 rpm for 85 min in 11 ml of a 15–50 % (w/v) sucrose gradient. The dotted line represents the background radioactivity, which was subtracted for comparison of the amounts of bound radioactivity. Data taken from ref. 5.

mately twofold lower in fasted rats than in normal rats, while it was approximately fourfold higher in refed rats than in normal rats. Various lines of evidence indicated that the observed binding of the labelled antibody to polysomes occurred in a specific and quantitative manner through recognition of the nascent peptide chains of acetyl-CoA carboxylase present on polysomes.[5]

Alternatively, acetyl-CoA carboxylase-synthesizing polysomes were quantitated by translating liver polysomes in the cell-free protein-synthesizing system derived from rabbit reticulocytes in the presence of L-[4,5-^{3}H]leucine. The completed enzyme, which was isotopically labelled, was measured by indirect immunoprecipitation followed by dodecylsulfate-polyacrylamide gel electrophoresis of the dissociated immunoprecipitate. The results of such an experiment, presented in Table I, showed that polysomes from fasted rats synthesized approximately one-third as much acetyl-CoA carboxylase as did polysomes from normal rats, whereas polysomes from refed rats produced an approximately threefold larger amount of the enzyme than did polysomes from normal rats. The synthesis of total protein was essentially unaffected after the dietary manipulation.

The results of analogous studies on alloxan-diabetic rats[5] and genetically obese hyperglycemic mice (C57BL/6J-*ob*),[7] together with the data just described, are summarized in Table II. The hepatic content of acetyl-CoA carboxylase-synthesizing polysomes correlates well with the rate of hepatic acetyl-CoA carboxylase synthesis *in vivo*, which was measured by administration of [^{3}H]leucine into animals followed by determination of isotope incorporation into the enzyme isolated by direct immunoprecipitation. This indicates that the different rates of acetyl-CoA carboxylase synthesis can be ascribed to changes in the amount of translatable messenger RNA coding for this enzyme.

TABLE I

EFFECTS OF DIETARY CONDITIONS ON THE AMOUNT OF ACETYL-CoA CARBOXYLASE SYNTHESIZED BY CELL-FREE TRANSLATION OF RAT LIVER POLYSOMES*1

Rat	[^3H]*leucine incorporation**2	
	Acetyl-CoA carboxylase (cpm)	*Total protein* ($cpm \times 10^{-4}$)
Normal	248	172
Fasted	72	162
Refed	730	188

*1 Data taken from ref. 6.

*2 Per 2.5 A_{254} units of polysomes.

TABLE II

CORRELATION BETWEEN HEPATIC CONTENT OF ACETYL-CoA CARBOXYLASE-SYNTHESIZING POLYSOMES AND RATE OF HEPATIC ACETYL-CoA CARBOXYLASE SYNTHESIS *in vivo*

Animal		*Content of specific polysomes**1	*Rate of enzyme synthesis in vivo**2
Rat	Normal*3	1	1
	Fasted	1/2–1/3	1/2
	Refed	3–4	4
	Alloxan-diabetic	1/2	1/2
Mouse	Normal*3	1	1
	Obese	2	3

*1 Data taken from refs. 5–7.

*2 Data taken from refs. 8 and 9.

*3 Values for normal animals are taken as 1.

An attempt was next made to gain insight into the question, which metabolite is responsible for the regulation of synthesis of acetyl-CoA carboxylase. Long-chain fatty acid would be a possible candidate in view of the fact that it is the end product of the synthetic pathway in which this enzyme is involved. In fact, our previous investigation with hepatocytes of the JTC-25·P3 line, cultured in a chemically defined medium, has demonstrated that the addition of long-chain fatty acid to the medium results in a reduction in the rate of acetyl-CoA carboxylase synthesis and therefore in a decrease in the enzyme content.[10] A similar repression of acetyl-CoA carboxylase by exogenous long-chain fatty acid was also observed with *Saccharomyces cerevisiae*.[11] The question arises then, whether this repression is mediated by fatty acid itself or by a compound metabolically derived from it. For the purpose of answering this question, mutants defective in acyl-CoA synthetase [acid:CoA ligase (AMP-forming), EC 6.2.1.3], would be very useful, because this enzyme catalyzes the initial step required for further metabolism of exogenous fatty acid. To isolate the mutants, we used the yeast *Candida lipolytica* as well as *S. cerevisiae*, a simple eukaryotic organism. A great advantage of *C. lipolytica* is that it can grow not only on glucose but also on long-chain fatty acid or alkane as a sole carbon source, so that much larger variations in the cellular content of acetyl-CoA carboxylase are expected in this yeast than in cultured hepatocytes or *S. cerevisiae*. In fact, the acetyl-CoA carboxylase content of *C.*

lipolytica cells grown on oleic acid is one-sixth to one-seventh that of glucose-grown cells.[12] Moreover, [^{3}H]leucine incorporation studies combined with immunochemical techniques have shown that the decrease in the enzyme content is due to diminished synthesis of the enzyme as in the case of cultured hepatocytes.[12]

The rationale for the isolation procedure of acyl-CoA synthetase mutants was based on the fact that this enzyme becomes indispensable only when *de novo* synthesis of fatty acids is blocked,[13] because the fatty acid synthetase complex from yeast produces fatty acyl-CoA rather than free fatty acid, as demonstrated by Lynen's group.[14] Under conditions where *de novo* synthesis of fatty acids is inhibited by the antibiotic cerulenin,[15] mutants incapable of growing in the presence of fatty acids were selected. In this manner, we were able to isolate *C. lipolytica* mutants, including strains L-5 and L-7, which exhibited essentially no acyl-CoA synthetase activity.[16] Spontaneous revertants, which were isolated with a reasonably high frequency, exhibited activities comparable to that of the wild-type strain. Available evidence indicates that these mutants arise from a single mutation and that strain L-7 at least is a structural gene mutant.[16] A surprising and unexpected finding was that these mutants normally grew on fatty acid or *n*-alkane as a sole carbon source. This riddle has been solved as follows.

In the experiment whose results are shown in Table III, cells were grown on pentadecanoic acid, an odd-chain-length fatty acid, as a sole carbon source, and the fatty acid composition of cellular lipids were then analyzed by gas-liquid chromatography. Nearly all the fatty acids of the wild-type as well as the revertant cells were of odd-numbered chain lengths (17:1, 15:0, 17:2, *etc.*), whereas the mutant cells contained almost exclusively even-chain-length fatty acids (18:1, 18:2, 16:1, 16:0, *etc.*) Control cells of all strains grown on tetradecanoic acid, an even-chain-length fatty acid, as a sole carbon source contained almost solely even-chain-length fatty acids. These data indicate that the mutant cells unlike, the wild-type and revertant cells, cannot incorporate exogenous fatty acid as a whole into cellular lipids, but utilize the fatty acid that is synthesized *de novo* from acetyl-CoA, which is produced by degradation of exogenous fatty acid. Therefore, exogenous fatty acid must somehow be activated in the mutant cells to be degraded.

On the basis of the results just described, four possible mechanisms of fatty acid activation were considered as follows: First, thioesterification of fatty acid catalyzed by an additional acyl-CoA synthetase which is still unknown; secondly, ω-oxidation to dicarbo-

TABLE III

RELATIVE CONTENT OF ODD-CHAIN-LENGTH FATTY ACIDS IN *C. lipolytica* CELLS GROWN ON FATTY ACID*1

Strain	*Odd-chain-length fatty acids in cells grown on*	
	Pentadecanoic acid (%)*2	*Tetradecanoic acid* (%)*2
Wild-type-*3	94.7	2.3
Mutant L-5	6.1	0.6
Mutant L-7	5.8	0.4
Revertant RL7–8	93.2	1.4

*1 Data taken from ref. 16.

*2 The sum of the amounts of the cellular fatty acids detected is taken as 100 %.

*3 NRRL Y-6795.

xylic acid followed by thioesterification at either carboxyl group; thirdly, ω-oxidation to semialdehyde followed by CoA-dependent dehydrogenation; and finally, α-oxidation to α-keto acid followed by CoA-dependent oxidative decarboxylation. These possibilities could be distinguished from one another by cultivating cells on either [1-^{14}C]- or [10-^{14}C] oleic acid and then determining how much ^{14}C has been incorporated into the carboxyl carbon of the cellular fatty acids with the aid of the Schmidt reaction. The results obtained have clearly demonstrated that the first mechanism is valid, thus predicting the presence of an additional acyl-CoA synthetase operating even in the mutant cells, which apparently exhibit no enzyme activity under normal assay conditions.[16]

This prediction has been fulfilled by the discovery of a second acyl-CoA synthetase, which almost absolutely requires phosphatidylcholine for its activity. In the experiment whose results are shown in Fig. 2, the particulate fraction derived from the wild-type and from the mutant cells, grown either on oleic acid or on glucose as a sole carbon source, was assayed for acyl-CoA synthetase activity in the presence and absence of phosphatidylcholine. The mutant strain L-7 evidently lacked the phosphatidylcholine-independent activity. The phosphatidylcholine-dependent activity was found in oleic acid-grown cells of both the wild-type and the mutant strain, but essentially not on glucose-grown cells, indicating its inducible nature.

More conclusive evidence for the presence of two distinct acyl-CoA synthetases was provided by the successful separation of the phosphatidylcholine-independent and the phosphatidylcholine-dependent enzyme from each other. In the experiment presented in Table IV, the particulate fraction from oleic acid-grown wild-type cells, which possess both enzymes, was treated with 5 mM Triton X-100, and the mixture was then subjected to high-speed centrifugation. The resulting supernatant and precipitate as well as the original

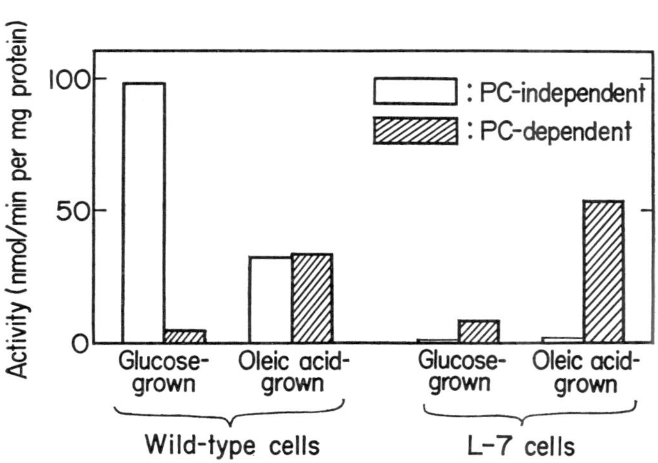

Fig. 2. Phosphatidylcholine-independent and phosphatidylcholine-dependent acyl-CoA synthetase activities in the particulate fraction derived from wild-type and mutant (L-7) cells grown on glucose or oleic acid. PC, phosphatidylcholine; PC-independent activity, activity measured without PC; PC-dependent activity, activity measured with PC *minus* activity measured without PC. Data taken from ref. 17.

TABLE IV
SEPARATION OF TWO ACYL-CoA SYNTHETASES FROM OLEIC ACID-GROWN WILD-TYPE CELLS BY TRITON X-100 TREATMENT*1

Fraction	*Phosphatidylcholine-independent activity (nmol/min)*	*Phosphatidylcholine-dependent activity (nmol/min)*
Particulate fraction*2	676	681
Supernatant*3	714	64
Precipitate*3	65	427

*1 Data taken from ref. 17.
*2 Equivalent to 25 mg of protein.
*3 Resulting from centrifugation at 105,000 × *g* of the particulate fraction treated with 5 mM Triton X-100.

particulate fraction were assayed for phosphatidylcholine-independent and the phosphatidylcholine-dependent activity. The results showed that the phosphatidylcholine-independent enzyme was solubilized by Triton X-100, whereas the phosphatidylcholine-dependent enzyme remained in the precipitate. The relatively low recovery of the phosphatidylcholine-dependent enzyme was due to its susceptibility to Triton X-100.[17] Thus, the two acyl-CoA synthetases were clearly separated from each other. Furthermore, evidence has been obtained to indicate that the two enzymes are localized in different subcellular fractions. We designate the phosphatidylcholine-independent enzyme as acyl-CoA synthetase I and the phosphatidylcholine-dependent enzyme as acyl-CoA synthetase II. The reaction product of both enzymes was identified as acyl-CoA. Thus, the mutant strains are defective in acyl-CoA synthetase I, but possess acyl-CoA synthetase II. It is evident from the phenotype of the mutant strains that acyl-CoA synthetase I is responsible for the formation of acyl-CoA to be utilized for the synthesis of cellular lipids, while acyl-CoA synthetase II provides acyl-CoA that is degraded *via* β-oxidation to yield acetyl-CoA.

It is to be noted here that the use of the *C. lipolytica* mutants lacking acyl-CoA synthetase I for the production of single-cell protein[18] appears to be of great advantage from a nutritional point of view, because their cellular lipids contain almost exclusively even-chain-length fatty acids, which occur naturally, even when they are grown on odd-chain-length hydrocarbons. To our knowledge, this group of mutants is the first organism reported that exhibits this ability.

The experiment represented in Table V deals with our original question, whether the repression of acetyl-CoA carboxylase is mediated by fatty acid itself or a metabolite derived from it. Wild-type, mutant and revertant cells were grown either on glucose or on oleic acid as a sole carbon source, and the cellular content of acetyl-CoA carboxylase was determined by activity measurements and immunochemical titrations. Acetyl-CoA carboxylase is repressed in the wild-type as well as in the revertant cells grown on oleic acid. In contrast, no such repression occurred in the mutant cells. (Similarly, *S. cerevisiae* mutants lacking acyl-CoA synthetase, in contrast to the wild-type strain, exhibited no repression of acetyl-CoA carboxylase upon addition of fatty acid.[13]) These results indicate that the activation of exogenous fatty acid by acyl-CoA synthetase I is required for the repression of acetyl-CoA carboxylase, thus supporting the view that the repressive effect is mediated by the direct or indirect product formed by acyl-CoA synthetase I.

TABLE V

LACK OF REPRESSION OF ACETYL-CoA CARBOXYLASE IN MUTANTS DEFECTIVE IN ACYL-CoA SYNTHETASE I

Strain	*Acetyl-CoA carboxylase*	
	Glucose-grown (nmol/min per mg protein)	*Oleic acid-grown (nmol/min per mg protein)*
Wild-type	19.6	2.9
Mutant L-5	21.0	17.8
Mutant L-7	23.3	16.5
Revertant RL7-8	23.9	3.1

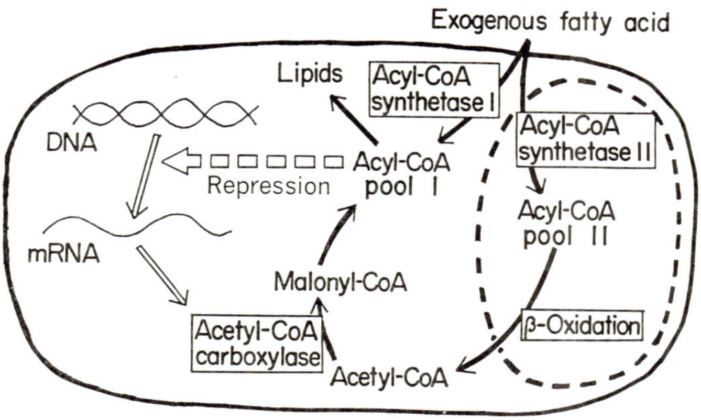

Fig. 3. Proposed mechanism of repression of acetyl-CoA carboxylase.

The conclusion drawn from the studies presented above is schematically shown in Fig. 3. In view of the different subcellular localizations of acyl-CoA synthetases I and II, it is reasonable to assume that there are two distinct acyl-CoA pools. Acyl-CoA pool I, which represents the product of acyl-CoA synthetase I, is utilized for the synthesis of cellular lipids, while acyl-CoA pool II, which is provided by acyl-CoA synthetase II, is exclusively degraded *via* β-oxidation to yield acetyl-CoA. Because no repression of acetyl-CoA carboxylase occurs in the mutant cells lacking acyl-CoA synthetase I, acyl-CoA pool I or a further metabolite derived from it must be the mediator of the repressive effect on acetyl-CoA carboxylase. This repression is assumed to be effected at the transcriptional level on the basis of the good correlation observed between the hepatic content of acetyl-CoA carboxylase-synthesizing polysomes and the rate of hepatic synthesis *in vivo* of this enzyme, although the possibility of translational control cannot be excluded. On the other hand, acyl-CoA pool II is not involved in the regulation of acetyl-CoA carboxylase synthesis. This regulatory mechanism is of teleological significance to maintain homeostasis of lipogenesis.

REGULATION OF FATTY ACID DISTRIBUTION IN GLYCEROLIPIDS

It is well known that in naturally occurring glycerolipids the C-1 position of the glycerol moiety is occupied principally by saturated fatty acids, while the C-2 position is occupied mainly by unsaturated fatty acids.[19,20] This asymmetric distribution of fatty acids appears to be of great importance for the functions of biological membranes. The formation of the non-random fatty acid distribution can be regarded as a kind of regulatory process, but the enzymic mechanism responsible for the specific introduction of fatty acids into glycerolipids remained obscure. We have attempted to answer this important question by isolating individual acyltransferases involved in glycerolipid synthesis and determining the acyl-donor and acyl-acceptor specificities of the isolated acyltransferases.[21–26]

Figure 4 shows the separation of glycerolphosphate acyltransferase (acyl-CoA: *sn*-glycerol-3-phosphate O-acyltransferase, EC 2.3.1.15), 1-acylglycerolphosphate acyltransferase (acyl-CoA: 1-acyl-*sn*-glycerol-3-phosphate O-acyltransferase, EC 2.3.1.51), 1-acylglycerophosphorylcholine acyltransferase (acyl-CoA: 1-acyl-*sn*-glycero-3-phosphorylcholine O-acyltransferase, EC 2.3.1.23), and diacylglycerol acyltransferase (acyl-CoA: 1,2-diacyl-*sn*-glycerol O-acyltransferase, EC 2.3.1.20). Rat liver microsomes were solubilized with Triton X-100, passed through Sepharose 2B and then subjected to sucrose density gradient centrifugation. Glycerolphosphate acyltransferase, which was found in the middle of the gradient, was clearly separated from 1-acylglycerolphosphate

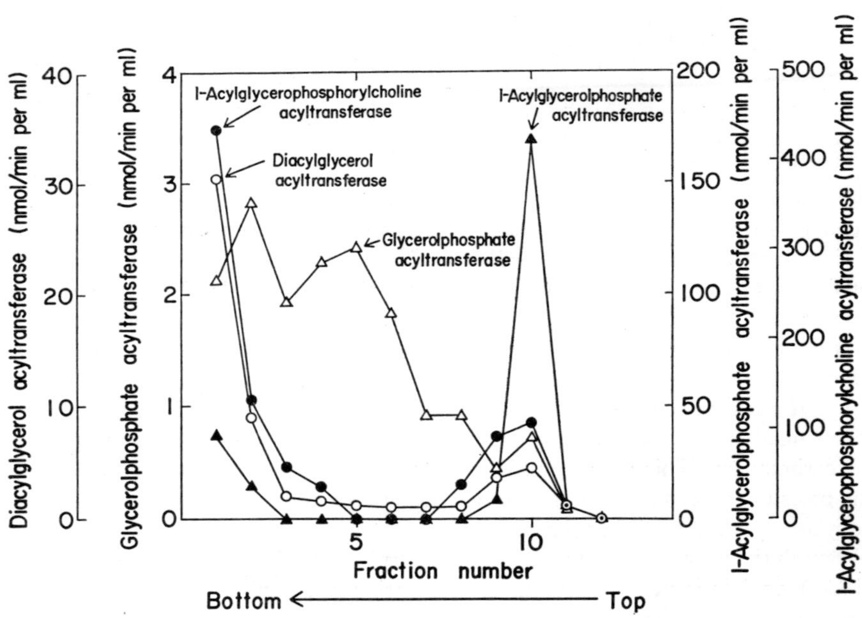

Fig. 4. Separation of the acyltransferases from rat liver microsomes by sucrose density gradient centrifugation. Microsomes solubilized with 8 mM Triton X-100 were subjected to Sepharose-2B chromatography and then centrifuged at 65,000 rpm for 7 hr in a two-layered sucrose gradient consisting of 0.3 ml of 2 M sucrose and 3.4 ml of a 0.5–1.1 M sucrose gradient. Data taken from ref. 25.

acyltransferase, remaining near the top of the gradient, and from 1-acylglycerophosphorylcholine acyltransferase and diacylglycerol acyltransferase, both of which sedimented to the bottom of the gradient. Although the latter two enzymes were not separated from each other, these enzymes were distinguishable with respect to sensitivity both to heat and to sulfhydryl-binding reagents.[25] Thus, it is evident that microsomes contain distinct acyltransferases responsible for the acylation of the different acyl acceptors.

The acyl-donor specificities of the four separated acyltransferases are schematically shown in Fig. 5. Glycerolphosphate acyltransferase introduces saturated acyl-CoA thioesters, especially palmityl-CoA, into the C-1 position, whereas unsaturated acyl-CoA thioesters are almost ineffective. 1-Acylglycerolphosphate acyltransferase exhibits a significant preference for monoenoic and dienoic acyl-CoA thioesters like oleyl-CoA and linoleyl-CoA, although saturated acyl-CoA thioesters are also utilized to some extent. It is noteworthy that arachidonyl-CoA is almost ineffective. In contrast, arachidonyl-CoA is the most effective acyl donor for 1-acylglycerophosphorylcholine acyltransferase. This enzyme also utilizes linoleyl-CoA and oleyl-CoA but is essentially inactive with saturated acyl-CoA thioesters. The acyl-donor specificities of 1-acylglycerolphosphate acyltransferase and 1-acylglycerophosphorylcholine acyltransferase are virtually not affected by the acyl constituent of the respective acyl acceptors. In contrast to the three acyltransferases just described, diacylglycerol acyltransferase exhibits a broad acyl-donor specificity, utilizing all acyl-CoA thioesters tested.

Figure 6 schematically shows the acyl-acceptor specificities of 1-acylglycerolphosphate acyltransferase and 1-acylglycerophosphorylcholine acyltransferase with respect to the

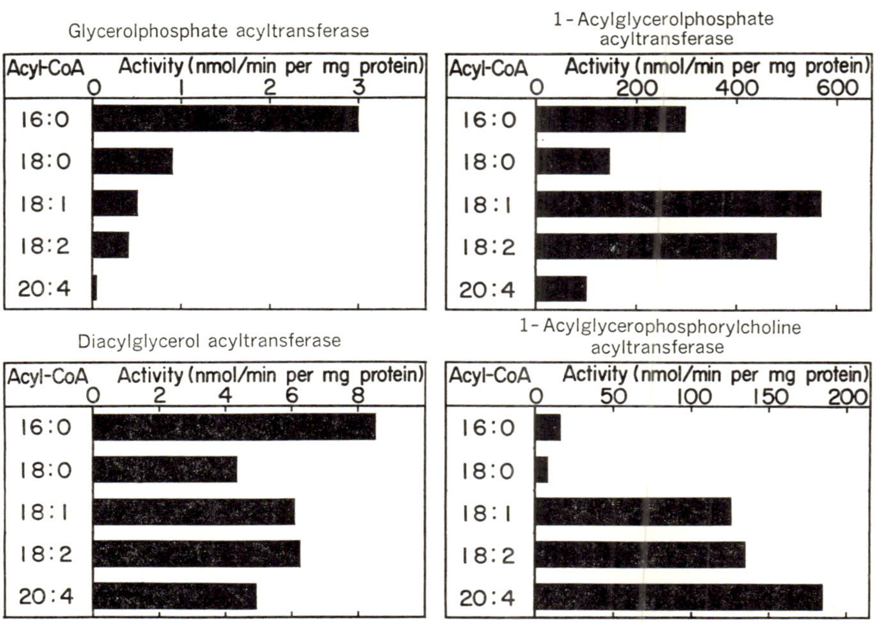

Fig. 5. Acyl-donor specificities of the acyltransferases. Results obtained with varying concentrations of acyl donor (and acyl acceptor in some cases) are schematically presented. Data taken from refs. 22, 24, 25–26.

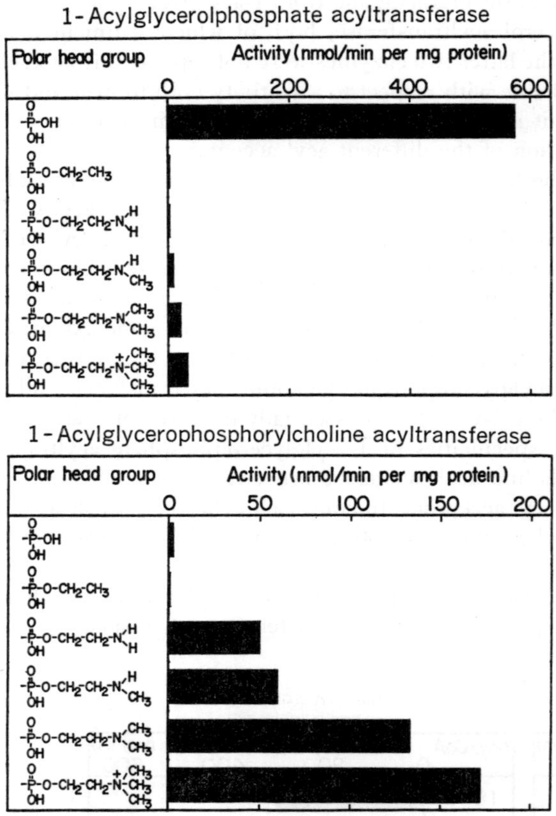

Fig. 6. Acyl-acceptor specificities of 1-acylglycerolphosphate acyltransferase and 1-acylglycerophosphorylcholine acyltransferase with respect to the polar head group. Results obtained with varying concentrations of acyl acceptor and acyl donor (oleyl-CoA for 1-acylglycerolphosphate acyltransferase and arachidonyl-CoA for 1-acylglycerophosphorylcholine acyltransferase) are schematically presented. Data taken from ref. 26.

polar head group. 1-Acylglycerolphosphate acyltransferase is highly specific for 1-acyl-*sn*-glycerol 3-phosphate. All other 1-acylglycerophospholipid analogues tested are ineffective. On the other hand, 1-acylglycerophosphorylcholine acyltransferase acts on several 1-acylglycerophospholipid analogues, 1-acyl-*sn*-glycero-3-phosphorylcholine being the best acyl acceptor. 1-Acyl-*sn*-glycero-3-phosphoryldimethylethanolamine is also utilized fairly efficiently, and 1-acyl-*sn*-glycero-3-phosphorylmonomethylethanolamine and 1-acyl-*sn*-glycero-3-phosphorylethanolamine to some extent, while 1-acyl-*sn*-glycerol 3-phosphate and 1-acyl-*sn*-glycero-3-phosphorylethanol are ineffective. The possibility that the 1-acylglycerophosphorylcholine acyltransferase preparation used may contain a group of enzymes which are responsible for the acylation of the different acyl acceptors has not been excluded. Anyhow, the acyl-donor specificity of this enzyme is not influenced by the polar basic group of the acyl acceptor.[26] Furthermore, the activities of 1-acylgly-

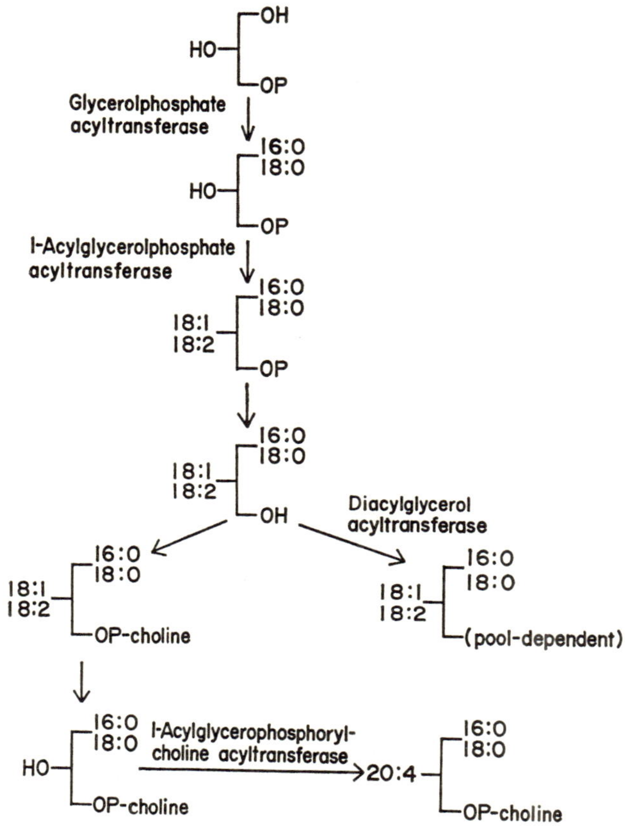

Fig. 7. Specific introduction of fatty acids into glycerolipids based on the substrate specificities of the acyltransferases.

cerolphosphate acyltransferase and 1-acylglycerophosphorylcholine acyltransferase are hardly affected by the acyl constituent of the respective acyl acceptors.[26]

Our results on the substrate specificities of the acyltransferases involved in glycerolipid synthesis are summarized in Fig. 7. The C-1 position of *sn*-glycerol 3-phosphate is first acylated with saturated acyl-CoA such as palmityl-CoA or stearyl-CoA. The C-2 position of the 1-acyl-*sn*-glycerol 3-phosphate formed is then acylated mainly with monoenoic or dienoic acyl-CoA such as oleyl-CoA or linoleyl-CoA to produce phosphatidic acid. 1-Acylglycerolphosphate acyltransferase, which catalyzes this reaction, strictly selects 1-acyl-*sn*-glycerol 3-phosphate as acyl acceptor and does not introduce arachidonyl-CoA at this step. Since this enzyme can utilize any 1-acyl-*sn*-glycerol 3-phosphate derivative regardless of which fatty acid is bound to the C-1 position, the 1-acyl-*sn*-glycerol 3-phosphate containing saturated fatty acid, which is formed by the action of glycerolphosphate acyltransferase, is simply further acylated at the C-2 position. The phosphatidic acid thus formed should therefore contain saturated fatty acid at the C-1 position and monoenoic or dienoic fatty acid at the C-2 position. Since diacylglycerol acyltransferase exhibits a broad acyl-donor specificity, the C-3 position of 1,2-diacyl-*sn*-glycerol can be acylated by any acyl-CoA thioester present in the pool. From what has been discussed thus far, it is evident that the non-random fatty acid distribution in monoenoic and dienoic species of glycerolipids is accomplished at the step of *de novo* synthesis of phosphatidic acid. On the other hand, glycerophospholipids in animal tissues are known to contain large amounts of arachidonic acid.[19] In this context, the substrate specificity of 1-acylglycerophosphorylcholine acyltransferase appears to be of great importance. This enzyme strictly recognizes the polar basic group at the C-3 position of the acyl acceptor and utilizes arachinodyl-CoA as the best acyl donor. This finding strongly supports the view that a portion of the newly synthesized glycerophospholipids is once deacylated at the 2-position and then reacylated with arachidonyl-CoA to form tetraenoic species of glycerophospholipids. Thus, it is concluded that the substrate specificities of the acyltransferases make an essential contribution to the specific introduction of fatty acids into glycerolipids, effecting the non-random fatty acid distribution in naturally occurring glycerolipids.

ACKNOWLEDGMENTS

This investigation was supported in part by research grants from the Ministry of Education, Science and Culture of Japan, the Mitsubishi Foundation, the Toray Science Foundation, the Foundation for the Promotion of Research on Medicinal Resources, the Japanese Foundation of Metabolism and Diseases, the Japan Heart Foundation, and the Japanese Medical Association.

REFERENCES

1 S. Numa, S. Nakanishi, T. Hashimoto, N. Iritani, and T. Okazaki, in R. S. Harris, J. A. Loraine, P. L. Munson, and E. Diczfalusy, *Vitamins and Hormones*, Academic Press, New York, vol. 28, 1970, p. 213.
2 S. Numa, in R. H. Adrian *et al.*, *Ergebnisse der Physiologie*, Springer-Verlag, Berlin, vol. 69, 1974, p. 53.
3 S. Numa and S. Yamashita, in B. L. Horecker and E. R. Stadtman, *Current Topics in Cellular Regulation*, Academic Press, New York, vol. 8, 1974, p. 197.
4 J. M. Taylor and R. T. Schimke, *J. Biol. Chem.*, 249 (1974) 3597.
5 S. Nakanishi, T. Tanabe, S. Horikawa, and S. Numa, *Proc. Natl. Acad. Sci. U. S.*, 73 (1976) 2304.
6 S. Horikawa, S. Nakanishi, and S. Numa, *FEBS Lett.*, 74 (1977) 55.
7 T. Tanabe, S. Horikawa, S. Nakanishi, and S. Numa, *FEBS Lett.*, 66 (1976) 70.
8 S. Nakanishi and S. Numa, *Eur. J. Biochem.*, 16 (1970) 161.
9 S. Nakanishi and S. Numa, *Proc. Natl. Acad. Sci. U. S.*, 68 (1971) 2288.
10 K. Kitajima, S. Tashiro, and S. Numa, *Eur. J. Biochem.*, 54 (1975) 373.
11 T. Kamiryo and S. Numa, *FEBS Lett.*, 38 (1973) 29.
12 M. Mishina, T. Kamiryo, A. Tanaka, S. Fukui, and S. Numa, *Eur. J. Biochem.*, 71 (1976) 301.
13 T. Kamiryo, S. Parthasarathy, and S. Numa, *Proc. Natl. Acad. Sci. U. S.*, 73 (1976) 386.
14 F. Lynen, I. Hopper-Kessel, and H. Eggerer, *Biochem. Z.*, 340 (1964) 95.
15 S. Ōmura, *Bacteriol. Rev.*, 40 (1976) 681.
16 T. Kamiryo, M. Mishina, S. Tashiro, and S. Numa, *Proc. Natl. Acad. Sci. U. S.*, 74 (1977) 4947.
17 M. Mishina, T. Kamiryo, S. Tashiro, and S. Numa, *Eur. J. Biochem.*, 82 (1978) 347.
18 R. I. Mateles and S. R. Tannenbaum, *Single-Cell Protein*, The MIT Press, Cambridge, Mass., 1968.

19 L. L. M. VAN DEENEN, in J. JÄRNEFELT, *Regulatory Functions of Biological Membranes*, Elsevier, Amsterdam, 1968, p. 72.
20 B. ÅKESSON, *Eur. J. Biochem.*, 9 (1969) 463.
21 S. YAMASHITA, K. HOSAKA, and S. NUMA, *Proc. Natl. Acad. Sci. U. S.*, 69 (1972) 3490.
22 S. YAMASHITA and S. NUMA, *Eur. J. Biochem.*, 31 (1972) 565.
23 S. YAMASHITA, K. HOSAKA, and S. NUMA, *Eur. J. Biochem.*, 38 (1973) 25.
24 S. YAMASHITA, N. NAKAYA, Y. MIKI, and S. NUMA, *Proc. Natl. Acad. Sci. U. S.*, 72 (1975) 600.
25 K. HOSAKA, U. SCHIELE, and S. NUMA, *Eur. J. Biochem.*, 76 (1977) 113.
26 Y. MIKI, K. HOSAKA, S. YAMASHITA, H. HANDA, and S. NUMA, *Eur. J. Biochem.*, 81 (1977) 433.

MECHANISM OF CHOLESTEROL-LOWERING EFFECTS OF POLYUNSATURATED FATS

J. GANGULY, RANAJIT PAUL, C. S. RAMESHA, AND P. BALARAM

Department of Biochemistry and Molecular Biophysics Unit, Indian Institute of Science, Bangalore (India)

Atherosclerosis is a disease of the intima of the aorta caused by the formation of lipid-containing lesions which proliferate in the lumen of the artery, eventually leading to obstruction of blood flow. Thrombosis is the end result of such degenerative changes of the intima, and ischemic heart disease usually results from thrombic obstruction that occurs in the coronary artery lesions. It has been widely recognized that a direct relationship exists between serum lipid levels and atherosclerosis, and that blood cholesterol levels are usually elevated in patients suffering from atherosclerosis. Moreover, according to Smith,[1] precipitation of lipids from specific serum lipoproteins may be a key factor in atherosclerosis in humans. Recognition of such a direct relationship between atherosclerosis and blood cholesterol levels has led to an extensive search for agents which can effectively lower blood cholesterol levels, and consequently many hypolipidemic drugs are being extensively used for the treatment of ischemic heart disease. But in many cases they show serious side effects.

Probably a more physiological approach to this problem would be use of natural dietary factors, and against this background the effect of different dietary fats on blood cholesterol levels assumes considerable significance, because overwhelming evidence has accumulated in the literature establishing the fact that the nature of dietary fats exerts profound influence on the blood cholesterol levels in various species of animals. Thus Kinsell *et al.*[2] had demonstrated that blood cholesterol levels are lowered in humans when plant fats containing very high proportions of unsaturated fatty acids are substituted for animal fats in the diet. It has also been demonstrated that oral or intravenous administration of lecithin isolated from soyabean or sunflower seeds containing very high proportions of linoleic acid prevents hyperlipemia in rats and humans.[3,4]

Clearly, these observations are of far-reaching clinical importance and therefore attempts have been made by many workers to find explanations for the mechanisms through which the blood cholesterol levels are lowered by highly unsaturated fats. Four possibilities have been considered in this respect; they are as follows:

1) Reduced absorption of cholesterol;
2) Reduced synthesis of cholesterol;
3) Increased excretion of cholesterol and its catabolites through bile and feces;
4) Redistribution of cholesterol from blood to other tissues.

Abbreviations: GPC, glycerylphosphoryl choline; α-GP, α-glycerophosphate; ANS, anilino-δ-naphthalene sulphonate; HDL, high density lipoprotein.

But the evidence from various laboratories from time to time has never been sufficient to establish any one of them, and, in fact, the results have been rather widely divergent.[5-13]

EFFECT OF DIETARY FATS ON THE BILIARY EXCRETION OF CHOLESTEROL

Since bile is the major route of excretion of cholesterol and its catabolites, attempts were made in our laboratory to correlate the excretion of cholesterol through the bile of rats fed polyunsaturated fats with the hypocholesterolemic effects of such fats. The following sets of experiments were designed for this purpose.[14]

Effect of highly unsaturated and less unsaturated fats

Groups of young rats were given *ad lib.* a normal diet (Hindusthan Lever Pellet) together with 10% safflower oil or coconut oil, for 30 days, after which cannulae were established in the bile ducts of these rats and the rates of bile flow were measured every 30 min. The bile was collected for 3 hr, following which the rats were sacrificed and the blood, liver, and bile were analyzed.

Table I shows that feeding of safflower oil led to striking increase in bile flow and reduced blood cholesterol levels but an increase in the liver cholesterol values, as compared to the feeding of coconut oil. At the same time the concentration of cholesterol per ml of bile as well as the total amounts of cholesterol excreted in 3 hr were markedly higher in the safflower oil-fed rats, while the bile salt values did not show any consistent difference in the bile of the two groups.

In separate experiments, where small amounts of 4-^{14}C-cholesterol dissolved in safflower oil or coconut oil were given to such rats 6 hr before cannulation, the radioactivity recovered in the bile salts and in the cholesterol of the bile was consistently higher in the safflower oil-fed rats (Table II).

Analysis of the fatty acid composition of the cholesteryl esters of the liver revealed striking increase in the relative proportions of unsaturated fatty acids in the safflower oil-fed rats, while no such significant differences in the unsaturation of the liver phospho-

TABLE I

EFFECT OF FEEDING SAFFLOWER OIL OR COCONUT OIL FOR 30 DAYS ON THE RATE OF BILE FLOW AND EXCRETION OF CHOLESTEROL THROUGH BILE IN RATS

Oil fed	*Serum cholesterol (μmol/ml)*	*Liver cholesterol (μmol/ml)*	*Bile*			
			Volume (ml/hr)	*Cholesterol (μmol/3 hr)*	*Bile acid (μmol/3 hr)*	*Phospholipids (μmol/3 hr)*
Safflower	2.40± 0.059*1	10.80± 0.81	0.548± 0.02	0.805± 0.051	15.83± 1.42	11.16± 1.18
				(0.595± 0.038)*2	(12.31± 1.50)	(7.30± 0.66)
Coconut	3.48± 0.084	8.67± 0.85	0.481± 0.02	0.502± 0.036	15.63± 1.33	11.58± 0.785
				(0.402± 0.022)	(12.86± 1.18)	(7.38± 0.311)

*1 S. E. of the mean.

*2 Figures in parentheses, values expressed per ml.

TABLE II

EXCRETION OF RADIOACTIVE CHOLESTEROL AND BILE SALTS IN THE BILE OF RATS GIVEN 4-^{14}C-CHOLESTEROL DISSOLVED IN OIL

Bile cannulation was done 6 hr after ^{14}C-cholesterol administration and collection of bile was for 3 hr.

Oil fed	*Cholesterol (cpm)*	*Bile salt (cpm)*
Safflower	855±58*1	2,191±161
	(664±42)*2	(1,388±88)
Coconut	622±46	1,661±85
	(471±41)	(1,164±83)

*1 S. E. of the mean.
*2 Figures in the parentheses, values expressed per ml.

TABLE III

FATTY ACID COMPOSITION OF LIPIDS IN LIVER AND BILE OF RATS FED SAFFLOWER AND COCONUT OIL FOR 30 DAYS

Fatty acid	*Liver cholesteryl ester*		*Liver phospholipids*		*Bile phospholipids*	
	Safflower oil	*Coconut oil*	*Safflower oil*	*Coconut oil*	*Safflower oil*	*Coconut oil*
C_{12}:0	2.54	2.30	—	—	—	—
C_{14}:0	4.30	4.29	—	—	—	—
C_{16}:0	26.55	31.95	16.26	21.47	40.99	48.04
C_{18}:0	11.04	12.36	39.92	42.71	11.67	13.30
C_{18}:1	16.58	34.37	8.40	10.35	5.77	13.30
C_{18}:2	38.88	15.51	21.62	13.98	41.55	25.01
C_{20}:4	—	—	13.77	11.47	—	—

lipids were noticed in the two groups. In sharp contrast, the fatty acids of the biliary phospholipids revealed a perceptible difference in that, while linoleic acid was the major fatty acid in the safflower oil-fed rats, the coconut oil-fed animals showed palmitic acid as the major fatty acid (Table III).

Effect of highly unsaturated and less unsaturated lecithin

In another set of experiments, groups of young rats were given the pellet diet *ad lib.* and either no phospholipid or 500 mg of soya phospholipid (EPL) or egg phospholipid per rat per day for 7 days. At the end of 7 days, the bile was similarly collected for 3 hr, after which the animals were sacrificed and the blood, liver, and bile were analyzed. Here, the blood cholesterol level was lower in the control (receiving no phospholipid) and soya phospholipid-fed rats as compared to the egg phospholipid-fed animals, while the liver cholesterol values were comparable in all the groups. But it was most significant that feeding of either type of phospholipid markedly stimulated the rate of bile flow, which was highest in the EPL-fed animals. The total amounts of cholesterol excreted in 3 hr were also appreciably higher in the rats given EPL, while the concentration of cholesterol per ml of bile did not show much difference in the rats receiving EPL and egg phospholipids.

Here also, the fatty acids of the cholesteryl esters and triglycerides of the liver were more unsaturated in the rats given EPL, while the fatty acid composition of the liver phospholipids showed little difference in the two groups. In striking contrast, the fatty acids of the biliary phospholipids revealed perceptible changes in that there were markedly higher proportions of linoleic acid in the bile of rats given EPL, as compared to the other two groups.

ABSORPTION OF DIETARY LECITHIN

The most important aspects of these experiments were that feeding of unsaturated lipids led to considerable increase in the rate of bile flow and in the unsaturation of biliary phospholipids also in increased excretion of cholesterol through the bile. These considerations led us to investigate the mode of absorption of dietary phospholipids and the possible contributions of dietary fatty acids and phospholipids to the synthesis of biliary phospholipids.

Although the mechanism of intestinal absorption of triglycerides has attracted extensive attention of many investigators for a long period of time, there has been relatively little work on absorption of phospholipids. While earlier workers had demonstrated that dietary phospholipids undergo extensive hydrolysis in the lumen of the small intestine, more recent work of Scow *et al.*[15] and of Nilsson[16] with lymph-cannulated rats has shown that about 80% of the radioactivity of the orally administered fatty acid-labelled lecithin can be accounted for in the lymph triglycerides, the rest of the radioactivity being recovered in the lymph lecithin. On the other hand, very recently Parthasarathy *et al.*[17] have demonstrated that during digestion in the intestine the dietary lecithin is extensively hydrolyzed to free fatty acids, GPC and α-GP, after which the free fatty acids and α-GP are reassembled into triglycerides *via* the Kennedy pathway.

The physicochemical state of the lipids during digestion of fats in the intestine has also attracted some attention of earlier workers. Lipids as such are insoluble in water; in order that enzymes and cells in general can deal with them effectively, they have to be rendered water-soluble. Hofmann and Borgstrom[18] had put forward the idea that during digestion of a fatty meal the products of lipolysis appear in human intestine in the form of water-clear micellar aggregates, thereby making the dietary lipids water-soluble. But later on,

TABLE IV

LIPID COMPOSITION OF THE FAT AND MICELLAR PHASES IN THE INTESTINE OF RATS FED 20 μMOL OF BILE SALTS AND 20 μMOL OF CHOLESTEROL IN 0.5 ML GROUNDNUT OIL DISPERSED IN 1 ML WATER WITH EPL*1

Free fatty acid and cholesterol were present in appreciable amounts in both micellar and fat phases.

EPL fed (*µmol*)	*Micellar phase**2 (*µmol*)				
	MG	*DG*	*TG*	*LPC*	*PC*
30	0.0492	0.073	0.024	0.0234	0.088
40	0.0901	0.057	0.042	0.0392	0.176
Fat phase					
30	0.0194	0.199	0.295	0.010	0.031
40	0.0192	0.211	0.308	0.0135	0.0392

*1 Soya lecithin.

*2 MG, monoglycerides; DG, diglycerides; TG, triglycerides; LPC, lysophosphatidyl choline; PC, phosphatidyl choline.

Porter and Saunders[19] showed that the methods employed by Hofmann and Borgstrom[20] for the isolation of the aqueous phase of the intestinal contents give rise to several artefacts and at the same time successfully used the technique of ultrafiltration for such purpose.

By isolating the micellar phase of the intestinal contents of rats by the ultrafiltration technique described by Porter and Saunders,[19] it has been demonstrated by us that, following feeding of soya lecithin or egg lecithin in groundnut oil together with bile salts, as compared to the fat phase, the micellar phase contained very high proportions of monoglycerides but much fewer diglycerides, while almost all of the triglycerides were recovered in the fat phase. The phospholipids, on the other hand, exhibited a rather different pattern in that, both lecithin and lysolecithin were present in much higher proportions in the micellar phase than in the fat phase, with the concentration of lecithin being much higher than that of lysolecithin in the micellar phase (Table IV).

INFLUENCE OF DIETARY LECITHIN ON BILIARY LECITHIN

Although a normal diet contains considerable amounts of phospholipids, the possibility of significant contributions of the dietary phospholipids to the synthesis of biliary phospholipids has been largely ignored by earlier workers. Therefore attempts were made in our laboratory to study the pattern of excretion of dietary labelled free fatty acids or phospholipids through the bile of rats. In the experiments where 1-^{14}C-linoleic acid was given to bile duct-cannulated rats, nearly 0.1% of the fed radioactivity was recovered in 3 hr in the biliary lecithin, which was in fact the only lipid in the bile to carry the fed radioactivity. It was also observed in these trials that the specific radioactivity of the biliary lecithin was markedly higher than in the liver lecithin, which obviously meant that the exogenous fatty acid was preferentially incorporated into the biliary lecithin. These findings of ours are in general agreement with those of Balint *et al.*,[21] who had claimed that separate pools exist in the liver for the synthesis of biliary and liver lecithin.

In similar experiments where β(1-^{14}C-linoleoyl)-lecithin was given, the bulk of the radioactivity present in the biliary lipids was recovered in the lecithin fraction, with virtually all of the radioactivity of the biliary lecithin being retained at the β-position (Table V). Such a situation can arise if the exogenous lecithin molecule escapes the attack of phospholipase A_2 in the intestine and is consequently absorbed intact. Alternatively, following attack of phospholipase A_2 the lysolecithin formed may be reacylated with the same fatty acid which is split off by the enzyme. But it has already been shown that large amounts of lecithin appear in the micellar state in the intestine of rats given lecithin, which would

TABLE V

DISTRIBUTION OF ^{14}C-FATTY ACID IN THE α- AND β-POSITIONS OF BILIARY LECITHIN IN RATS GIVEN 20.0 μMOL OF β-(1-^{14}C-LINOLEOYL) LECITHIN*

Time after feeding (min)	*β-Fatty acid (cpm)*	*α-Fatty acid (cpm)*
90	1,200	170
150	1,930	150
210	1,960	130
270	1,500	200
330	1,557	150

* Sp. activity = 80,000 cpm/μmol.

TABLE VI

^{14}C- AND ^{32}P-RADIOACTIVITIES IN THE BILIARY LECITHIN IN RATS GIVEN β-(1-^{14}C-LINOLEOYL) LECITHIN-^{32}P WITH A $^{14}C/^{32}P$ RATIO OF 1

Bile collection started 30 min after administration of the doubly-labelled lecithin. Recovery in 300 min: $^{14}C=0.3\%$ of dose, $^{32}P=0.1\%$ of dose.

Time (min)	^{14}C *(cpm/sample)*	^{32}P *(cpm/sample)*	$^{14}C/^{32}P$
60	863	131	6.58
120	1,056	327	3.35
180	1,638	514	3.18
240	1,139	608	1.87
300	1,264	756	1.67

strongly suggest that some proportions of exogenous lecithin are probably absorbed intact. Such a possibility was supported by the results of our experiments on biliary excretion of exogenous doubly-labelled lecithin. In these experiments, where rats were given β(1-^{14}C-linoleoyl)-lecithin-^{32}P with a $^{14}C/^{32}P$ ratio of 1, at the initial stages of collection of bile the $^{14}C/^{32}P$ ratio of the biliary lecithin was nearly 7, which declinced to a value of nearly 1 at the termination of the experiments at 5 hr (Table VI). These results therefore showed that some proportions of the dietary lecithin are not only absorbed intact, but are transported all the way through the bile in the intact form. The relative loss of ^{32}P against ^{14}C in the biliary lecithin, however, was probably due to base-exchange reactions as suggested by Kanoh,[22] Weiss,[23] and others.

PHYSICO-CHEMICAL STUDIES OF THE BILE MICELLE

Cholesterol is insoluble in water and it exists in the bile in the form of mixed micelles together with phospholipids and bile salts. Small[24] had concluded from X-ray and NMR studies that phospholipid: bile salt mixed micelles are disc-shaped bimolecular leaflets of lecithin molecules which form the core of the micelle. The ends of the discs are covered by the hydrophilic choline [$N^{+}(CH_3)_3$] groups, while the sides consist of hydrocarbon alkyl chains. The steroid nucleus of the bile salt molecule is hydrophobically associated with the alkyl chain of the lecithin molecule while its hydrophilic parts orient towards the aqueous phase. It has been suggested that, being highly hydrophobic in nature, cholesterol associates itself with the hydrocarbon residues of the phospholipids of the micelles.

The marked increase in the unsaturation of the fatty acids of the biliary lecithin and the increased concentrations of cholesterol of the bile of rats given unsaturated fats led us to compare the mode of packing of the lipids in the bile micelles of rats receiving unsaturated and saturated fats, and these investigations were further extended to an examination of the artificial model micelles made of cholesterol, sodium deoxycholate and lecithin of different fatty acid composition.

The NMR spectra of natural bile fluid of rats closely resembled those of the model micelles prepared with bile salt, cholesterol, and lecithin. The bile salt molecules in the micelles appeared rigidly packed, while the phospholipid molecules were in a fluid state which was evident from the overwhelming contributions of the NMR signals of phospholipids. The natural bile micelles seem to be quite stable: Heating, sonication, or treatment with protease or phospholipase A_2 failed to effect any perceptible changes in the gross appearance of the spectra. Addition of ANS, however, perturbed the micelles and led to the appearance of steroid signals and an upfield shift of the choline methyl signals. The only significant difference observed in the NMR spectra of the bile from rats fed saturated and unsaturated fats was the increase in the line-width of the choline resonance in the case of the latter samples. Similar broadening of the choline resonance was also observed in model phospholipid: bile salt mixed micelles following incorporation of increasing amounts of cholesterol. These NMR studies have also shown that mixed micelles containing unsaturated phospholipids exhibit greater lipid mobility than those containing dipalmitoyl lecithin. Further, incorporation of cholesterol led to greater restriction of the fluidity of the phospholipids in the unsaturated phospholipid micelles as compared to the micelles containing dipalmitoyl lecithin, thereby suggesting more effective packing of cholesterol in the micelles containing unsaturated phospholipids.

Parallel studies using fluorescent probes like ANS, pyrene, and dansyl cadaverine have lent further support to our conclusions that the matrix of mixed micelles made of polyunsaturated lecithin is more disordered than those prepared from less unsaturated lecithin. Similar conclusions were drawn from a comparative study of the bile of chickens, goats, and sheep. Analysis of the fatty acid composition of the lecithin of these bile samples revealed that, compared to sheep and goat bile, the lecithin of chicken bile is more unsaturated and contains more cholesterol per unit volume of bile. At the same time, it was also found that the matrix of chicken bile micelles is considerably more fluid than that of sheep and goat bile micelles. All these observations are in conformity with our views that cholesterol is more effectively packed in the matrix of the micelles of polyunsaturated lecithin.

PHYSIOLOGICAL IMPLICATIONS

The physiological implications of these findings and the overall picture that has emerged regarding the cholesterol-lowering effects of polyunsaturated lipids are schematically presented in Fig. 1 and are briefly discussed below.

It is clear from our work that intake of polyunsaturated lipids in the form of safflower oil or soya phospholipid leads to a striking increase in the rate of bile flow and in the unsaturation of the biliary phospholipids; these in turn solubilize more cholesterol, as a consequence of which higher amounts of cholesterol are excreted through the bile. On the other hand, earlier workers have shown that considerable amounts of cholesterol are excreted into the intestine, where they undergo extensive bacterial modification and are eventually excreted through the feces.[25]

Let us now consider the effects on tissue cholesterol. Cholesterol is transported in the blood by the circulating lipoproteins, and numerous studies have shown that the plasma lipoproteins, especially the HDL, play an important role in the efflux of cholesterol from arterial smooth muscle cells.[26,27] Thus it has been demonstrated that the cholesterol of the arterial smooth muscle cells can freely exchange with the cholesterol of the pre-existing lipoproteins in the fluid environment. In this context it would be pertinent to recall here that in recent years increased fluidity of the lipoprotein matrix has been demonstrated in animals given unsaturated fats,[28] which would obviously mean that, in atherosclerotic animals, feeding of unsaturated fats should lead to a net transfer of cholesterol from the arterial cells to the HDL which have become more fluid due to increase in the unsaturation of its lipids. Indeed, it has been claimed that intravenous infusion of polyunsaturated

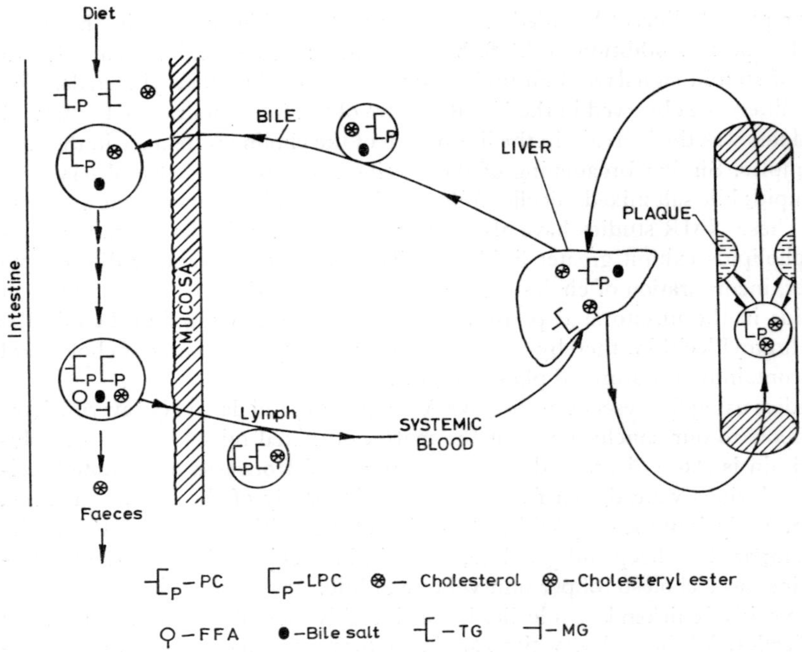

Fig. 1. Dynamics of cholesterol in animal body.

phospholipids in animals can reverse atherosclerosis by removing the lipids deposited in the aorta.[29,30] As we have noted much of the cholesterol thus removed from the tissues is eventually eliminated through the feces *via* bile.

Yet another point which deserves special mention here is that in our work we have failed to notice any significant increase in the conversion of cholesterol to bile salts or in the excretion of bile salts in the rats given polyunsaturated lipids. On the other hand, markedly higher amounts of cholesterol were excreted through the bile of such rats, so that under such conditions the sterol is actually removed as cholesterol and not as its catabolites.

Another equally important point which should be mentioned here regards the solubility of cholesterol in the bile micelles, which is rather critical, because an increase in the ratio of cholesterol: phospholipids or cholesterol: bile salts leads to precipitation of cholesterol causing the formation of gall stones. Therefore it follows that any treatment which enhances the solubility of cholesterol in bile (*e.g.*, an increase in the unsaturation of the biliary phospholipids) should not only prevent gall stone formation but should also dissolve the cholesterol of gall stones. In fact, Dam *et al.*[31] were able to dissolve such gall stones in hamsters by giving margarine rich in linoleic acid.

ACKNOWLEDGMENT

This work was supported by a grant from the Department of Science and Technology, Government of India, New Delhi. R. P. wishes to thank the Council of Scientific and Industrial Research, New Delhi, for the award of a Junior Research Fellowship. We thank Dr. Hans Genthe of Nattermann International, Cologne, Germany, for supply of EPL.

REFERENCES

1 E. B. Smith, R. Paoletti, and D. Kritchevsky, *Advances in Lipid Research*, Academic Press, New York, vol. 12, 1974, p. 1.
2 L. W. Kinsell, J. Partridge, L. Boling, S. Margen, and G. Michaels, *J. Clin. Endocrinol.*, 12 (1952) 909.
3 H. Schon, *Med. Klin.*, 54 (1959) 1394.
4 V. Blaton, F. Soeteway, D. Vandamme, B. Declercq, and H. Peeters, *Artery*, 2 (1976) 309.
5 S. O. Byers and M. Friedman, *Proc. Soc. Expt. Biol. Med.*, 98 (1958) 523.
6 J. D. Wilson and M. D. Siperstein, *Am. J. Physiol.*, 196 (1959) 596.
7 R. F. Mcgovern and F. W. Quackenbush, *Lipids*, 8 (1973) 470.
8 T. F. Kellogg, *J. Lipid Res.*, 15 (1974) 574.
9 T. Gerson, F. B. Shorland, and Y. Adams, *Biochem. J.*, 81 (1961) 584.
10 R. Reiser, M. C. Williams, M. F. Sorrels, and N. L. Murty, *Arch. Biochem. Biophys.*, 102 (1963) 276.
11 P. Wood, Y. Lee, and L. Kinsell, *Fed. Proc.*, 26 (1967) 261.
12 S. S. Pawar and H. C. Tidwell, *Am. J. Physiol.*, 213 (1967) 1350.
13 P. J. Nestel, in R. Paoletti and D. Kritchevsky, *Advances in Lipid Research*, Academic Press, New York, vol. 8, 1970, p. 1.
14 R. Paul and J. Ganguly, *Chem. Phys. Lip.*, 17 (1976) 315.
15 R. O. Scow, Y. Stein, and O. Stein, *J. Biol. Chem.*, 242 (1967) 4919.
16 A. Nilsson, *Biochim. Biophys. Acta*, 152 (1968) 379.
17 S. Parthasarathy, P. V. Subbaiah, and J. Ganguly, *Biochem. J.*, 140 (1974) 503.
18 A. F. Hofmann and B. Borgstrom, *Fed. Proc.*, 21 (1962) 43.
19 H. P. Porter and D. R. Saunders, *Gastroenterology*, 60 (1971) 997.
20 A. F. Hofmann and B. Borgstrom, *J. Clin. Invest.*, 43 (1964) 247.
21 J. A. Balint, D. A. Beeler, D. H. Treble, and H. L. Spitzer, *J. Lipid Res.*, 8 (1967) 486.
22 H. Kanoh and K. Ohno, *Biochim. Biophys. Acta*, 306 (1973) 203.
23 S. B. Weiss, S. W. Smith, and E. P. Kennedy, *J. Biol. Chem.*, 231 (1958) 53.
24 D. M. Small, in P. P. Nair and D. Kritchevsky, *The Bile Acids*, Plenum Press, New York, vol. 1, 1971, p. 249.
25 C. H. Gray, D. C. Nicholson, and R. V. Quincey, in C. F. Code, *Alimentary Canal*, American Physiological Society, Washington, D. C.,vol. V, 1968, p. 2483.
26 Y. Stein, M. C. Glangeaud, M. Fainaru, and O. Stein, *Biochim. Biophys. Acta*, 380 (1975) 106.
27 R. L. Jackson, O. Stein, A. M. Gotto, and Y. Stein, *J. Biol. Chem.*, 250 (1975) 7204.
28 J. D. Morrisett, R. Segura, O. D. Taunton, H. J. Pownall, R. L. Jackson, and A. M. Gotto, *Biophys. J.*, 15 (1975) 217a.
29 V. H. Peters, V. Blaton, F. Soetewey, B. Declercq, and D. Vandamme, *Munch. Med. Wochenschr.*, 115 (1973) 1358.
30 C. W. M. Adams and Y. H. Abdulla, in G. Schettler, *Phospholipide*, George Thieme Verlag, Stuttgart, 1972, p. 44.
31 H. Dam, I. Prange, and F. Christensen, *Z. Ernaehrungswiss.*, 6 (1965) 97.

MICROSOMAL ELECTRON TRANSFER SYSTEM IN LIPID METABOLISM

TERUO ONO,* TAKAKO OKAYASU, KENSUKE KAMEDA, AND YOH IMAI
Department of Biochemistry, Hokkaido University School of Medicine, Sapporo (Japan)

Recent progress in lipid metabolism in liver microsomes has revealed that a key enzymatic reaction is often related to "oxygenase" or to the interaction of an electron transfer system with molecular oxygen. Among numerous examples of this reaction type, we will discuss in this paper only the microsomal electron transfer system in relation to lipid metabolism, in particular the system which does not require cytochrome P-450 as a direct oxidase.

DESATURATION OF FATTY ACID

It has been well known since the early works of Schoenheimer and Stetten (1936–1940) that polyunsaturated fatty acids such as linoleic acid are not biosynthesized in the animal body, but a monounsaturated fatty acid such as oleic acid is formed from a corresponding saturated acid. However a long time was needed to reach the next step: Understanding that such desaturation is performed not by dehydrogenase but by "oxygenase." In 1960, Bloomfield and Bloch first described a yeast extract that could form palmitoleic acid from palmitic acid by means of an oxygenase-like reaction in the presence of molecular oxygen and reduced pyridine nucleotide. Imai in our laboratory also demonstrated that rat liver homogenates catalyzed aerobically the Δ^9-desaturation of stearic to oleic acid. He also reported that activity of the Δ^9-desaturation of stearic acid in liver microsomal preparation was significantly decreased both in fasting and alloxan-treated diabetic rats, but the rate of ω-oxidation of the acid in the same microsomal preparation was stimulated under such conditions. These early observations have stimulated the preparation of the concerned enzymes and the investigation for desaturation mechanisms in living cells.

Wakil and coworkers[1] in 1969 found that hen liver microsomes, when extracted with aqueous acetone, lost the ability to desaturate stearoyl-CoA to oleate, and that decreased activity was restored by addition of lipid micelles prepared from membranous lipids. They had already shown that microsomal NADH-cytochrome *c* reductase system required lipid micelles.[2] Noting the similar requirement for NADH and lipids between the Δ^9-desaturase and NADH-cytochrome *c* reductase, Wakil and coworkers[1] suggested that the two systems might share a common electron transfer pathway or carrier. Several workers in our laboratory have solubilized the individual enzyme components of NADH-cytochrome *c* reductase as well as NADH-cytochrome b_5 reductase from lipid-depleted microsomes of

* The present adress: Department of Biochemistry, Niigata University School of Medicine, Niigata, Japan.

the liver. In a reconstruction study, they also confirmed that both reductase systems required lipid micelles for complete reduction.[3-5] In contrast to cytochrome P-450-mediated monoxygenase reactions, Sato and coworkers found that Δ^9-desaturation of stearoyl-CoA was insensible to carbon monoxide but was inhibited by cyanide.[6] Based on this and other observations, they concluded that a cyanide-sensitive factor which was non-hemoprotein was functional in the Δ^9-desaturase system as the terminal oxidase.[6,7] Strittmatter and coworkers[8] in 1974 isolated the terminal oxidase from rat liver microsomes. We have also partially purified the terminal Δ^9-desaturase from liver microsomes of rats fed with high stearate diet after one day starvation, and the specific activity at the reconstruction system was elevated about 80-fold compared to that of the original fortified microsomes.

Thus the Δ^9-desaturation of stearoyl-CoA to oleate in liver microsomes has been known to be catalyzed by multienzyme components, consisting of NADH-cytochrome b_5 reductase, cytochrome b_5, Δ^9-desaturase (a non-heme iron protein), and a lipid micelle. On the other hand, it was also reported, not in the reconstituted system but in intact microsomes, that NADPH also provided the electrons to Δ^9-desaturase *via* the other microsomal electron transport components which included flavoprotein NADPH-cytochrome *c* (P-450) reductase, instead of NADH cytochrome b_5 reductase, and cytochrome b_5.[9]

Meanwhile, the pathway for biosynthesis of polyunsaturated fatty acids in animals has been also investigated by many workers. Nugteren in 1962 proved that liver microsomes desaturated labeled linoleic acid into γ-linolenic acid. Satomi in our laboratory observed such a process is quite active at fetal and new born age.[10] The Δ^6-desaturation of linoleic acid has a physiological importance since the reaction is involved in the biosyntheses of arachidonic acid and prostaglandins. Several reports have provided evidence that Δ^6-desaturase is different from Δ^9-desaturase by experiments on dietary induction, circadian rhythm, and hepatomas with different growth rates. It is well known that high

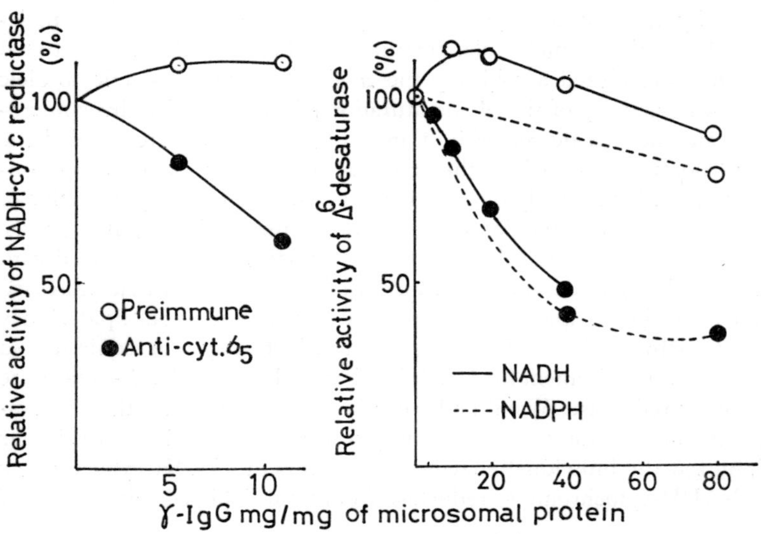

Fig. 1. Effects of anti-cytochrome b_5 on activities of microsomal NADH-cytochrome *c* reductase and Δ^6-desaturase.

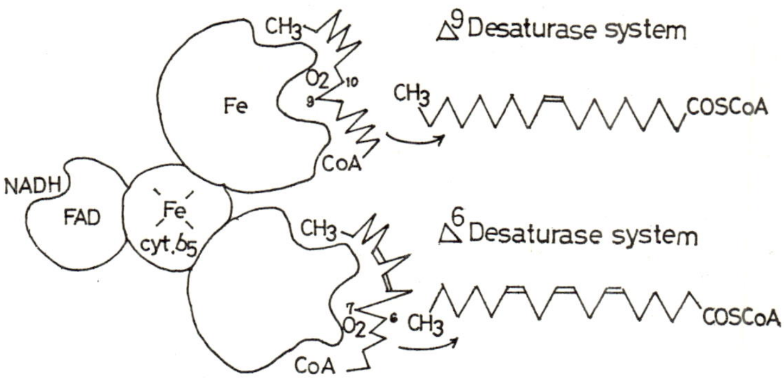

Fig. 2. Scheme of fatty acid desaturation systems in microsomes.

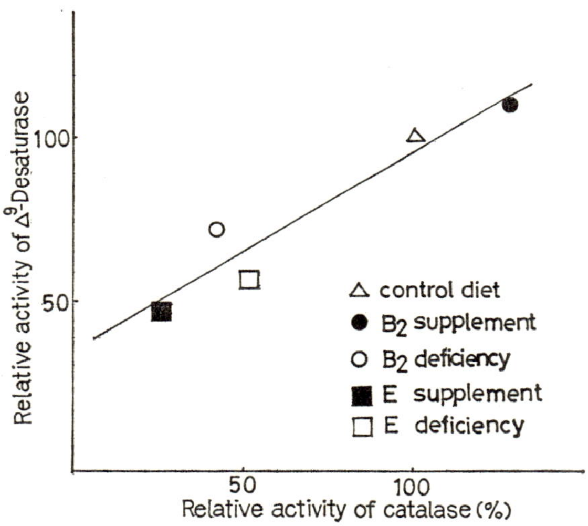

Fig. 3. Correlation between Δ^9-desaturase and catalase in microsomes.

carbohydrate diets caused an increase of microsomal Δ^9-desaturase activity. In contrast to this, high protein diets caused an increase of Δ^6-desaturase activity. The effect of antibodies against the hydrophilic parts of cytochrome b_5 and NADPH-cytochrome c reductase on microsomal Δ^6-desaturase activity provided evidence that cytochrome b_5 involved in desaturation was initiated either by NADPH or NADH (Fig. 1). It is possible that the same electron carrier, cytochrome b_5, participates in both Δ^6- and Δ^9-desaturation systems in intact microsomes (Fig. 2).[11] However, we still don't know the reason why the antibody against NADPH-cytochrome c reductase did not inhibit the microsomal Δ^6-desaturase activities initiated by NADPH.

Brenner and cowokers[12] observed that when microsomes were extracted by low ionic strength solutions, the extracted microsomes lost most of the Δ^9-desaturase activity, and that a protein factor restored full desaturation activity when the extract was added to the depleted microsomes. The protein factor itself, however, had no desaturation activity.

Baker *et al.*[13] also reported that catalase stimulates microsomal desaturation of 1-alkyl-2-acyl-*sn*-3-glycero-phosphoethanolamine, that provides ethanolamine plasmalogen, and the mechanism may be analogous to acyl CoA desaturation. We have observed that the modified catalase activity in microsomes *in vivo* induced by either vitamin B_2 or vitamin E affects the microsomal Δ^9-desaturase activities (Fig. 3). Compared to glutathione peroxidase, catalase may have a more important role in removing hydrogen peroxide in microsomes, since the catalase level was much higher than that of glutathione peroxidase.[15] It is suggested that the multienzymes of Δ^9-desaturase system, which are bound to the microsomal membrane, are in danger of being affected with oxidative change of membrane constituents by hydrogen peroxide, since rat liver has hydrogen peroxide generating systems such as superoxide dismutase and xanthine oxidase.[16]

LIPID PEROXIDATION

Microsomal NADPH-dependent lipid peroxidation was first described by Hochstein and Ernster. May and McCay observed that polyunsaturated fatty acids in microsomal lipids are decreased in the course of NADPH-dependent lipid peroxidation. Pederson *et al.*[17] tried to solubilize a microsmal enzyme of lipid peroxidation by bromelain digestion, and the enzyme was characterized as NADPH-cytochrome *c* reductase. Like the NADPH-dependent lipid peroxidation in microsomes,[18] the purified NADPH-cytochrome *c* reductase required ferric iron and EDTA or ADP for the optimal lipid peroxidation. While NADPH-cytochrome *c* reductase, prepared by detergent solubilization from microsomes, has the ability to catalyze ω-hydroxylation of fatty acids *via* cytochrome P-450, that obtained by protease digestion cannot support ω-hydroxylation.[19] Therefore, we compared the potential for methyl-γ-linolenate peroxidation of protease- and detergent-solubilized preparations. Measured by malondialdehyde formation, however, there was no difference in methyl-γ-linolenate peroxidation between the two reductase preparations, when compared at the same degree of cytochrome *c* reduction. ESR spectrum suggested that ferric iron is reduced to ferrous iron during the lipid peroxidation.[20] It seems likely that the specific binding of lipid to reductase may not be involved in the peroxdation process, but that reductase and ferric iron may play an important role in the generation of specific oxygen species which are required for lipid peroxidation. As for oxygen species, several workers reported the participation of singlet oxygen, superoxide anion and hydroxyl radical for lipid peroxidation, in either enzymatic or non-enzymatic oxidation systems.[21-23] It should be noted, however, that there were no significant differences between enzymatic and non-enzymatic oxidation systems as regards oxygenated products from methyl-γ-linolenate, in both systems, the main oxygenated products contained the oxygen atom at the C-6 and/or C-13 position when hydrogenated trimethyl derivatives were identified by gas chromatography and mass spectrometry.[20,24] In such NADPH-dependent lipid peroxidation, esterified forms of unsaturated fatty acids are far more favorable as substrates, compared to carboxyl free acids.

Some oxygenases in microsomes are known to be tightly associated with NADPH-cytochrome *c* reductase, and NADPH-dependent peroxidation seems physiologically toxic to maintain membrane structures and functions. It is interesting, therefore, to survey the way peroxide scavenging systems are involved in enzyme activity of microsomes. Tappel and Zalkin[25] reported that lipid peroxidation in mammalian tissues fed with a vitamin E-deficient diet is increased when compared with that of the control diet. On the other hand, El-Khatib *et al.*[26] could not detect the formation of lipid peroxides in subcellular fractions under vitamin E-deficient conditions, though vitamin E, a biological antioxidant, seems to protect membrane lipid peroxidation. We observed that NADPH-dependent microsomal lipid peroxidation measured by either malondialdehyde or conjugated diene formation indicated no difference between vitamin E-deficient diet and vitamin E-supplemented diet (Fig. 4). This discrepancy may be partially explained by the difference in the levels of various microsomal enzymes which are modified with a vitamin E deficiency, since *in vitro* addition of superoxide dismutase is known to inhibit the lipid peroxidation when using purified NADPH-cytochrome *c* reductase as the reconstructed assay system.[27] The addition of either catalase or superoxide dismutase *in vitro* is also known to inhibit the reaction catalyzed by xanthine oxidase.[28] However, at either microsomal catalase or superoxide dismutase levels, we could not detect any statistically significant differences between vitamin E deficiency and vitamin E supplementation.[29] Among microsomal enzymes investigated, the activity of microsomal glutathione peroxidase is only significantly increased in the vitamin E-deficient liver. Since glutathione peroxidase catalyzes the conversion of reduced glutathione to oxidized glutathione in the presence of hydrogen peroxide, we tested the *in vitro* effect of reduced glutathione and oxidized glutathione on NADPH-dependent microsomal lipid peroxidation. The rate of malondialdehyde formation in microsomes was inhibited by the additon of either reduced glutathione or oxidized glutathione, and the extent of inhibition was proportional to the added amount of glutathione. The inhibitory effect of oxidized glutathione was further intensified by the addition of glutathione reductase. Therefore, the low level of NADPH-dependent lipid peroxidation observed in microsomes of vitamin E-deficient rats may be attributed to the redox states of the glutathione generating system caused by high glutathione peroxidase

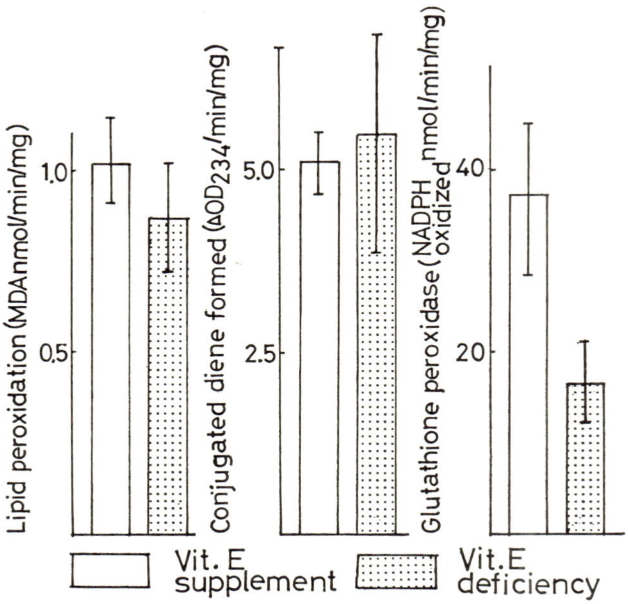

Fig. 4. Effect of dietary vitamin E on microsomal lipid peroxidation and glutathione peroxidase.

activity. Christophersen[30] reported that glutathione peroxidase catalyzed the reaction of hydroperoxy linolenic acid to the corresponding hydroxy fatty acid in the presence of reduced glutathione. McCay *et al.*[31] also suggested the possibility that glutathione peroxidase prevents free radical attack on membranous polyunsaturated lipid, by estimating the varied composition of fatty acids in microsomes during the lipid peroxidation assay. Those findings would suggest that glutathione peroxidase in microsomes may play a physiologically important role in the peroxidation of membrane lipid.

SQUALENE EPOXIDATION

In 1957, Tchen and Bloch first demonstrated the introduction of molecular oxygen into the aliphatic squalene structure to form the 3β-hydroxyl group of the steroidal nucleus. This is the first step in the process of *de novo* cholesterol biosynthesis, since squalene is known to be the end product under anaerobic conditions. Until 1966, this transformation was considered to occur in synchrony with cyclization to lanosterol. However, a stepwise mechanism was presented by the discovery of 2,3-oxidosqualene as an intermediate in the squalene cyclization. Then 2,3-oxidosqualene lanosterol cyclase was first isolated from microsomes and the cofactor requirement was tested. Yamamoto and Bloch presented evidence that the combination of microsomes and $105{,}000 \times g$ supernatant was responsible for converting squalene into 2,3-oxidosqualene in the presence of molecular oxygen and NADPH.[32] The supernatant was resolved into three components: A protein factor (mol. wt. 44,000), phosphatidylserine and FAD.[33] As regards microsomal components, Ono and Bloch observed that microsomes alone could act as the squalene epoxidase even when Triton X-100 and FAD were fortified in place of the supernatant components.[34] The supernatant protein might act internally within the microsomal system, facilitating the access of substrate to specific enzyme sites.[35] The supernatant protein factor is not catalytic, since the squalene epoxidase system after being solubilized does not respond to the supernatant.[34]

The activity of squalene epoxidase was decreased in liver microsomes of rat when fed with diets deficient of vitamin B_2, even under the FAD fortified assay condition, but the epoxidase activity was increased with vitamin B_2-supplemented diets. The same tendency was also observed on the NADPH-cytochrome *c* reductase activity in microsomes. When incubated with Triton X-100, microsomal squalene epoxidase required FAD for manifestation of enzyme activity. Solubilized microsomal squalene epoxidase with Triton X-100 was resolved into two fractions by DEAE-cellulose chromatography.[34] One fraction contained the NADPH-cytochrome *c* reductase, and the activity of NADH-ferricyanide reductase was found in the other. From the former fraction, we solubilized NADPH-cytochrome *c* (P-450) reductase with deoxycholate. By stepwise purification, the specific activity of the reductase was increased. When each reductase preparation was used as a reconstruction member, the increase in squalene epoxidase activity was parallel to that of reductase activity. Rabbit antisera were prepared to the purified NADPH-cytochrome *c* reductase which was solubilized with trypsin; and the antisera inhibited in microsomes concomitantly NADPH-cytochrome *c* reductase activity and squalene epoxidase activity.[36] These observations strongly suggested that one of the two components of the microsomal squalene epoxidase system is identical with the detergent-solubilized NADPH-cytochrome *c* (P-450) reductase. Recently we obtained a highly purified preparation of NADPH-cytochrome *c* (P-450) reductase by affinity chromatography with 2′,5′-ADP Sepharose

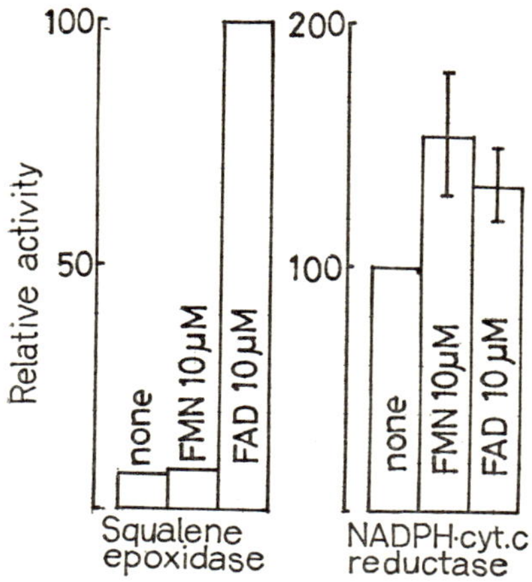

Fig. 5. *In vitro* effect of flavins on microsomal squalene epoxidase and NADPH-cytochrome *c* reductase.

4B, and confirmed further that NADPH-cytochrome *c* (P-450) reductase is a component of the microsomal squalene epoxidase system. As described above, squalene epoxidase requires FAD absolutely, and the enzyme activity was highest at the concentration of 10 μM FAD. *In vitro* addition of the same 10 μM FAD also stimulated microsomal NADPH-cytochrome *c* reductase activity 1.5 times in the presence of Triton X-100 (Fig. 5). Since NADPH-cytochrome *c* (P-450) reductase is known to contain one mol of both FAD and FMN per mol of enzyme,[37] the absolute requirement of FAD for microsomal squalene epoxidase may partially be explained by the fortified effect of dissociable FAD on the reductase. However, it should be noted that in contrast to FAD, FMN was not required for squalene epoxidase activity, even though FMN stimulated at most 1.8 times the microsomal NADPH-cytochrome *c* reductase activity at a concentration of 10 μM (Fig. 5). These results suggested that the requirement of FAD in squalene epoxidase system involves not only NADPH-cytochrome *c* (P-450) reductase but also the other component, presumably the epoxidase fraction.

The mixed-function oxidases of liver microsomes which catalyze the hydroxylation of a wide variety of substrates have been shown to consist of a flavoprotein indicated as NADPH-cytochrome P-450 reductase, cytochrome P-450 species and a phosphatidylcholine.[38] Since NADPH-cytochrome *c* (P-450) reductase is one of the components of microsomal squalene epoxidase, it is interesting to see whether the epoxidase fraction is identical with cytochrome P-450 species. Yamamoto and Bloch reported that carbon monoxide did not inhibit microsomal squalene epoxidase activity under the inhibitory conditions on aniline hydroxylase.[32] The same result was observed in the reconstituted system of squalene epoxidase. Two preparations of the epoxidase fraction revealed that squalene epoxidase activity did not depend on the cytochrome P-450 content.[34] Thus, at the present time, no evidence has been found for participation of cytochrome P-450 species in squalene epoxidation. It is reported that a certain porphyrin mutant of yeast, lacking all respiratory cytochromes, has retained the ability to synthesize lanosterol.[39,40] Therefore, it is not likely that the epoxidase fraction is identical with the cytochrome P-450 species.

The epoxidase fraction was first considered to contain NADH-ferricyanide reductase.[34] However, NADPH is more likely to support the reaction than NADH. The NADH-ferricyanide reductase was separated from the epoxidase fraction by further DEAE-cellulose chromatography in the presence of deoxycholate. These facts might suggest that NADH-ferricyanide reductase is not involved in the squalene epoxidase system, recovery of the epoxidase fraction being only 10% by this procedure. Since the epoxidase fraction was less well characterized in the previous paper,[34] we engaged in the further purification of this fraction. Though the epoxidase fraction was unstable in ionic detergents such as deoxycholate, we finally found the original epoxidase fraction to be fairly stable for potassium cholate solubilization if the ionic detergent medium was fortified with 0.1 mM of FAD. Starting from this treated soluble fraction, the DEAE-cellulose chromatography resulted in an epoxidase fraction which was completely separated from NADH-ferricyanide reductase, at a reasonable good yield (over 55%). The specific activity of the purified epoxidase fraction was elevated 55 times compared to that of the original epoxidase fraction. SDS gel electrophoresis still revealed four major bands in the purified epoxidase fraction, but cytochrome P-450 content in these was less than 0.05 nmol/mg of protein. FAD stabilized the epoxidase fraction in cholate medium, suggesting that the epoxidase fraction may have a dissociable FAD group. We still don't know the catalytic prosthetic group of the epoxidase fraction; however, the additions of either EDTA (1 mM), cyanide (5 mM), superoxide dismutase or catalase have no effect on the activity of the reconstituted squalene epoxidase system.

Until recently our knowledge of the NADPH-cytochrome P-450 reductase has been limited, since cytochrome P-450 species are achieved as the only terminal oxidases in NADPH-dependent mixed function oxygenases of liver microsomes. We believe that the squalene epoxidase system affords the first presentation on a terminal oxidase which is distinct from hemoproteins such as cytochrome P-450 species, and is linked to a flavoprotein indicated as NADPH-cytochrome P-450 reductase (Fig. 6). Discovery of those chemically distinguishable enzymes linked to NADPH-cytochrome P-450 reductase may widen the scope of the physiological role of the microsomal electron transport chain and its interaction between the reductase and terminal oxidases.

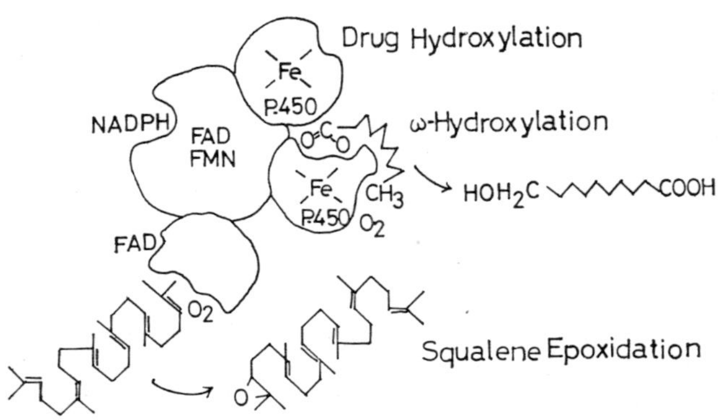

Fig. 6. Scheme of NADPH-cytochrome *c* reductase involved reactions in microsomes.

REFERENCES

1 P. D. Jones, P. W. Holloway, R. O. Peluffo, and S. J. Wakil, *J. Biol. Chem.*, 244 (1969) 744.
2 P. D. Jones and S. J. Wakil, *J. Biol. Chem.*, 242 (1967) 5267.
3 T. Ishibashi and Y. Imai, *Tohoku J. Exp. Med.*, 118 (1976) 365.
4 S. Ozaki, T. Ohnishi, and Y. Imai, *Proc. Japan. Conf. Biochem. Lipids*, 14 (1972) 115.
5 T. Ohnishi, Y. Yamazaki, and Y. Imai, *Arch. Biochem. Biophys.*, 167 (1975) 488.
6 N. Oshino, Y. Imai, and R. Sato, *Biochim. Biophys. Acta*, 128 (1966) 13.
7 N. Oshino, Y. Imai, and R. Sato, *J. Biochem.*, 69 (1971) 155.
8 P. Strittmatter, L. Spatz, D. Corcoran, M. J. Rogers, B. Setlow, and R. Redline, *Proc. Natl. Acad. Sci. U. S.*, 71 (1974) 4565.
9 N. Oshino and T. Omura, *Arch. Biochem. Biophys.*, 157 (1973) 395.
10 S. Satomi and Y. Imai, *Biol. Neonate*, 22 (1971) 1.
11 T. Okayasu, T. Ono, K. Shinojima, and Y. Imai, *Lipids*, 12 (1977) 267.
12 A. Catala, A. M. Nervi, and R. R. Brenner, *J. Biol. Chem.*, 250 (1975) 7481.
13 R. C. Baker, R. L. Wykle, J. S. Lockmiller, and F. Snyder, *Arch. Biochem. Biophys.*, 177 (1976) 299.
14 T. Okayasu, K. Kameda, T. Ono, and Y. Imai, *Biochim. Biophys. Acta*, in press.
15 P. Nicholls, *Biochim. Biophys. Acta*, 279 (1972) 306.
16 P. B. Rowe and J. B. Wyngaarden, *J. Biol. Chem.*, 241 (1966) 5571.
17 T. C. Pederson, J. A. Beuge, and S. D. Aust, *J. Biol. Chem.*, 248 (1973) 7134.
18 E. D. Wills, *Biochem. J.*, 113 (1969) 315.
19 A. Y. Lu, K. W. Junk, and M. J. Coon, *J. Biol. Chem.*, 244 (1969) 3714.
20 H. Sano, T. Ono, M. Yamazaki, and Y. Imai, *Japan. J. Agric. Chem.*, 50 (1976) 469.
21 M. M. King, E. K. Lai, and P. B. McCay, *J. Biol. Chem.*, 250 (1975) 6496.
22 K. Sugioka and M. Nakano, *Biochim. Biophys. Acta*, 423 (1976) 203.
23 K. Fong, P. B. McCay, and J. L. Poyer, *J. Biol. Chem.*, 248 (1973) 7792.
24 A. Wakizaka and Y. Imai, *Hokkaido J. Med. Sci.*, 49 (1974) 536.
25 A. L. Tappel and H. Zalkin, *Arch. Biochem. Biophys.*, 80 (1959) 333.
26 S. El-Khatib, U. A. Chenau, M. P. Carpenter, R. E. Trucco, and R. Caputto, *Nature*, 201 (1964) 188.
27 T. C. Pederson and S. D. Aust, *Biochem. Biophys. Res. Commun.*, 48 (1972) 789.
28 E. W. Kellog and I. Fridovich, *J. Biol. Chem.*, 250 (1975) 8812.
29 K. Kameda, T. Okayasu, T. Ono, and Y. Imai, *J. Nutr. Sci., Vitaminol.*, in press.
30 B. O. Christophersen, *Biochim. Biophys. Acta*, 176 (1968) 463.
31 P. B. McCay, D. D. Gibson, K. Fong, and R. Hornbrook, *Biochim. Biophys. Acta*, 431 (1976) 459.
32 S. Yamamoto and K. Bloch, *J. Biol. Chem.*, 245 (1970) 1670.
33 H-H. Tai and K. Bloch, *J. Biol. Chem.*, 247 (1972) 1670.
34 T. Ono and K. Bloch, *J. Biol. Chem.*, 250 (1975) 1571.
35 Y. A. Saat and K. Bloch, *J. Biol. Chem.*, 251 (1976) 5155.
36 T. Ono, S. Ozasa, F. Hasegawa, and Y. Imai, *Biochim. Biophys. Acta*, 486 (1977) 401.
37 T. Iyanagi and H. S. Mason, *Biochemistry*, 12 (1973) 2297.
38 H. W. Strobel, Y. H. Lu, J. Heidema, and M. J. Coon, *J. Biol. Chem.*, 245 (1970) 4851.
39 M. Band, R. A. Woods, and J. M. Haslam, *Biochem. Biophys. Res. Commun.*, 56 (1974) 324.
40 E. G. Gollub, P. Trocha, P. K. Lilu, and D. B. Sprinson, *Biochem. Biophys. Res. Commun.*, 56 (1974) 471.

SOME ASPECTS OF DIETARY STARCH UTILIZATION IN THE MAMMALIAN DIGESTIVE TRACT

J. JOHN MARSHALL AND WILLIAM J. WHELAN

Laboratories for Biochemical Research, Howard Hughes Medical Institute and Departments of Biochemistry and Medicine, University of Miami School of Medicine, Miami, Florida (U.S.A.)

The principal features of the starch degradation process in the mammalian digestive tract are well established.[1] Thus, depolymerization of starch molecules takes place first of all under the action of salivary and pancreatic α-amylases,[2] followed by hydrolysis of the resulting oligosaccharides by α-glucosidases present in the brush border of the intestinal epithelial cells.[3,4] This latter process results in the production of glucose which is assimilated through the wall of the intestine to provide metabolic energy. However, in regard to the finer aspects of the process, a number of questions still need to be answered, including the following:

a) How is granular starch (as opposed to cooked starch) rendered susceptible to α-amylase action? Most starches in their native (granular) form are resistant to the action of purified α-amylases *in vitro*.[5] Apparently, *in vivo*, the starch granule is either physically denatured or modified in some other manner (enzymic?) to render it susceptible to α-amylase action.

b) While the action of the intestinal α-glucosidases can account for the breakdown of linear oligosaccharides, the mechanism whereby the branched*[3] oligosaccharides that arise from α-amylolysis of the amylopectin component of starch is not clear. The nature of the enzyme(s) responsible for the hydrolysis of the α-1,6-glucosidic linkage(s) in these oligosaccharides, and the specificity of the enzyme(s), is not known. Enzymes have been isolated from intestinal mucosa that can hydrolyze isomaltose[3,6]; however, the role of such enzymes in the degradation of starch is not clear since isomaltose itself has never been demonstrated to be a primary product of starch breakdown.

c) A related question, which does not yet appear to have been addressed, is whether any enzymes besides α-amylase and the intestinal α-glucosidases are involved in the degradation of starch in the digestive tract.

With these questions in mind we have initiated a study aimed at elucidating the full details of the starch breakdown process in the mammalian digestive tract. Herein we present some of our recent findings related to the second and third of the above questions.

* The term branched is used to indicate starch-derived oligosaccharides containing one or more α-1,6-glucosidic linkages, which constitute the branch points in starch. The term is used for convenience only and it should be recognized that some of the so-called branched oligosaccharides do not contain a disubstituted glucose unit and are therefore, strictly speaking, linear.

PANCREATIC α-GLUCOSIDASES

The pancreas of mammalian species produces a number of proteolytic enzymes with different specificities that act jointly in the breakdown of proteins.[7] While the pancreas also produces large quantities of α-amylase in response to the ingestion of dietary starch, the possibility of its producing other enzymes involved in the starch degradation process does not appear to have been considered.

We have therefore tested pancreas extracts and secretions for amylolytic enzymes, other than α-amylase, that might be involved in the breakdown of starch and the further hydrolysis of starch-derived oligosaccharides. Crude extracts of human and hog pancreas were found to hydrolyze maltose. This activity was not significantly diminished following inhibition of α-amylase with phaseolamin, the proteinaceous inhibitor of α-amylase from kidney beans,[8] nor by removal of α-amylase by binding to a cross-linked glycogen adsorbent.[9] These latter observations showed the observed action on maltose to be due to an α-glucosidase rather than being an artefact caused, for example, by α-amylase action on the higher oligosaccharides that commonly contaminate commercial maltose preparations.[10] Chromatography of a cross-linked-glycogen-treated pancreas extract on a column of Sephadex G-100 separated the α-glucosidase activity into two fractions which differed in pH optimum, one having maximum activity around pH 4.6 and the other, around pH 6.6. A survey of extracts of pancreatic tissue from a number of different species all showed the presence of both acid and neutral α-glucosidase activities and the same activities were also present in the secretion collected from a patient fitted with a pancreatic fistula following surgery of the pancreas (Table I). We therefore conclude that the presence of α-glucosidases is common to the pancreas of mammalian species and that, in the case of the human, at least, these activities are secreted by the pancreas into the small intestine.

TABLE I
α-AMYLASE AND α-GLUCOSIDASE ACTIVITIES IN PANCREAS EXTRACTS AND SECRETIONS*1

Origin of extract or secretion	*α-Amylase activity (units/mg)*	*α-Glucosidase activity**2	
		pH 4.6	*pH 6.6*
Extracts			
Pig	6.7	4.5	8.2
Rat	19.9	0.5	0.07
Human	11.9	2.8	0.3
Guinea pig	8.3	0.1	0.4
Dog	20.7	0.3	1.0
Chicken	32.1	0.2	8.8
Rabbit	22.5	3.0	1.0
Mouse	12.7	0.3	0.2
Cow	7.9	0.6	1.7
Secretion			
Human*3	33.0	6.0	7.0

*1 J. J. Marshall, W. J. Whelan, and W. Woloszczuk, unpublished results.

*2 Activities are expressed as nmol maltose hydrolyzed per min per mg of protein in crude homogenates of pancreatic tissue or secretion.

*3 Values are the mean of the activities in three samples collected at different times on a single day.

The two α-glucosidases were isolated from pancreatin, a crude enzyme preparation from hog pancreas. Chromatography of a pancreatin extract on a column of DEAE-cellulose, eluted with a gradient of salt, separated the two forms of the enzyme, and also served to remove α-amylase, which does not bind to DEAE-cellulose. The acid α-glucosidase was further purified by fractionationwith cold acetone, followed by chromatography on Sephadex G-100. Like other such α-glucosidases, the enzyme is retarded by interaction with the gel matrix, and methyl α-glucoside was used to recover it from the column after all other non-enzymic protein had been eluted. Subsequent chromatography on Sepharose 4B gave an α-glucosidase peak across which the specific activity was constant, thus indicating homogeneity.

Purification of the neutral α-glucosidase was effected by ammonium sulfate fractionation, the majority of the enzyme being precipitated between 45–65% saturation. The redissolved precipitate, after dialysis, was chromatographed on hydroxylapatite, followed by chromatography on Sepharose 4B. The neutral α-glucosidase purified in this way appeared homogeneous by polyacrylamide gel electrophoresis.

The purification details for both enzymes are presented in Table II.

The actions of both of these purified enzymes on a variety of oligosaccharide and polysaccharide substrates are presently under study. Both enzymes are able to hydrolyze, in addition to maltose, maltotriose and higher oligosaccharides, starch and α-limit dextrins. The acid α-glucosidase acts on starch at about half the rate of its action on maltose; the neutral α-glucosidase has much less ability to bring about hydrolysis of starch and α-limit dextrins. With large amounts of enzyme and extended incubation periods, complete hydrolysis of starch can be achieved by the acid α-glucosidase. However, complete degrada-

TABLE II

PURIFICATION OF PORCINE PANCREATIC α-GLUCOSIDASES*1

Step	*Protein (mg)*	*Activity**2 (units × 10³)*	*Specific activity (units/mg × 10³)*	*Purification factor*	*Yield (%)*
a. Neutral α-glucosidase					
1. Crude extract	80,000	164,000	2.1	1	100
2. Dialysis	25,560	118,800	4.7	2.3	72
3. Heat treatment (55°, 10 min)	24,600	94,800	3.9	1.9	58
4. DEAE-cellulose chromatography	1,170	49,050	41.9	20	30
5. Ammonium sulfate fractionation	816	39,200	47.8	23	24
6. Hydroxylapatite chromatography	21	13,000	620	300	8
7. Sepharose 4B chromatography	0.24	10,200	41,670	20,000	6
b. Acid-α-glucosidase					
1. Crude extract	80,000	127,000	1.6	1	100
2. Dialysis	25,560	88,800	3.5	2.2	70
3. Heat treatment (55°, 10 min)	24,600	68,400	2.8	1.7	54
4. DEAE-cellulose chromatography	600	39,000	65.0	41	31
5. Acetone fractionation	437	30,800	71.0	45	24
6. Sephadex G-100 chromatography	5	20,000	4,000	2,500	16
7. Sepharose 4B chromatography	0.54	16,200	31,480	20,000	13

*1 J. J. Marshall, W. J. Whelan, and W. Woloszczuk, unpublished results.

*2 Measured against maltose at pH 6.6 (neutral α-glucosidase) or pH 4.6 (acid α-glucosidase).

tion of starch by the neutral enzyme has not been demonstrated. α-Limit dextrins are degraded at approximately 20% and 10% of the rate of maltose by the neutral and acid α-glucosidases, respectively. However, although the initial rate of enzyme action on α-limit dextrins is significant, the rate of hydrolysis slows down markedly after 20–30% conversion into glucose, particularly in the case of the neutral α-glucosidase. This observation, together with the extremely poor action of both enzymes on substrates such as panose and isomaltose, indicates that the specificity of the enzymes is directed toward α-1,4-glucosidic linkages. We therefore conclude that if these enzymes are involved in starch breakdown in the digestive tract, and the neutral enzyme at least should be active under the physiological conditions in the small intestine, their primary function is likely to be in the conversion of linear oligosaccharides produced by α-amylase action, into glucose. However, they might also be involved in initiating the breakdown of α-limit dextrins, possibly serving to expose terminal α-1,6-linked glucose units that are then susceptible to the action of another enzyme with specificity designed for the hydrolysis of the latter structural feature.

Further studies on the pancreatic α-glucosidases are in progress, aimed at determining the complete substrate specificities of the enzymes and defining the extent of their involvement in starch digestion. Efforts are also being made to investigate whether the secretion of the pancreatic α-glucosidases in response to the ingestion of dietary starch parallels that of α-amylase.

BREAKDOWN OF α-LIMIT DEXTRINS BY INTESTINAL MUCOSAL α-GLUCOSIDASES

Intestinal mucosal α-glucosidases are membrane-bound and the purification and characterization of these enzymes requires their prior solubilization. In an effort to establish the most effective procedure for solubilization of the enzyme(s) in porcine intestine responsible for α-limit dextrin breakdown, we have compared[11] the effectiveness of a number of procedures that have previously been used for solubilization of intestinal α-glucosidases.

TABLE III

SOLUBILIZATION OF PORCINE INTESTINAL α-GLUCOSIDASES*[1]

Method of solubilization	*Percentage solubilization**[2]				
	Glucoamylase	*Maltase*	*Limit dextrinase*	*Sucrase*	*Isomaltase*
Homogenization	12	11	5	10	10
Sonication	6	12	11	7	10
Autolysis	23	12	32	6	5
Papain treatment	53	47	25	40	45
Deoxycholate treatment	86	45	41	20	27
Deoxycholate + sonication	55	45	44	19	23
Digitonin treatment	10	10	10	8	8
Digitonin + sonication	54	48	55	42	39
Triton X-100 treatment	94	90	100	90	90
Freeze-thaw treatment (10 cycles)	66	60	65	8	9

*[1] From ref. 11.

*[2] Percentage solubilization refers to the percentage of the total enzyme activity found in the supernatant solution after centrifugation at 105,000 *g* for 60 min.

TABLE IV

PURIFICATION OF PORCINE INTESTINAL LIMIT DEXTRINASES*1

Step	*Form of enzyme**3	*Protein (mg)*	*Activity**2 *(units × 10³)*	*Specific activity (units/mg × 10³)*	*Purification factor*	*Yield (%)*
1. Freeze-thaw solubilized enzyme preparation		2,190	56,000	26	1	100
2. DEAE-cellulose	I	200	22,000	110	4	39
chromatography	II	241	14,000	58	2	26
3. Ammonium sulfate	I	82	19,000	232	8	34
fractionation	II	52	14,000	269	10	25
4. Sephadex G-200	I	51	19,000	373	13	34
chromatography	II	31	10,000	323	12	17
5. Sepharose 4B	I	30	15,000	500	18	26
chromatography	II	22	10,000	455	16	18
6. Hydroxylapatite	I	0.5	13,000	26,000	929	23
chromatography	II	0.4	9,000	22,500	804	17

*1 J. J. Marshall, R. Datema, and W. J. Whelan, unpublished results.

*2 Measured against α-limit dextrins.

*3 The designations I and II refer to two forms of the limit dextrinase obtained by DEAE-cellulose fractionation and then purified separately.

TABLE V

SUBSTRATE SPECIFICITY OF LIMIT DEXTRINASES PURIFIED FROM PORCINE INTESTINAL MUCOSA*1

Substrate	*Relative rate of hydrolysis**2	
	I	*II*
Maltose	100	100
α-Limit dextrins	72	75
Starch	21	16
Isomaltose	1	0.5
Sucrose	0.2	0

*1 J. J. Marshall, R. Datema, and W. J. Whelan, unpublished results.

*2 I and II designate the two forms of the enzyme purified according to the scheme shown in Table IV.

Table III shows the solubilization of various α-glucosidase activities using a number of different procedures. The most effective process for bringing about solubilization of all the α-glucosidases is the use of Triton X-100, which solubilizes about 90–100% of the activity towards starch, maltose, α-limit dextrins, sucrose, and isomaltose, these activities being conveniently referred to as glucoamylase, maltase, limit dextrinase, sucrase, and isomaltase, respectively. However, the most interesting and useful procedure for bringing about enzyme solubilization is repetitive freeze-thaw treatment. In this way, after 10 freeze-thaw cycles, 65% of the limit dextrinase activity was solubilized, together with similar amounts of glucoamylase and maltase. This process resulted in minimal (less than 10%) solubilization of sucrase and isomaltase. Immediately, a distinction between limit dextrinase and isomaltase becomes apparent; *i.e.*, although all α-limit dextrins contain one or more α-1,6-glucosidic linkages, clearly isomaltase is not the principal enzyme involved in the breakdown of these complex oligosaccharides. This finding is in contrast with the conclusions of Gray.[4]

By using repeated freeze-thaw treatment a solubilized preparation of porcine intestinal mucosal limit dextrinase was obtained. Conventional protein purification procedures were used to isolate two forms of a limit-dextrin-hydrolyzing activity from the crude solubilized enzyme preparation. The two forms of the enzyme appear to differ only in charge properties, as evidenced by their separation on DEAE-cellulose but their identical behavior on other chromatographic media. The purification details for the two enzymes is given in Table IV.

A study of the substrate specificity of the two α-limit dextrinase fractions (Table V) showed this to be identical for each; both enzymes hydrolyze maltose and α-limit dextrins rapidly and starch relatively slowly. A study of the time course of α-limit dextrin hydrolysis showed the substrate to be incompletely converted into glucose. Typically, hydrolysis essentially ceased after about 30% conversion into glucose. This observation, together with the lack of significant action on isomaltose, has led us to recognize that the "α-limit dextrinases" we have isolated are α-1,4-glucosidases, possibly corresponding to one or more of the maltases described by Semenza.[3] We therefore infer that the breakdown of α-limit dextrins in the small intestine involves at least two types of enzyme, the first being that which we have isolated, and which removes susceptible terminal α-1,4-linked glucose units. The nature of the products resulting from the action of this enzyme is not yet known. However, it might be speculated that these will be either linear or branched oligosaccharides containing an α-1,6-linked glucosyl unit as A-chain, for example 6^3-α-glucosylmaltotriose or 6^3-α-glucosylmaltotetraose. Our future studies will be aimed at determining the structures of the resistant oligosaccharides arising from the action of intestinal limit dextrinase on α-limit dextrins, and establishing the pathway(s) whereby these resistant oligosaccharides are further broken down.

ACKNOWLEDGMENTS

This work was supported by NIH Grant GM 17733. We acknowledge the assistance of Drs. Catharine Sturgeon, Gail Partington, Wolfgang Woloszczuk, and Roelf Datema in the experimental work reported. J. J. Marshall is an Investigator of Howard Hughes Medical Institute.

REFERENCES

1 G. M. Gray, *Gastroenterology*, 58 (1970) 96.
2 G. Semenza, *Handbook of Physiology—Alimentary Canal*, American Physiological Society, Washington, D. C., vol. 5, 1968, p. 2637.
3 G. Semenza, *Handbook of Physiology—Alimentary Canal*, American Physiological Society, Washington, D. C., vol. 5, 1968, p. 2543.
4 G. M. Gray, *Am. Chem. Soc. Symp. Series*, 15 (1977) 181.
5 G. J. Walker and P. M. Hope, *Biochem. J.*, 86 (1963) 452.
6 A. Dahlqvist, *Acta Chem. Scand.*, 14 (1960) 72.
7 I. T. Beck, *Am. J. Clin. Nutr.*, 26 (1973) 311.
8 J. J. Marshall and C. M. Lauda, *J. Biol. Chem.*, 250 (1975) 8030.
9 J. J. Marshall and W. Woloszczuk, *Carbohyd. Res.*, 61 (1978) 407.
10 J. Lehrfeld, *Carbohyd. Res.*, 19 (1971) 400.
11 J. J. Marshall, C. M. Sturgeon, and W. J. Whelan, *Anal. Biochem.*, 82 (1977) 435.

THE SUCRASE-ISOMALTASE COMPLEX, A LARGE DIMERIC AMPHIPATHIC PROTEIN FROM THE SMALL-INTESTINAL BRUSH BORDER MEMBRANE: ITS POSITIONING AND IMPLICATIONS AS TO ITS BIOSYNTHESIS

G. SEMENZA
Laboratorium für Biochemie der ETH-Zürich, Zürich (Switzerland)

The two subunits of the small intestinal sucrase-isomaltase complex (a maltase-sucrase and a maltase-isomaltase), although not identical, have a considerable degree of homology,[1-3] and are apparently subjected to the same or to related biological control mechanism(s), as shown by the constancy of the sucrase/isomaltase ratios in random samples of human peroral biopsies,[4] by their simultaneous[5,6] or almost simultaneous[7] appearance in development and their simultaneous absence in sucrose-isomaltose malabsorption,[8,9] a *mono*-factorial genetic desease.[10] Much is known, also, of their hormonal and dietary control and on the effects, sometimes apparently contradictory, of inhibitors of protein synthesis.[11-13] However, up to now virtually nothing is known as to the actual mechanism of biosynthesis of this membrane protein.

Clearly, any hypothesis on the biosynthesis of a membrane protein has to take into account the positioning of the protein in the membrane fabric. One of the best known membrane protein, glycophorin, spans the erythrocyte plasma membrane, with most of the protein, including the N-terminal region and the sugar residues, protruding on the outside of the membrane. A hydrophobic segment occurs in the polypeptide chain not far from the C-terminal; it presumably interacts with the paraffinic chains of the bilayer lipids and helps in anchoring glycophorin to the fabric. The C-terminal region is located at the cellular side of the plasma membrane.[14] Accordingly, the biosynthetic mechanism generally assumed for this kind of membrane proteins suggests that they are synthetized in the rough endoplasmic reticulum, and that the nascent polypeptide chain enters "head on" (*i.e.*, beginning with the N-terminal) the intracisternal space. The protein is not eventually released into the intracisternal space, but is kept in place, spanning across the membrane, by its hydrophobic area. (Glycosylation follows in the Golgi apparatus.) Since the intracisternal space corresponds topologically to the extracellular space, the polypeptide chain is now in its final, correct, positioning (for a review, see ref. 15).

A perhaps different mode of biosynthesis and assembly into the membrane could be envisaged in principle, for cytochrome b_5. This protein is reported to bind spontaneously to *pre-formed* lipid vesicles.[16] It might, therefore, be synthetized like an ordinary, water-soluble, protein and interact with the membrane *after* complete biosynthesis.

In the case of small-intestinal sucrase-isomaltase complex, neither of these two relatively straight forward biosynthetic mechanisms applies. As a matter of fact, even *a priori* considerations lead us to expect a more complicated biosynthetic mechanism: Sucrase-isomaltase has a mol. wt. of about 220,000, *i.e.*, several times larger than glycophorin or cytochrome b_5; and, contrary to these proteins, it is composed of two subunits.

The data which are summarized and discussed below deal with the positioning of sucrase-isomaltase in the small-intestinal brush border membrane. While many details are still missing, the broad features emerge rather clearly and allow some meaningful questions on the biosynthesis of this protein to be asked. It is quite possible that the conclusions reached for sucrase-isomaltase may hold true for other large integral membrane proteins also, such as aminopeptidase, which has a similar size and possibly similar positioning in the membrane, at least as far as it can be judged from the data presently available.[17]

MOST OR ALL OF THE SUCRASE-ISOMALTASE MOLECULES PROTRUDE TOWARDS THE LUMINAL SIDE OF THE BRUSH BORDER MEMBRANES

The sucrase-isomaltase complex is a building block or firmly bound to the brush border membrane[2,18]. It cannot be solubilized by washings with either high or low ionic strength, with or without EDTA, *etc.* Thus, this protein can be operationally defined as "interinsic."

It corresponds to about 9% of the total brush border membrane protein: Isolated and essentially pure brush border membranes have a sucrase-specific activity approximately equal to 1.2 units $\cdot$ mg^{-1} protein,[19] as compared to the 14 units $\cdot$ mg^{-1} protein of the homogeneous sucrase-*iso*-maltase complex.[20]

The following observations allow a gross localization of the sucrase-isomaltase complex in the native membranes:

i) Negative stain electron microscopy of small intestine or of brush borders isolated therefrom reveal "bugs" or "lollipops" at the outer (luminal) side of the brush border membrane.[21,22] These bodies have been identified as digestive enzymes, including the sucrase-isomaltase complex. Even if—as in the case of mitochondrial F_1—these "bugs" may not protrude in the native membrane as much as they do in negative-stained preparations, their appearance at least indicates that the sucrase-isomaltase tends to protrude to the outside of the membrane.

ii) It is possible to obtain brush border membrane vesicles most of which must be closed, as shown by the dependence of their inner space from the osmolarity of the medium.[19] Lytic concentrations of Triton X-100 do not lead to any increase in sucrase activity, showing that sucrose has equally free access to the hydrolytic catalytic sites of lysed and of intact brush border vesicles.[19]

iii) Finally, and perhaps most important of all, it is possible to solubilize essentially all the sucrase-isomaltase of these brush border membrane vesicles by controlled papain treatment, without increasing the permeability of these vesicles for small mol. wt. substrates.[23,24] Therefore, since papain presumably does not diffuse through the membrane (and thus does not act from the inside) either before or during the proteolytic digestion, we must conclude that all, or essentially all, sucrase-isomaltase molecules must be accessible to papain from the outer, luminal side.

IS THERE ANY FUNCTIONAL INTERACTION BETWEEN THE CATALYTIC SITES OF THE SUCRASE-ISOMALTASE COMPLEX AND THE HYDROPHOBIC LAYER OF THE NATIVE BRUSH BORDER MEMBRANE?

The experimental evidence up to now leads to a negative answer to this question.

i) Solubilization of the complex by either Triton or papain treatment does not change (Table I) the K_m values, or the extent of activation by Na^+, or the K_{cat} of the enzyme (the latter is shown by the essentially quantitative yields of the solubilization procedures).

ii) Changes in temperature, which should affect at least partially the state of fluidity of the brush border membrane lipids (the transition temperature as determined by fluorescence polarization is reported to be approximately 26° (ref. 25) produce the same changes in V_{max} values in papain-solubilized and in membrane-bound sucrase: In both cases the Arrhenius plots correspond to an activation energy of 10 kcal·mol^{-1} above 13° and of 16.5 kcal·mol^{-1} below.[2] Similar resultswere obtained with solubilized and membranebound isomaltase (H. Braun, unpublished results, 1977).

We conclude that the portion of the sucrase-isomaltase complex which anchors it to the membrane fabric is not necessary for the catalytic function of the enzyme.

This is in keeping with the observation that at least some portions of the catalytic sites of this enzyme complex must be in hydrophilic areas: upon affinity labeling of the sites with conduritol B-epoxide, followed by tryptic digestion, one can isolate a peptide which carries both the label bound to the β-COO$^-$ of Asp and some of the sugar residues of the glycoprotein.[26,27]

TABLE I

SOME KINETIC PARAMETERS OF MEMBRANE-BOUND AND OF PAPAIN-SOLUBILIZED SUCRASE-ISOMALTASE FROM RABBIT SMALL-INTESTINAL BRUSH BORDERS*1

	Membr. bd.	*Papain-solub.*	*Triton-solub.*
pH optimum of sucrase and isomaltase	6.8	6.8	6.8
K_m for sucrose	8.4 mM	8.5 mM	8.4 mM
K_m for palatinose	4.3 mM	4.3 mM	N.D.*2
Na^+ activation of sucrase and of isomaltase	*ca.* 30%	*ca.* 30%	*ca.* 30%

*1From various papers from the author's laboratory.
*2N.D., not determined.

WHAT MACROMOLECULAR DIFFERENCES EXIST BETWEEN TRITON-SOLUBILIZED AND PAPAIN-SOLUBILIZED SUCRASE-ISOMALTASE COMPLEX?

Or in other words, what is the mechanism of solubilization of this protein by papain treatment?

The complex can be solubilized from the brush border membrane by either of two procedures.[28,29] As obtained by controlled papain solubilization, the complex has the hydrodynamic properties indicated in Table II. The frictional ratio (1:31) corresponds to a revolution ellipsoid with a hydration of 30% and an axial ratio of about 1:4. The isolated native isomaltase has a frictional ratio of 1.36: Thus, the isomaltase moiety is even less

TABLE II

MOLECULAR PROPERTIES OF THE SUCRASE ISOMALTASE COMPLEX AND THE ISOMALTASE FROM RABBIT SMALL INTESTINE AS OBTAINED AFTER PAPAIN SOLUBILIZATION*1

Conditions	*Parameter*	*Sucrase isomaltase complex*	*Isomaltase*
Native, at low ionic strength	$s^0_{20,w}$(S)	9.60	6.35
	$D^0_{20,w}$(F)	4.05	4.90
	$\bar{v}$ (ml/g) found	0.739	N.D.
	calcd.	0.726	0.721
	Molecular weight	221,000	121,000*2 113,000*3
	f/f_0	1.31	1.36
Native, at high ionic strength	$s^0_{20,w}$(S)	14.66	
	Molecular weight	424,000*2,4	
Denatured, in guanidine hydrochloride and mercaptoethanol	$s^0_{20,w}$(S)	3.59	
	$D^0_{20,w}$(F)	2.99	
	Molecular weight	112,000*2	

*1 From ref. 30.

*2 Assuming a $\bar{v}$ value of 0.739 ml/g.

*3 Calculated with the $\bar{v}$ value of 0.726 ml/g obtained from the amino acid and carbohydrate analysis.

*4 Calculated assuming that the complex and its dimer have the same degree of hydration and shape.

spherical than the whole complex. With the same assumptions as for the complex the axial ratio of the isomaltase subunit would be approximately 1:5.[30]

When isolated by detergent solubilization, the sucrase-isomaltase complex has, *in the presence of detergent*, essentially the same molecular size as when isolated after controlled proteolytic digestion. This is shown by similar sedimentation constant and by the similar behavior on Sepharose columns (Stokes' radius for both, *ca.* 7 nm). However, in the absence of detergents, the sucrase-isomaltase complex forms aggregates of rather regular shape, as shown by electron microscopy. Gel filtration and sedimentation analysis also show that the Triton-solubilized sucrase-isomaltase complex forms aggregates in the absence of detergents (Stokes' radius, *ca.* 15 nm). Their size is not detectably affected by the ionic strength of the buffer, which indicates that the interaction among the Triton-solubilized sucrase-isomaltase complexes is not electrostatic in nature.

The specific sucrase and isomaltase activities of these aggregates are identical with those of the (non-aggregating) papain-solubilized sucrase-isomaltase complex. Thus, the substrates must have free access to the catalytic sites, which we already know are located in hydrophilic areas.

When mixed with *pre-formed* monolamellar egg lecithin liposomes, the aggregates of Triton-solubilized sucrase-isomaltase do not interact detectably with them. Thus, the (presumably hydrophilic) surface of the aggregates does not interact strongly with the polar heads of lecithins. This is at variance with what is known for cytochrome b_5 (ref. 16) and makes a spontaneous post-translational insertion of sucrase-isomaltase into the membrane an improbable mode of assembly, but of course does not rule it out: The possible roles of some membrane lipids and/or protein(s) have not been investigated thus far.

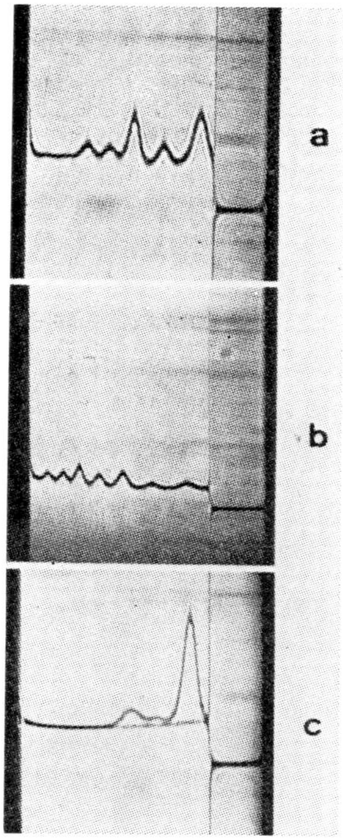

Fig. 1. Ultracentrifugal Schlieren pattern of lipoprotein complex reconstituted from egg lecithin and sucrase-isomaltase (lecithin conc. 0.037 M, lecithin/protein wt. ratio 4, solvent used: 0.1 M NaCl); sedimentation (from right to left) at 50, 740 rpm and 20°; phase plate angle 70°, time 41.3 min; the peak at the extreme right represents pure lecithin vesicles with $s_{20,w}=2.9$ S; the other 4 peaks represent lipoprotein complexes (I, II, III, and IV, cf. Table II) in order of increasing apparent sedimentation coefficients; I: $s_{20,app}=7.61$ S; II: $s_{20,app}=10.3$ S; III: $s_{20,app}=14.4$ S; IV: $s_{20,app}=17.2$ S (a). Schlieren pattern of lipoprotein complex reconstituted from egg lecithin and sucrase-isomaltase (lecithin conc. 0.016 M, lecithin/protein wt. ratio 1.4, solvent: 0.1 M NaCl); sedimentation at 50,740 rpm and 20°, phase plate angle 75°, time 42 min (b). Schlieren pattern of lipoprotein complex shown in Fig. 1a after papain treatment; sedimentation at 50,740 rpm and 20°; phase plate angle 60°, time 39.9 min. In addition to free lipid with a sedimentation coefficient $s_{20,w}=2.9$ S (right hand peak), the "papain" form of sucrase-isomaltase is identified as fastest migrating peak with an apparent sedimentation coefficient $s_{20,app}=10.0$ S (c). From ref. 41.

If, on the contrary, however, cholate is present when liposomes are mixed with Triton-solubilized (*i.e.*, "hydrophobic") sucrase-isomaltase, and then the cholate is removed by gel filtration (a procedure which, in the absence of protein, leads to the formation of a very homogeneous population of monolamellar liposomes having a diameter of 300 Å,[31] sucrase-isomaltase does interact with lecithin, with generation of liposome populations carrying 0, 1, 2, 3, 4 *etc.* molecules of Triton-sucrase-isomaltase per liposome.[32] Apparently, therefore, this protein can interact with liposomes in the course of their formation *only*, *i.e.*, with *nascent* liposomes (Fig. 1 and Table III). The lipid portion of these sucrase-isomaltase carrying liposomes is very similar to protein-free liposomes:

TABLE III

SEDIMENTATION BEHAVIOR OF THE LIPOPROTEIN COMPLEX (Fig. 1 a) RECONSTITUTED FROM LECITHIN AND SUCRASE-ISOMALTASE*1

*Lipoprotein fraction**2	$s_{20,app}$ *S*	$s_{20,w}$ *S**3	s_x/s_I*4	s_x/s_I*4	$M\times10^{-6}$ (*dalton*)*6	$\bar{v}$ (*ml/g*)*6
I	7.61	7.50	1.0	1.0	2.92	0.9656
II	10.87	10.90	1.43	1.45	3.14	0.9497
III	14.4	14.7	1.89	1.96	3.36	0.9360
IV	17.2	18.0	2.26	2.40	3.58	0.9237

*1 From ref. 41.

*2 Schlieren peaks 2–5 of Fig. 1a (see legends).

*3 Sedimentation coefficient $s_{20,w}$ calculated from the following equation

$$s_{20,w}=\frac{M(1-\bar{v}\,\rho_{20})}{\rho\pi N r\eta}$$

where M and $\bar{v}$ are given in the table, ρ_{20} is the density of water at 20°, N is Avogadro's number, r is the Stokes' radius determined from gel filtration (r=135 Å) and η is the viscosity of water at 20° (η=0.01 poise).

*4 Ratio of experimental sedimentation coefficients, x=I, II, III, IV.

*5 Calculated ratios of sedimentation coefficients using values in 3rd column.

*6 Particle weight of lipoprotein complex calculated on the basis that 1–4 sucrase-isomaltase molecules are present per lecithin vesicle (see below) of 5,500 lipid molecules. The partial specific volumes were calculated from the lipid-protein weight ratio in each lipoprotein complex, using the partial specific volume of lecithin volume of lecithin $\bar{v}$=0.984 ml/g^{-1} and of sucrase-isomaltase $\bar{v}$=0.793 ml/g^{-1}.

It has essentially identical non-specific permeability, the same NMR and ESR spectra (the latter with N→O fatty acid derivatives), the same volume of the internal cavity (0.47 µl/µmol of lecithin). In addition, and perhaps most significant of all properties measured, titration of the lecithin polar heads by ^{1}HMR and ^{31}PMR with negatively or positively charged shift reagents, respectively, yields identical results with protein-free as with sucrase-isomaltase-carrying liposomes, which (considering that the size of the protein molecule is similar to that of the liposome moiety) indicates again lack of interaction between sucrase-isomaltase and the polar heads of lecithins. The protein molecules are oriented asymmetrically; in fact: (i) Addition of lytic concentrations of Triton do not produce any large increase in sucrase or isomaltase activity, and (ii) papain treatment removes almost totally the sucrase-isomaltase activity from these liposomes (leaving behind, associated with the lipids, a hydrophobic peptide). The sucrase-isomaltase so removed is indistinguishable from the complex solubilized from native brush border membranes by papain treatment. (The asymmetry of the protein in sucrase-isomaltase carrying liposomes is not absolute, however: Triton treatment of papain-digested liposomes does lead to a sizable increase in sucrase activity. It can be calculated that some 5–10% of the original sucrase-isomaltase-lipid-vesicles must have carried the catalytic sites oriented towards the inside.) Papain-solubilized sucrase-isomaltase does not interact with either nascent or pre-formed liposomes.[41]

Summing up: The major macromolecular difference between Triton-solubilized and papain-solubilized sucrase-isomaltases is the ability of the former to aggregate and to interact with *nascent* liposomes. There are some indications that the forces involved in these processes are hydrophobic in nature: In addition to some of the observations mentioned above, it can be mentioned that high ionic strength does not dissociate either the aggregates of Triton-sucrase-isomaltase or the artificial protein-lipid vesicles. Only detergents, including non-ionic ones, can do so.

THE CHEMICAL DIFFERENCE(S) BETWEEN TRITON-SOLUBILIZED AND PAPAIN-SOLUBILIZED SUCRASE-ISOMALTASE

Controlled papain treatment of the native brush border membrane, of Triton-solubilized sucrase-isomaltase complex or of artificial sucrase-isomaltase lipid vesicled does not change the catalytic properties of the enzyme, while changing radically its capability to aggregate. SDS-PAGE of Triton-solubilized sucrase-isomaltase yields two clearly separated bands (Fig. 2), with apparent mol. wt.-values of 120,000 (sucrase) and of 140,000 (isomaltase), respectively. Papain-solubilized sucrase-isomaltase yields, under the same conditions, two bands, one of which (sucrase) shows unchanged electrophoretic mobility (and thus presumably mol. wt.), and the other (isomaltase) an increased mobility corresponding to an apparent mol. wt. of about 123,000. At the same time, a peptide is produced (not shown in the figure). Although its mol. wt. could not be determined with security, due to its tendency to aggregate, it should not be too different from the difference in mol. wt.-values of the two isomaltases (140,000—123,000=17,000). Thus, it seems certain that papain treatment of the native (or of the detergent-solubilized sucrase-isomaltase) splits off a piece of the polypeptide chain of the isomaltase subunit. The next questions are: From which area of the isomaltase subunit does this polypeptide (which, incidentally,

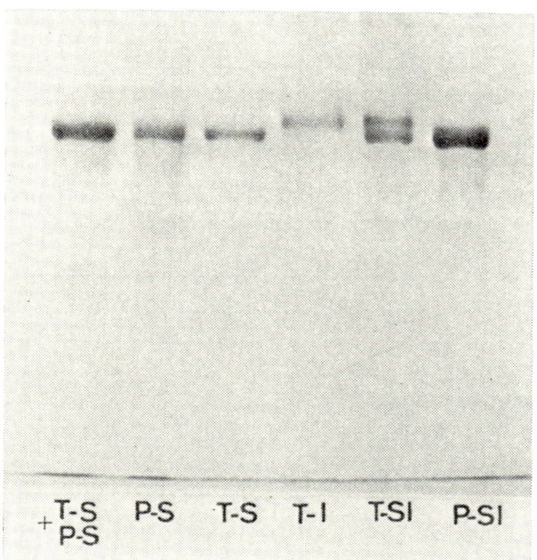

Fig. 2. SDS-polyacrylamide gel electrophoresis of papain-solubilized, Triton-solubilized sucrase-isomaltase complex and of the individual subunits from either form of the complex. P-SI, papain-solubilized sucrase-isomaltase complex; T-SI, Triton-solubilized sucrase-isomaltase complex; T-S and T-I, sucrase subunit (and isomaltase subunit, respectively) from Triton-solubilized sucrase-isomaltase complex; P-S, sucrase subunit from papain-solubilized sucrase-isomaltase complex. From ref. 42.

has a rather hydrophobic composition) arise? Is the sucrase subunit also modified by papain, or not? Table IV compares the aminoacids released from carboxypeptidase Y from Triton-solubilized and from papain-solubilized sucrase-isomaltase complex. Clearly, there are no differences. This observation, along with the observation that the isolated sucrase and isomaltase subunits are equally well degraded under these conditions, while not establishing the sequence at the C-terminals, provides nevertheless evidence that papain digestion does *not* split the polypeptide chains of either sucrase or isomaltase subunit in their C-terminal areas. As to the N-terminals, they were identified (by dansylation) in papain-solubilized, Triton-solubilized sucrase-isomaltase and in the isolated subunits from the latter. Clearly, papain solubilization does not change the N-terminal of sucrase, whereas it does so at the N-terminal of the isomaltase subunit. The microheterogeneity of the N-terminal in papain-isomaltase can presumably be explained by the rather broad substrate specificity of this protease (Table V).

Thus, the sucrase subunit is unchanged by papain, as shown by unchanged apparent mol. wt., unchanged C-terminal and unchanged N-terminal. Furthermore, these data show unequivocally that the peptide formed during papain treatment of native sucrase-

TABLE IV

LIBERATION OF AMINO ACID RESIDUES BY THE ACTION OF CARBOXYPEPTIDASE Y ON TRITON-SOLUBILIZED OR PAPAIN-SOLUBILIZED SUCRASE-ISOMALTASE COMPLEX*

Twelve nmol (approx. 2.6 mg) of either T-SI or P-SI were incubated with CPY (100:1 by weight) at 25° for 3 hr, in 0.05 M Na phosphate buffer, pH 6.5, in the presence of 0.056 M SDS. The data are expressed as moles of amino acid(s) released per nmol of P-SI or T-SI, respectively.

Amino acid	*From P-SI*	*From T-SI*
Ser+Asn+Gln	1.07	0.92
Ile	0.56	0.51
Trp	0.46	0.44
Thr	0.34	0.35
Leu	0.30	0.22
Phe	0.14	0.21
Val	0.08	0.05

* From ref. 42.

TABLE V

AMINO-ENDS OF SMALL-INTESTINAL SUCRASE-ISOMALTASE COMPLEX*

By dansylation. The complex was obtained from brush border membranes of rabbit small intestine.

Protein	*N-terminal(s)*
Triton X-100 solubilized SI	Ile, Ala
Papain-solubilized SI	Ile, (Glu, Gly, Thr)
Sucrase subunit from Triton-solubilized SI	Ile
Isomaltase subunit from Triton-solubilized SI	Ala

H_2N-Ala . . . (Glu, Gly, Thr)——Ⓘ

Papain

H_2N-Ile——Ⓢ

* From ref. 42.

TABLE VI

AMINO ACID SEQUENCE AT THE N-TERMINAL OF THE ISOMALTASE SUBUNIT FROM TRITON-SOLUBILIZED SUCRASE-ISOMALTASE COMPLEX*

```
                                     (CHO)
                                       |
Ala-Val-Asn-Ala-Phe-Ser-Gly-Leu-Glu-Ile-Thr-Leu-Ile-Val
 1               5                   10
Leu-Phe-Val-Ile-Val-Phe-Ile-Ile-Ala-Ile-Ala-Leu-Ile-Ala
 15                  20                  25
Val-Leu-Ala-x-x-x-Pro-Ala-Val
    30              35
```

* From ref. 43.

isomaltase complex does not arise from the C-terminal area, but from the *N-terminal area* of the isomaltase subunit.

Since this portion of the isomaltase polypeptide chain is the only difference between Triton-solubilized and papain-solubilized sucrase-isomaltase, it must be responsible for (much of) the interactions leading to the aggregation of Triton-sucrase-isomaltase and the interaction anchoring this protein in the native brush border membrane.

As I have mentioned previously, the peptide liberated during papain treatment is rather hydrophobic in composition. More instructive is, however, the amino acid sequence of the N-terminal of the isomaltase subunit from the Triton-solubilized complex (ref. 43) (Table VI), from which the "hydrophobic peptide" should arise by papain treatment.

Clearly, this confirms the existence of a hydrophobic region at the N-terminal of this subunit and further substantiates the previous conclusion that the polypeptide segment responsible for (much of) the interaction anchoring the sucrase-isomaltase subunit to the membrane comes indeed from the N-terminal area of the isomaltase subunit. This is at variance with what is established for glycophorin,[14] in which the hydrophobic "anchor" is located not far from the C-terminal but it may hold true for brush border aminopeptidase.[33,34]

We do not know yet whether the N-terminal is located at the outer, luminal side of the membrane, or at the inner, cellular side. Attempts at establishing (by making use of the elegant method of Louvard *et al.*[17] whether or not the hydrophobic segment of isomaltase protrudes into the cellular side of the membrane have failed up to now.

It should be noted that if all the hydrophobic side chains of residues 10 to 31 of the isomaltase subunit interact with the hydrophobic layer of the membrane fabric, the entropic energy alone would be probably sufficient to keep the sucrase-isomaltase complex bound to the membrane.

Succinylation, maleinylation, citraconylation, and dimethylmaleinylation have been used to separate subunits and also to solubilize some membrane proteins (*e.g.*, refs. 35, 36, and references therein). In the case of sucrase-isomaltase we have reported previously that this treatment can be used to separate the two subunits.[37] When applied to the brush border membrane, citraconylation produces a preferential solubilization of sucrase subunit (Fig. 3), which again shows that the major interaction of the sucrase-isomaltase complex with the native brush border membrane takes place *via* the isomaltase subunit and/or that the interactions of sucrase with the membrane fabric are of different nature. An anchoring of the sucrase-isomaltase complex *via* the isomaltase subunit would also agree with the observations of Nishi and Takesue[38] that the precipitate of anti-isomaltase antibodies is located closer to the apparent "unit membrane" than that given by anti-sucrase antibodies.

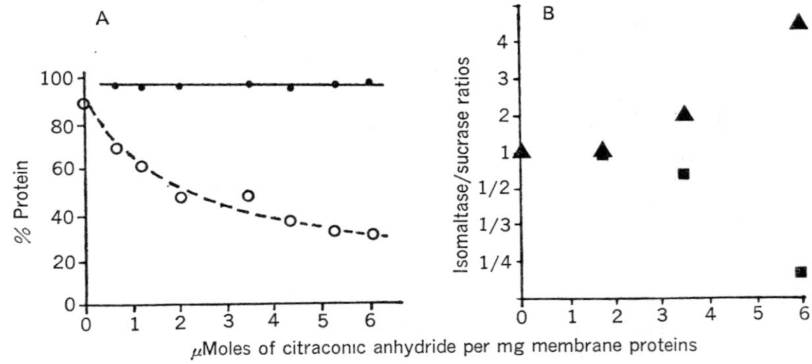

Fig. 3. Preferential solubilization of the isomaltase moiety by citraconylation of native brush border membrane vesicles. A, solubilization of membrane protein. ● recovery of protein in sediment+supernatant; ○ percent of protein left in the 100,000 *g* sediment. B, isomaltase/sucrase ratios in the sediment (▲) or in the supernatant (■), as determined by SDS-PAGE. From ref. 42.

SOME QUESTIONS ON THE BIOSYNTHESIS OF THE SUCRASE-ISOMALTASE COMPLEX

At the beginning of this review I mentioned briefly the current ideas as to the mechanism of biosynthesis of glycophorin and of similar small membrane proteins which span the membrane and have a hydrophobic area not far from the C-terminal of the chain. In considering possible biosynthetic mechanisms for the sucrase-isomaltase complex of small-intestinal brush borders, we must now take into consideration at least two major features: (i) Most (if not all) of the interaction anchoring this protein to the membrane involves a hydrophobic segment located not far from the *N-terminal* (rather than close to the C-terminal) of isomaltase; (ii) the sucrase subunit seems to interact with the membrane fabric mainly (if not exclusively) *via* the isomaltase subunit.

In this connection Blobel's "signal" hypothesis for the biosynthesis of export proteins must now be mentioned. He suggests that they are synthetized as pre-proteins, *i.e.*, the synthesis of the polypeptide chain of the final protein is preceded by the synthesis of a hydrophobic segment (the "signal") of some 16 amino acids. This segment, which is supposed to be material in the "gliding" of the polypeptide chain across the membrane of the rough endoplasmic reticulum, is then split off in the intracisternal space, either while later portions of the chain are being synthetized or after completion of the biosynthesis and release of the protein into the intracisternal space.[39,40] (The enzyme involved is given the name "signalase" or "clippase.")

The first question which can be asked is, therefore: Is the hydrophobic segment at the N-terminal area of the isomaltase subunit nothing else than a modified "signal," which was not split off due to its different amino acid sequence,[40] or to the lack of "clippase" in this tissue, or to other reasons; or is the biosynthesis of the hydrophobic segment in isomaltase preceded by the biosynthesis of the "signal" proper? Work is presently in progress to answer this question (for further discussion, see ref. 43).

Whatever function the hydrophobic segment at the N-terminal area of isomaltase may have in biosynthesis, it may either reassociate with the membrane from the outside or "stick" in it during biosynthesis, so that the nascent polypeptide chain would (temporarily, at least) from a loop.

Is there an additional hydrophobic region at the C-terminal area of isomaltase (or sucrase), at least during biosynthesis? We should keep in mind that small-intestinal brush borders are exposed to the action of a number of proteases. It is perfectly conceivable that the C-terminal area of either sucrase or isomaltase may originally span the membrane with the C-terminal at the cellular side, and that a protease (*e.g.*, trypsin or chymotrypsin) may split the chain at the luminal side, thereby creating a new C-terminal, now located outside the cell.

As I have mentioned at the start, the two subunits of the complex probably have extensive homology and are subjected to the same or to related biological control mechanism(s). They are thus likely to have arisen by gene duplication. How is sucrase synthetized so that it has eventually a peripheral position? At least two possibilities are at hand: (i) If the two genes are still closely associated, they may be transcribed without discontinuity leading to a single, common giant mRNA, which in turn may lead to a pro-sucrase-isomaltase complex composed of a single polypeptide chain beginning with the N-terminal of the isomaltase subunit and ending with the C-terminal of the sucrase subunit (+ perhaps additional pieces at the N- and C-terminals). Post-translational partial proteolysis of this hypothetical precursor could, among other things, lead to the formation of the two subunits, which would still remain assembled. (ii) Alternatively, the two subunits of the sucrase-isomaltase complex can arise from two mRNA's, and the two chains should then assemble during or after biosynthesis, for which coordination of the biosyntheses of the two subunits would be essential. Each of the two hypotheses has merits and demerits. It may be possible in the future to decide between them.

ACKNOWLEDGMENT

This work was supported in part by the Swiss National Science Foundation, Berne, and by Nestlé Alimentana, Vevey, Switzerland.

REFERENCES

1 G. Semenza, in L. Bolis and A. Leaf, *Membranes and Diseases*, Raven Press, New York, 1976, p. 243.

2 G. Semenza, in A. Martonosi, *The Enzymes of Biological Membranes*, Plenum Press, New York, vol. 3, 1976, p. 349.

3 G. Semenza, in M. Rechcigl, Jr., *Handbook Series in Nutrition and Food*, CRC Press, Inc., Ohio, Section B, 1979, in press.

4 S. Auricchio, A. Rubino, R. Tosi, G. Semenza, M. Landolt, H. Kistler, and A. Prader, *Enzym. Biol. Clin.*, 3 (1963) 193.

5 A. Rubino, F. Zimbalatti, and S. Auricchio, *Biochim. Biophys. Acta*, 92 (1964) 305.

6 A. Dahlqvist and T. Lindberg, *Clin. Sci.*, 30 (1966) 517.

7 K. Yamada, S. Moriuchi, and N. Hosoya, *J. Nutr. Sci. Vitaminol.*, 24 (1978) 177.

8 S. Auricchio, A. Rubino, A. Prader, J. Rey, J. Jos, J. Frézal, and D. Davidson, *J. Pediatr.*, 66 (1965) 555.

9 G. Semenza, S. Auricchio, A. Rubino, A. Prader, and J. D. Welsh, *Biochim. Biophys. Acta*, 195 (1965) 386.

10 K. R. Kerry and R. R. W. Townley, *Aust. Paediatr. J.*, 1 (1965) 223.
11 O. Koldovský, in M. Winick, *Nutrition and Development*, John Wiley & Sons, New York, 1972, p. 135.
12 K. M. Brown, *J. Exptl. Zool.*, 177 (1971) 493.
13 F. Moog, A. E. Denes, and P. M. Powell, *Dev. Biol.*, 35 (1973) 143.
14 S. F. Cotmore, H. Furthmayr, and V. T. Marchesi, *J. Mol. Biol.*, 113 (1977) 539.
15 D. D. Sabatini and G. Kreibich, in A. Martonosi, *The Enzymes of Biological Membranes*, Plenum Press, New York, vol. 2, 1976, p. 531.
16 P. W. Holloway and J. T. Katz, *Biochem. Biophys. Res. Commun.*, 54 (1973) 808.
17 D. Louvard, M. Semeriva, and S. Maroux, *J. Mol. Biol.*, 106 (1976) 1023.
18 G. Semenza, in C. F. Code, J. R. Brobeck, R. K. Crane, H. W. Davenport, M. I. Grossman, H. D. Janowitz, C. L. Prosser, and T. H. Wilson, *Handbook of Physiology—Alimentary Canal*, American Physiology Society, Washington, D.C., vol. V, 1968, p. 2543.
19 M. Kessler, O. Acuto, C. Storelli, H. Murer, M. Müller, and G. Semenza, *Biochim. Biophys. Acta*, 506 (1978) 136.
20 J. Kolínská and G. Semenza, *Biochim. Biophys. Acta*, 146 (1967) 181.
21 C. F. Johnson, *Science*, 155 (1967) 1670.
22 T. Oda and S. Seki, 6th Int. Congr. Electron Microscopy, Kyoto, 1966, p. 387 (abstr.).
23 G. Semenza, C. Tannenbaum, M. Kessler, G. Toggenburger, and L. Wahlgren, in G. Semenza and E. Carafoli, *Proceedings of the FEBS Symposium No. 42 on the Biochemistry of Membrane Transport*, Springer-Verlag, Heidelberg, 1977, p. 270.
24 C. Tannenbaum, G. Toggenburger, M. Kessler, A. Rothstein, and G. Semenza, *J. Supramol. Struct.*, 6 (1977) 519.
25 D. Schachter and M. Shinitzky, *J. Clin. Invest.*, 59 (1977) 536.
26 A. Quaroni, E. Gershon, and G. Semenza, *J. Biol. Chem.*, 249 (1974) 6424.
27 A. Quaroni and G. Semenza, *J. Biol. Chem.*, 251 (1976) 3250.
28 H. Sigrist, P. Ronner, and G. Semenza, *Biochim. Biophys. Acta*, 406 (1975) 433.
29 Y. Takesue, T. O. Yoshida, T. Akaza, and Y. Nishi, *J. Biochem.*, 74 (1973) 415.
30 H. Mosimann, G. Semenza, and H. Sund, *Eur. J. Biochem.*, 36 (1973) 489.
31 J. Brunner, P. Skrabal, and H. Hauser, *Biochim. Biophys. Acta*, 455 (1976) 322.
32 J. Brunner, H. Hauser, G. Semenza, and H. Wacker, in G. Semenza and E. Carafoli, *Proceeding of the FEBS Symposium No. 42 on the Biochemistry of Membrane Transport*, Springer-Verlag, Heidelberg, 1977, p. 105.
33 S. Maroux, D. Louvard, and J. Baratti, *Biochim. Biophys. Acta*, 321 (1973) 282.
34 S. Maroux and D. Louvard, *Biochim. Biophys. Acta*, 419 (1976) 189.
35 P. Lundahl and S. Hjertén, *Prot. Biol. Fluids*, 21 (1974) 27.
36 P. Lundahl, *Biochim. Biophys. Acta*, 379 (1975) 304.
37 H. Braun, A. Cogoli, and G. Semenza, *Eur. J. Biochem.*, 52 (1975) 475.
38 Y. Nishi and Y. Takesue, 32nd Annu. Meet. Japan. Sci. Electron Microscopy, Nagoya (1976) (abstr.)
39 G. Blobel and B. Dobberstein, *J. Cell Biol.*, 67 (1975) 835, 852.
40 A. Devillers-Thiery, T. Kindt, G. Scheele, and G. Blobel, *Proc. Natl. Acad. Sci. U.S.*, 72 (1975) 5016.
41 J. Brunner, H. Hauser, and G. Semenza, *J. Biol. Chem.*, 253 (1978) 7538.
42 J. Brunner, H. Hauser, H. Braun, K. J. Wilson, H. Wacker, B. O'Neill, and G. Semenza, *J. Biol. Chem.*, 254 (1979) in press.
43 G. Frank, J. Brunner, H. Hauser, H. Wacker, G. Semenza, and H. Zuber, *FEBS Lett.*, 96 (1978) 183.

UPTAKE AND UTILIZATION OF THIAMINE IN LIVING ORGANISMS

Y. NOSE, A. IWASHIMA, AND Y. WAKABAYASHI

Department of Biochemistry, Kyoto Prefectural University of Medicine, Kyoto, Japan

It is well known that microorganisms—not only mutants requiring a vitamin for the growth, but also the wild strains—can easily take up the exogenous vitamin and utilize it through conversion to coenzyme in a manner similar to higher animals. During the course of the studies of thiamine biosynthesis we found that the exogenous thiamine added to the growth medium of *E. coli* was rapidly taken up by the cells and that it repressed *de novo* synthesis of thiamine accompanied by a reduction of thiamine transport. It was therefore of interest to study the mechanism of the transport and utilization of thiamine in the biological systems (including higher animals) as compared with other vitamins.

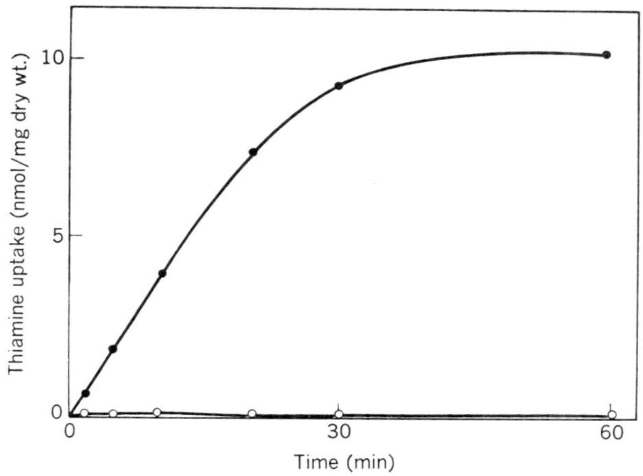

Fig. 1. Time course of [^{14}C]thiamine uptake and effect of temperature in yeast. Ten ml of yeast cell suspensions (81 μg dry wt./mg) in 0.05 M potassium phosphate buffer (pH 5.0) containing 0.1 M glucose, were preincubated for 15 min at 37°, and then [^{14}C]thiamine was added to the medium at 1 μM concentration, followed by further incubation at 37° (●) and 0° (○), respectively. The uptake of [^{14}C]thiamine was measured by counting radioactivities in the cells filtered on membrane filter at the indicated time.

Abbreviations: TDP, thiamine pyrophosphate; TMP, thiamine monophosphate; TTP, thiamine triphosphate.

GENERAL PROPERTIES OF THE THIAMINE UPTAKE SYSTEM IN MICROORGANISMS

Figure 1 shows the time course of [^{14}C]thiamine uptake by yeast cells. The uptake was linear for about 20 min, reaching maximum at 30 min. It was a temperature-dependent process and has an optimal pH at 4.5. A similar result was obtained with a mutant of *E. coli* auxotrophic for thiamine thiazole except that the optimal pH for the uptake was 6.5. The intracellular thiamine concentration in yeast incubated with [^{14}C]thiamine for 30 min was approximately 10,000 times higher than the extracellular thiamine concentration. Similarly, *E. coli* showed a concentrative uptake of thiamine in which a ratio of intracellular to extracellular thiamine concentration was 175 at the equilibrium state.

Both uptake systems showed a similar energy requirement, since omission of glucose in the medium or addition of the metabolic inhibitors such as DNP and cyanide caused a marked reduction in the amount of [^{14}C]thiamine transported in the cells. However, the intracellular form of [^{14}C]thiamine taken up was different in yeast and *E. coli* cells.

The thiamine was extracted from the cells incubated with [^{14}C]thiamine for 1 and 15 min with yeast cells and for 30 sec and 2 min with *E. coli* cells respectively and sub-

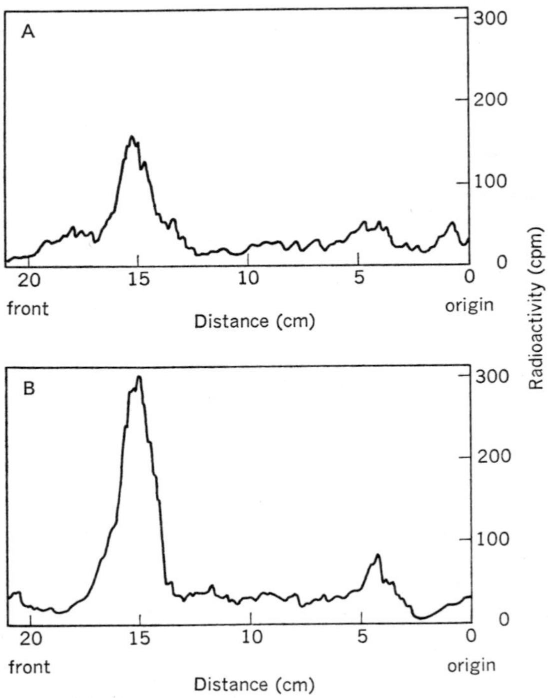

Fig. 2. Intracellular state of [^{14}C]thiamine transported by yeast. Samples of yeast cell suspensions (81 μg dry wt./ml) were exposed to 1 μM [^{14}C]thiamine for 1 min (A) and 15 min (B), respectively. Chromatographic analysis was performed for each samples extracted from the cells; Toyo filter paper No. 50, solvent system, isopropanol-0.5 M acetate buffer (pH 4.5)-water (65: 15: 20, by vol.). Radioactivities on the papers were scanned with, actigarph II, Nuclear Chicago.

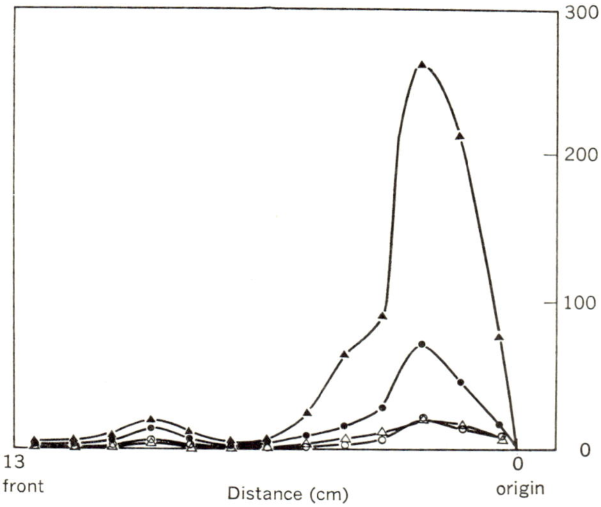

Fig. 3. Intracellular state of [^{14}C]thiamine transported by *E. coli*. Samples of cell suspensions of *E. coli* mutant were exposed to 1 μM [^{14}C]thiamine (25.1 mCi per mmol) for 30 sec and 2 min at 37° and 0°, respectively. Methods used for extraction of [^{14}C]thiamine taken up, and for chromatographic analysis are the same as described in Fig. 2 except for estimation of radioactivities. The paper was cut into small strips of 1-cm width and the radioactivities were counted differently in 10 ml of Bray's solution. ● 30 sec at 37°; ▲ 2 min at 37°; ○ 30 sec at 0°; △ 2 min at 0°.

TABLE I

REQUIREMENTS FOR THIAMINE MONOPHOSPHATE KINASE REACTION

Complete system, in a volume of 3 ml, contained: 100 μmol Tris-HCl, pH 7.5, 10 μmol ATP, 10 μmol $MgCl_2$, 1 mmol KCl, 30 nmol TMP, and the enzyme preparation (20–40% ammonium sulfate fraction, 1.7 mg protein).

Additions	*TDP formed (nmol/mg/30 min)*
Complete	0.762
Complete − TMP	0.023
Complete − ATP	0.010
Complete − Mg^{2+}	0.014
Complete − K^+	0.478
Complete − TMP + thiamine	0
Complete but boiled enzyme	0.020

jected to paper chromatography. As shown in Figs. 2 and 3, a major peak of the radioactivity of free thiamine at R_f of 0.72 was detected (Fig. 2). With *E. coli* cells a major radioactive peak mainly due to TDP was observed even after 30 sec incubation (Fig. 3). These results suggest that the thiamine transported into *E. coli* cells was rapidly converted to phosphorylated forms by thiamine phosphorylating enzyme in the cells, while in yeast cells [^{14}C]thiamine was accumulated as a free form without trapping by phosphorylation. A saturation kinetics of thiamine uptake by yeast cells showed an apparent K_m for thiamine

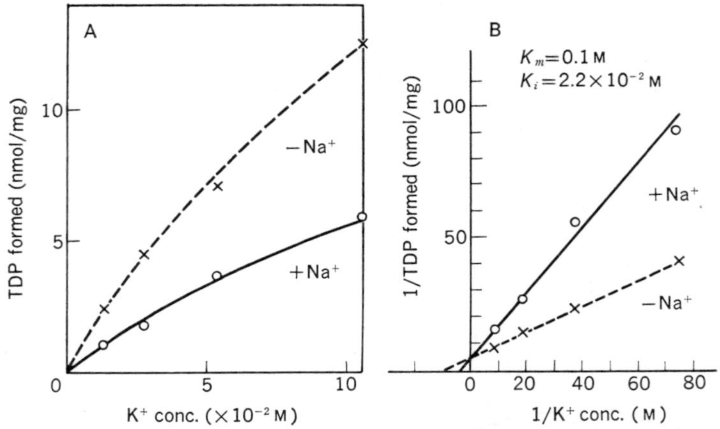

Fig. 4. Effect of K^+ and Na^+ on thiamine monophosphate kinase reaction. Partially purified enzyme was used. The reaction mixture was the same as described in Table I, except for varying K^+ concentrations and the addition of Na^+ (3.3×10^{-2}M) as indicated; × without Na^+; ○ with Na^+.

of 0.18 μM. These results show that the thiamine uptake by yeast cells occurred by a carrier-mediated active process. The accumulation of thiamine as a free form can be fairly understood from the difference between the K_m values for thiamine transport and thiamine pyrophosphokinase reaction. The K_m value for thiamine of the enzyme is 75 μM as reported by Kaziro,[1] and it is approximately 2 orders of magnitude higher than that of thiamine transport.

Since the accumulation of thiamine in *E. coli* showed a different characteristic from that of the yeast cells, we studied thiamine pyrophosphokinase of *E. coli* by estimating TDP formation from thiamine in the presence of ATP and Mg^{2+}.

As shown in Table I, TMP rather than thiamine was unexpectedly a better substrate for TDP synthesis by the crude extract from *E. coli* K-12.[2]

Figure 4 shows the marked stimulation of the enzyme by K^+ and a competitive inhibition with Na^+ which were not observed with thiamine pyrophosphokinase isolated so far.[3] This indicates that *E. coli* can utilize TMP synthesized *de novo* directly for TDP synthesis without producing free thiamine, and it would be also against one step pyrophosphorylation of thiamine to TDP as found in yeast and other organisms.

Subsequently we demonstrated an enzymatic synthesis of TMP from thiamine in the presence of ATP and Mg^{2+} by cell-free extract of *E. coli* K-12.[4] Thus, two new enzymes concerning TDP synthesis were found in *E. coli*, and these were recently approved by the Commission on Biochemical Nomenclature as follows[5]:

	K_m
TMP+ATP ⟶ TDP+ADP Thiamine monophosphate kinase (EC 2.7.4.16)	1.1 μM for TMP
Thiamine+ATP ⟶ TMP+ADP Thiamine kinase (EC 2.7.1.89)	2.8 μM for thiamine

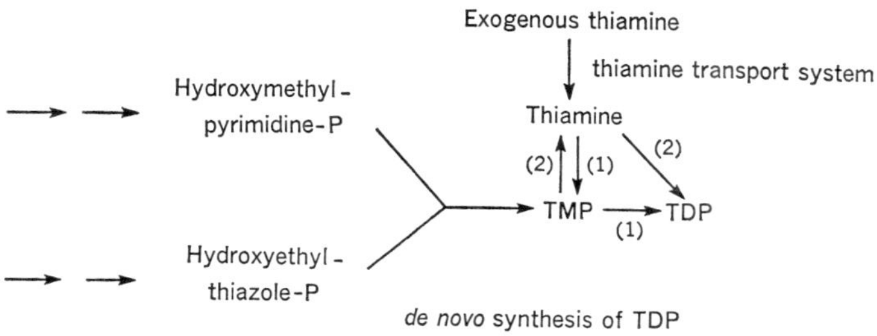

Fig. 5. Schema of thiamine uptake and utilization system in microorganisms.

The apparent K_m values for both enzymes are close to apparent K_m of 0.83 μM for thiamine of the transport in *E. coli*.[6] Figure 5 shows a summary of the pathways of TDP synthesis in several microorganisms.

TDP synthesis from TMP is different in *E. coli* and yeast as mentioned above. Recently, Kawasaki *et al.* have demonstrated that certain thermophilic bacteria synthesize TDP by the *E. coli* route and *Micrococcus denitrificans* by the yeast route.[7,8] Therefore, utilization routes of exogenous thiamine in these organisms are also different, dependent on their pathways of TDP synthesis *de novo*.

It is not clear, at present, whether *E. coli* take up thiamine by an active transport similarly to yeast cells or by a facilitated diffusion, followed by trapping as thiamine phosphates. Kawasaki *et al.* have demonstrated that two mutants of *E. coli*, thiamine kinase-less and thiamine monophosphate kinase-less, accumulated [^{35}S]thiamine as free thiamine and TMP in the cells, respectively, against a concentration gradient.[9] However, it remains to be further clarified whether this is the case for thiamine transport of the wild strain of *E. coli* and other bacteria.

PROPERTIES OF THIAMINE UPTAKE BY MAMMALIAN SYSTEMS

Thiamine uptake by mammalian tissues has been studied by several investigators using intestine and brain slices. They have described how thiamine is actively taken up by animal tissues at low concentrations of thiamine and rapidly converted to TDP by thiamine pyrophosphokinase in the cells.

Thiamine has been well accepted as a neurotropic vitamin, and its deficiency causes a dysfunction of the central nervous system. Therefore, we have principally employed rat brain slices for the study of thiamine uptake in animal tissues, and it seemed to be as important as the thiamine transport through the blood-brain barrier system. Brain slices, quickly prepared by cutting both hemispheres of rat brain, were incubated with [^{14}C] thiamine at 37° in Krebs-Ringer bicarbonate medium containing glucose under gassing with a mixture of O_2 and CO_2 (95: 5, v/v) usually for 60 min. The intracellular thiamine concentration was calculated by subtracting the extracellular space in the slices. The thiamine uptake by brain slices was a temperature- and energy-dependent process as previously reported by Sharma and Quastel.[10]

The ratio of intracellular to extracellular concentration of [^{14}C]thiamine (C_{ICF}/C_{ECF}) exceeded unity after 60 min incubation at low thiamine concentrations (0.1 to 2.0 μM). At 0.2 μM of the initial concentration of thiamine, the C_{ICF}/C_{ECF} was 3.8. This ratio de-

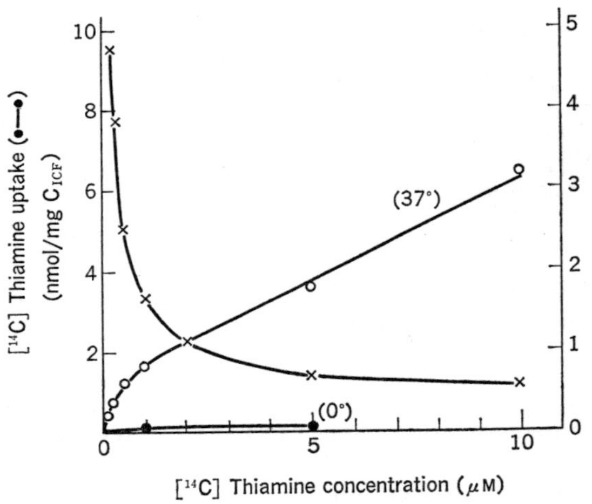

Fig. 6. Effect of [14C]thiamine concentrations on [14C]thiamine uptake.
×, the ratio of intracellular thiamine concentration (C_{ICF}) to extracellular thiamine concentration (C_{ECF}). From Nose *et al.*[11]

TABLE II

[14C]THIAMINE COMPOUNDS ACCUMULATED IN BRAIN SLICES*

Values in parentheses are the ratio of the intracellular to extracellular concentration.

Concentration of initial external [14C]*thiamine*	[14C]*thiamine uptake (nmol/ml C_{ICF})*		
	Total	*Free*	*Phosphorylated*
2×10^{-8}M	0.117	0.017	0.100
	(5.38)	(0.84)	
2×10^{-7}M	0.771	0.129	0.642
	(3.86)	(0.65)	
2×10^{-6}M	2.34	0.922	1.418
	(1.17)	(0.46)	

* From Nose *et al.*[11]

creased concurrently with the increase of external concentrations, and the shape of the uptake curve showed a saturable hyperbola at low external thiamine concentrations, but a linear relationship was observed at high thiamine concentrations (Fig. 6).

An apparent K_m of the uptake for thiamine gave 0.36 μM. It has already been reported that [14C]thiamine compounds transported into brain slices appear to a considerable extent in phosphorylated form.[10]

After 60 min incubation with several low concentrations of [14C]thiamine, the brain slices were homogenized, and [14C]thiamine compounds extracted were analyzed by paper chromatography. As shown in Table II, the [14C]thiamine compounds accumulated in the slices were found to be mostly phosphorylated form, and the ratio of intracellular to extracellular concentration of total thiamine exceeded unity. This ratio increased with a decrease in the external thiamine concentration. However, with respect to free thiamine, the C_{ICF}/C_{ECF} did not exceed unity in all cases. Thus [14C]thiamine transported appears

TABLE III

EFFECT OF THIAMINE DERIVATIVES AND ITS ANALOGS ON [^{14}C]THIAMINE UPTAKE

The brain slices were incubated for 1 hr at 37° at the initial [^{14}C]thiamine concentration of 2×10^{-7}M. Thiamine analogs (2×10^{-6}M) were added to the preincubated medium just before the addition of [^{14}C]thiamine. The rate of thiamine uptake was measured as described in the text.

Additions	*[^{14}C]thiamine uptake (nmol/ml CICF)*	*Inhibition (%)*
None	0.660	
TMP	0.330	50.0
TDP	0.342	48.2
Pyrithiamine	0.175	73.5
Oxythiamine	0.556	15.7
Chloroethylthiamine*1	0.150	77.2
Dimethialium*2	0.310	53.1

*1 3-2′-Methyl-4′-aminopyrimidyl-(5′)-methyl-4-methyl-5-chloroethyl thiazolium chloride hydrochloride.

*2 3-2′-Methyl-4′-aminopyrimidyl-(5′)-methyl-4,5-dimethyl thiazolium chloride hydrochloride.

TABLE IV

EFFECT OF THIAMINE ANALOGS ON CRUDE THIAMINE PYROPHOSPHOKINASE OF RAT BRAIN

Complete system, in a volume of 3 ml, contained: 100 μmol Tris-HCl, pH 7.5, 10 μmol ATP, 10 μmol $MgCl_2$, 6 nmol thiamine, and the enzyme preparation (a fraction precipitated by 0.5 to 0.6 $(NH_4)_2SO_4$ saturation from the crude extracts of rat brains).

Additions	*TDP formed (pmol/mg protein)*	*Inhibition (%)*
None	29.9	
Pyrithiamine	9.3	69.0
Oxythiamine	31.3	—
Chloroethylthiamine	22.3	25.3

to be rapidly trapped as phosphorylated form in the cells, which is very similar to that obtained with *E. coli* cells.[11]

Komai *et al.*[12,13] have reported another type of the thiamine uptake by small intestines of chick and rat, in which the ratio, with respect to free thiamine of the intracellular to extracellular [^{35}S]thiamine concentration, exceeded unity, indicating an active transport of thiamine itself. In order to determine whether a step of thiamine transport across the cell membrane of brain slices is an active process or the concentrative uptake only dependent on phosphorylation, the effects of thiamine analogs on [^{14}C]thiamine uptake were studied.

As shown in Table III the thiamine derivatives and analogs which showed inhibitory effects on the thiamine uptake by microbes inhibited the uptake by brain slices. The inhibitions by pyrithiamine and chloroethylthiamine were remarkable to almost the same extent, while oxythiamine showed a much weaker inhibitory effect. Therefore, the effects of these three analogs on the activity of thiamine pyrophosphokinase in rat brain homogenate were compared to determine the role of phosphorylation of thiamine in thiamine uptake by brain slices.

As shown in Table IV oxythiamine had almost no effect, as expected, but the degrees

TABLE V

PURIFICATION OF THIAMINE PYROPHOSPHOKINASE FROM PIG BRAIN

Fraction	*Total activity (nmol)*	*Total protein (mg)*	*Specific activity (nmol/mg/hr)*	*Yield (%)*
Crude extract	1,453.6	21,695	0.067	100
Heat treatment	778.3	3,151	0.247	53.5
$(NH_4)_2SO_4$ fraction (45–65% saturated)	1,136.4	1,095	1.04	78.2
DEAE-cellulose	878.5	98.2	8.95	60.4
TMP-agarose	545.5	0.067	8,145	37.5

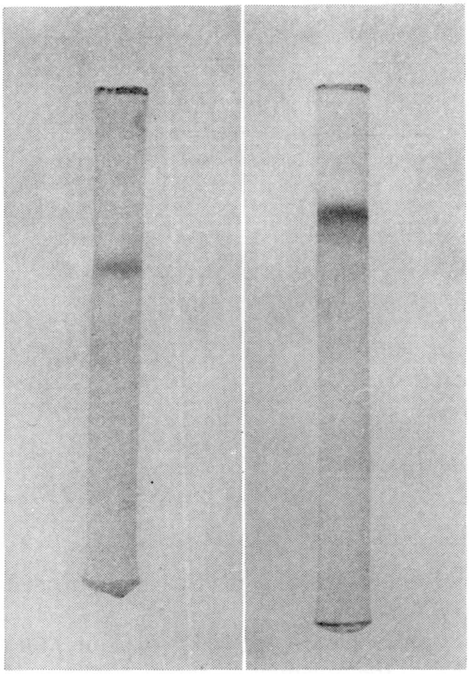

Fig. 7. Polyacrylamide gel electrophoresis of the purified thiamine pyrophosphokinase. Disc gel electrophoresis was carried out at pH 8.3 on 7.5% acrylamide according to the method of Davis. Four μg (left) and 20 μg (right) each of protein was run for 50 min. The current density was 4 mA/tube. Bands were stained with Coomassie blue.

of the inhibition by pyrithiamine and chloroethylthiamine were considerably different. This result suggests that [^{14}C]thiamine uptake by brain slices cannot be ascribed only to the phosphorylating activity in the cells, another specific mechanism, probably some carrier system in the cell membrane, might be involved. In order to understand better the relationship between the transport and the phosphorylation of thiamine, thiamine pyrophosphokinase was purified from pig brain. An affinity column chromatography using agarose coupled with thiamine monophosphate could be effectively applied to purify the enzyme from pig brain.

The enzyme was purified about 100,000-fold from the crude extract, which is homogenous on the polyacrylamide gel electrophoresis as shown in Fig. 7.

The inhibition of the purified enzyme by thiamine analog was very similar to that of the crude exzyme from rat brain. The K_m value for thiamine of the enzyme gave 0.4 μM, which was very close to the apparent K_m value for thiamine transport by rat brain slices. These results suggest that the thiamine uptake by brain slices is a process mediated with a membrane carrier specific for thiamine, and regulated by thiamine pyrophosphokinase activity. It has been accepted that thiamine phosphates in the brain consist of free thiamine, TMP, TDP, and TTP.[14] Among them, TTP is believed to be synthesized from TDP, and it has been examined by studies of subacute necrotizing encephalomyelopathy, a hereditary disease of infants. It is of interest to know whether [^{14}C]TTP can be synthesized from [^{14}C]thiamine taken up by the brain slices.

The [^{14}C]thiamine compounds in the brain slices after 1.5 hr incubation, were separated using column chromatography on Dowex 1×4 according to the method of Koike and Yusa.[15] Authentic TTP added to the sample (before the adsorption on Dowex column) was detected as a peak of OD_{245} around fraction No. 50 in the eluates. However, the radioactivity responsible for [^{14}C]TTP synthesized was negligible around this fraction. A large

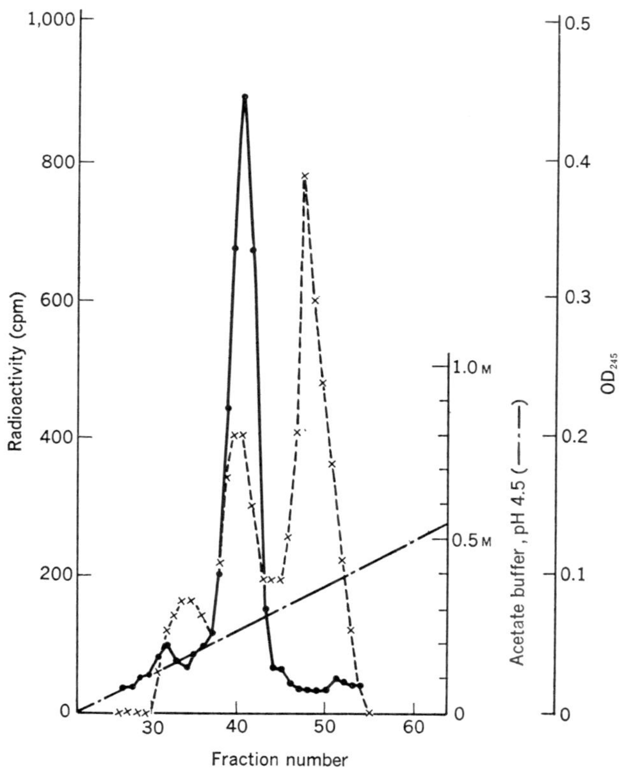

Fig. 8. Analysis of [^{14}C]thiamine compounds in brain slices by Dowex 1 column chromatography. Solid line, the radioactivity; dotted line, OD_{245}. From Nose *et al.*[11]

peak of the radioactivity was identified as [^{14}C]TDP formed, indicating that [^{14}C]TTP synthesis hardly ever occurred under the conditions employed.[11]

THIAMINE TRANSPORT AND THIAMINE-BINDING PROTEIN

As described above, the enzymatic mechanism of TDP synthesis from thiamine or TMP has been elucidated in both microorganisms and mammalian tissues, but the molecular mechanism of membrane transport of thiamine across the cell membrane, which is the first step of thiamine utilization, is still unknown. However, recently evidence has accumulated to imply that periplasmic binding proteins of gram-negative bacteria may be involved in the active transport of the molecules which they bind.[16]

With regard to a protein binding thiamine, Nishimune and Hayashi[17] first described the occurrence of a thiamine-binding protein in *E. coli*. Subsequently, we obtained a thiamine-binding protein in homogenous state from a thiazole requiring mutant of *E. coli* K-12, which shows a single band on polyacrylamide gel electrophoresis.[18] Several lines of indirect evidence have suggested that the thiamine-binding protein may participate in thiamine transport in *E. coli*. First, the activity of thiamine uptake by *E. coli* cells reduced with osmotic shock treatment was partially restored by the addition of shock fluid. Second, the rate of thiamine uptake repressed by thiamine added to the growth medium of *E. coli* was roughly proportional to the thiamine binding activity in shock fluid. However, the purified thiamine-binding protein showed a K_D value of 9.2 nM for thiamine much lower than K_m value for thiamine transport *in vivo*[19] and several inhibition kinetics by thiamine analogs also differed from those of thiamine uptake by the cells. Furthermore, a shock fluid prepared from a mutant of *E. coli* defective in thiamine uptake isolated by Kawasaki *et al.*[20] uses almost the same activity to bind thiamine as that of the parent strain. Thus, it seems that a periplasmic thiamine-binding protein is not involved, at least in the translocation step in thiamine transport in *E. coli*, but its role may be to recognize thiamine in the medium and increase the affinity of the transport system for thiamine by interacting with a membrane component.

On the other hand, the existence of a thiamine-specific transport carrier in yeast cells is also conceivable from the susceptibility to the inhibition of thiamine transport by thiamine analogs. Thiamine transport in yeast was effectively inhibited by several thiamine analogs both in *E. coli* and rat brain slices. Based on strong growth inhibition by pyrithiamine, we isolated two mutants of *Saccharomyces cerevisiae* resistant to this analog by nitrosoguanidine treatment.[21] These mutants were found to be deficient in the uptake of thiamine as well as pyrithiamine. This suggests the existence of a common carrier for both thiamine and pyrithiamine in yeast which is probably defective in the mutants.

Recently, we found thiamine binding activities in both soluble and membrane fractions of sonic extracts of *S. cerevisiae*.

Table VI shows a relationship between activities of these binding components and of thiamine transport in *S. cerevisiae*. The K_D of the membrane-bound component for thiamine (0.17 μM) was almost identical with the K_m of thiamine transport system (0.18 μM) in *S. cerevisiae*, whereas the K_D of the soluble component was 0.04 μM. The thiamine binding activity of the membrane-bound component was strongly inhibited by O-benzoylthiamine disulfide, which is a potent inhibitor of yeast thiamine transport,[22] but the soluble component was hardly affected by it. In addition, the binding activity was found to be markedly low in the membrane fraction from a thiamine transport mutant, but no difference

TABLE VI

THIAMINE TRANSPORT AND THIAMINE BINDING ACTIVITY IN *S. cerevisiae*

	Thiamine transport	*Thiamine binding activity*	
		Membrane fraction	*Soluble fraction*
K_m for thiamine	0.18 μM	0.17 μM*	0.04 μM*
Effect of thiamine analogs			
Pyrithiamine	Inhibited	Inhibited	Inhibited
O-benzoylthiamine disulfide	Inhibited	Inhibited	No effect
Addition of thiamine to growth medium	Reduced	Reduced	Reduced
Thiamine transport mutant	Markedly low	Markedly low	Same as parent strain

* K_D for thiamine.

was observed in the activity of the soluble fraction between the parent strain and the mutant. On the other hand, growth on the medium containing thiamine caused a remarkable reduction in the activities of the transport system and of the thiamine binding of both components. These results may indicate that the membrane-bound component rather than the component in soluble fraction might be involved directly in thiamine transport in yeast cells. The solubilization of the thiamine-binding component from yeast membrane is now being attempted.

In conclusion, it became fairly clear that the transport and utilization of thiamine in biological systems have a characteristic mechanism like those of the other nutrients. However, further investigations are required to understand the mechanism of membrane transport of thiamine in living organisms on the molecular levels. We hope that the findings described above will make some contribution to the solution of this interesting problem.

REFERENCES

1 Y. Kaziro, *J. Biochem.*, 46 (1959) 1523.
2 H. Nishino, A. Iwashima, and Y. Nose, *Biochem. Biophys. Res. Commun.*, 45 (1971) 363.
3 H. Nishino, A. Iwashima, and Y. Nose, *J. Nutr. Sci. Vitaminol.*, 19 (1973) 505.
4 A. Iwashima, H. Nishino, and Y. Nose, *Biochim. Biophys. Acta*, 258 (1972) 333.
5 E. C. Webb, personal communication (1976).
6 T. Kawasaki, I. Miyata, K. Esaki, and Y. Nose, *Arch. Biochem. Biophys.*, 131 (1969) 223.
7 T. Kawasaki and K. Yamada, unpublished data.
8 H. Sanemori, Y. Egi, and T. Kawasaki, *J. Bacteriol.*, 126 (1976) 1030.
9 T. Kawasaki and K. Yamada, *Biochem. Biophys. Res. Commun.*, 47 (1972) 465.
10 S. K. Sharma and J. H. Quastel, *Biochem. J.*, 94 (1965) 790.
11 Y. Nose, A. Iwashima, and H. Nishino, in C. J. Gubler, M. Fujiwara, and P. M. Dreyfus, *Thiamine*, John Wiley & Sons, New York, 1976, p. 157.
12 T. Komai and H. Shindo, *J. Vitaminol.*, 18 (1972) 55.
13 T. Komai, K. Kawai, and H. Shindo, *J. Nutr. Sci. Vitaminol.*, 20 (1974) 163.
14 Y. Itokawa and J. R. Cooper, *Biochim. Biophys. Acta*, 196 (1970) 274.
15 H. Koike and T. Yusa, *Methods Enzymol.*, 18A (1970) 105.
16 W. Boos, *Annu. Rev. Biochem.*, 43 (1974) 123.
17 T. Nishimune and R. Hayashi, *Biochim. Biophys. Acta*, 244 (1971) 573.
18 A. Matsuura, A. Iwashima, and Y. Nose, *Biochem. Biophys. Res. Commun.*, 51 (1973) 241.

19 Y. Nose, A. Iwashima, and A. Nishino, in C. J. Gubler, M. Fujiwara, and P. M. Dreyfus, *Thiamine*, John Wiley & Sons, New York, 1976, p. 105.
20 T. Kawasaki, I. Miyata, and Y. Nose, *Arch. Biochem. Biophys.*, 131 (1969) 231.
21 A. Iwashima, Y. Wakabayashi, and Y. Nose, *Biochim. Biophys. Acta*, 413 (1975) 243.
22 A. Iwashima, Y. Wakabayashi, and Y. Nose, *J. Bacteriol.*, (1977) in press.

METABOLISM OF FLAVINS

JUN OKUDA*1 AND KUNIO YAGI*2

*Department of Clinical Biochemistry, Faculty of Pharmacy, Meijo University**1 *and Institute of Biochemistry, Faculty of Medicine, University of Nagoya,**2 *Nagoya (Japan)*

Biochemical significance of an essential nutrient, riboflavin, is mainly ascribed to its coenzyme action after it is synthesized to FMN or FAD. Accordingly, the metabolism of flavins, especially the biosynthesis of flavin coenzymes in mammals, is important in both biochemical and nutritional viewpoints. For this reason, we have been working on this problem soon after the device of a method for separating determination of flavin nucleotides in mammalian tissues.[1] Later, isotope-labeled flavin aided to reveal the metabolism of flavins by observing exchange between administered flavin for pre-existing one. The data obtained in this line of experiments are documented in this communication.

BIOSYNTHESIS OF FLAVIN NUCLEOTIDES IN MAMMALIAN TISSUES

To elucidate the mode of biosynthesis of flavin nucleotides in mammals, [isoalloxazine-2-^{14}C]riboflavin (Radiochemical Centre, Amersham) was injected into a rat, and 1 hr after the injection, the radioactivity of flavins in each tissue was analyzed. As shown in Table I, the radioactivity was highest in the kidney, followed by the small intestine, liver, heart, stomach, spleen, and muscle.[2]

Then, the distribution of radioactivity and the specific radioactivity of flavin nucleotides in three organs, the kidney, small intestine, and liver, were measured. As shown in Table II, radioactive riboflavin was incorporated into both FMN and FAD in the kidney,

TABLE I

RADIOACTIVITY OF FLAVIN IN VARIOUS TISSUES AFTER THE ADMINISTRATION OF [^{14}C]RIBOFLAVIN

47.4 μmol (17.8 mg)/kg of [^{14}C]riboflavin (specific radioactivity: 3.7 cpm/nmol) was injected subcutaneously into a rat. One hr after the injection, the tissues were taken. The total amount of flavins is expressed in terms of riboflavin.

Tissues	*Total flavin* ($\mu g/g$)	*Radioactivity* (cpm/g)
Kidney	62.8	2,950
Small intestine	25.2	2,550
Liver	47.6	1,390
Heart	24.2	490
Stomach	5.95	230
Spleen	6.40	220
Muscle	2.38	120

TABLE II

INCORPORATION OF [^{14}C]RIBOFLAVIN INTO FLAVINS IN THE KIDNEY, LIVER, AND SMALL INTESTINE

540 μmol (20.3 mg)/kg of [^{14}C]riboflavin (specific radioactivity: 128.6 cpm/nmol) was injected subcutaneously into a rat. One hr after the injection, the organs were taken. The amount of each flavin is expressed in terms of riboflavin.

Tissues	*Distribution of radioactivity* (%)			*Specific radioactivity* (*cpm/nmol*)		
	FAD	*FMN*	*Riboflavin*	*FAD*	*FMN*	*Riboflavin*
Kidney	39.3	28.5	32.2	8.68	22.29	23.01
Liver	47.2	25.0	27.8	5.11	17.63	28.57
Small intestine	12.9	19.5	67.6	17.67	45.38	66.05

TABLE III

INCORPORATION OF [^{14}C]RIBOFLAVIN INTO FLAVIN NUCLEOTIDES IN PERFUSED LIVER OF RAT

The amount of each flavin is expressed in terms of riboflavin.

Flavin	*Before perfusion*	*After perfusion (1 hr)*	
	μg/g	*μg/g*	*cpm/μg*
FAD	19.1	19.6	2,090
FMN	6.5	9.3	2,830
Riboflavin	2.9	2.6	10,700

liver, and small intestine.[2] This result definitely indicates that FMN and FAD can be synthesized from riboflavin in mammalian body. However, it is not certain whether the biosynthesis was carried out in each organ. To check the possibility of the coenzyme synthesis in each organ, a perfusion experiment using an isolated liver was made. The liver isolated from a rat was perfused with 1.5 times diluted 100 ml of rat blood containing 100 μg of [isoalloxazine-2-^{14}C]riboflavin for 1 hr by using the apparatus described by Katz *et al.*[3] After the perfusion, 58.6% and 5.3% of the original radioactivity were found in the liver and in the bile collected, respectively. Flavin in the bile was found to be riboflavin, which is circulated through so-called entero-hepatic circulation.[4] Then, flavins in the perfused liver were analyzed, and radioactivity was found to be incorporated into FAD, FMN in the liver as shown in Table III.[5] This indicates that the biosynthesis of flavin nucleotides from riboflavin occurs in each organ.

Considering that each organ can synthesize flavin coenzymes from riboflavin, the data shown in Table II are interpreted. From the table, it can be seen that radioactivities in riboflavin, FMN, and FAD in these organs are different from each other, but it is common in each organ that the order of the specific radioactivities is: riboflavin>FMN>FAD. This means that the process of biosynthesis is: riboflavin→FMN→FAD.

Now a question arises whether or not FMN and FAD synthesized can be transported from one organ to another. For this purpose, incorporation of radioactivity into riboflavin, FMN, and FAD of the liver of mouse after the injection of the double-labeled [isoalloxazine-2-^{14}C, ^{32}P]FMN or [isoalloxazine-2-^{14}C,adenine-2,8-^{14}C]FAD was studied.[6]

Ninety min after the injection of [isoalloxazine-2-^{14}C, ^{32}P]FMN into a mouse, radioactivity of each flavin in the liver was analyzed. [^{14}C]Radioactivity in the isoalloxazine part of the injected [isoalloxazine-2-^{14}C, ^{32}P]FMN was found to be incorporated markedly

TABLE IV

INCORPORATION OF ^{14}C AND ^{32}P RADIOACTIVITIES INTO FLAVIN NUCLEOTIDES IN THE LIVER OF MOUSE UPON INJECTION OF DOUBLE-LABELED [^{14}C, ^{32}P]FMN

Double-labeld [^{14}C, ^{32}P]FMN (25 μg in terms of riboflavin) was injected in to a mouse. Specific radioactivities of the isoalloxazine nucleus and phosphorus in injected [^{14}C, ^{32}P]FMN were 104.2 cpm/nmol (F-^{14}C) and 254.6 cpm/nmol (P-^{32}P) respectively.

Flavin	Specific radioactivity			
	F-^{14}C		*P-^{32}P*	
	cpm/nmol	*%**	*cpm/nmol*	*%**
FAD	9.5	9.1	0.62	0.24
FMN	26.57	25.5	0.97	0.38
Riboflavin	81.5	78.2	—	

*Per cent of specific radioactivity found to that of injected [^{14}C, ^{32}P]FMN.

TABLE V

INCORPORATION OF ^{14}C RADIOACTIVITIES INTO FLAVIN NUCLEOTIDES IN THE LIVER OF MOUSE UPON INJECTION OF DOUBLE-LABELED [^{14}C]FAD

Double-labeled [^{14}C]FAD (25 μg in terms of riboflavin) was injected into a mouse. Specific radioactivities of the isoalloxazine and adenine nuclei in injected [^{14}C]FAD were 251.0 cpm/nmol (F-^{14}C) and 407.9 cpm/nmol (A-^{14}C) respectively.

Flavin	Specific radioactivity			
	F-^{14}C		*A-^{14}C*	
	cpm/nmol	*%**	*cpm/nmol*	*%**
FAD	28.28	11.3	7.51	1.84
FMN	57.98	23.1	—	
Riboflavin	170.30	67.8	—	

*Per cent of specific radioactivity found to that of injected [^{14}C]FAD.

into FMN and FAD in the liver, while incorporation of [^{32}P]radioactivity of the injected double-labeled FMN into flavin nucleotides was almost negligible, as shown in Table IV. In the case of double-labeled FAD, radioactivity in the isoalloxazine part of the injected [isoalloxazine-2-^{14}C,adenine-2,8-^{14}C]FAD was also markedly incorporated into FMN and FAD in the liver, however, only small amounts of the adenine part of double-labeled FAD was incorporated into FAD of the liver, as can be seen in Table V.

These results indicate that the injected FMN and FAD are easily hydrolyzed and resynthesized so that the phosphorus and the adenine moiety of the double-labeled FMN and FAD were diluted with cold phosphorus and adenine in the liver.

As it is well known that FAD of succinate dehydrogenase, monoamine oxidase, and sarcosine dehydrogenase bind covalently with the protein at 8α-position of the isoalloxazine nucleus, we studied the incorporation of [^{14}C]riboflavin into the covalently bound flavins in the liver of rat. After the injection of 1 mg/kg body weight of [^{14}C]riboflavin into a rat, the radioactivities of both dissociable and covalently bound flavins in the liver were analyzed. The liver homogenate (10%) was heated at 80°, and the precipitate was washed firstly with 5% trichloroacetic acid and then with acetone, and subjected to the determination of radioactivity of covalently bound flavin. As shown in Fig. 1, the incorporation of the radioactivity into covalently bound flavin was already detectable 30 min

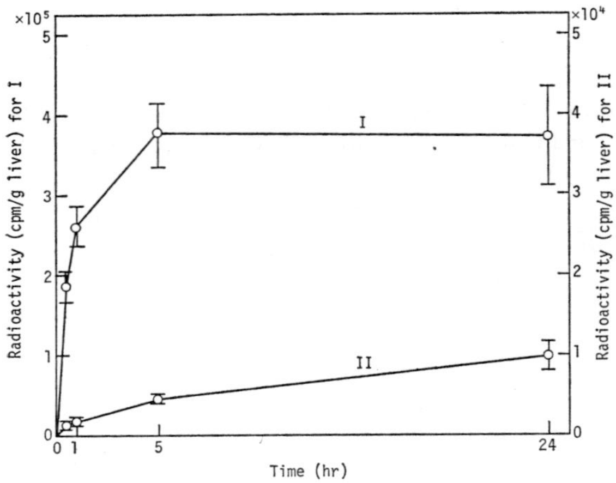

Fig. 1. Incorporation of radioactive riboflavin into flavins in rat liver. One mg/kg body weight of [2-^{14}C] riboflavin (specific radioactivity: 76.4 μCi/mg) dissolved in 0.9% NaCl (200 μg/ml) was injected into a rat through a tail vein. Curve I, radioactivity of total flavins; curve II, radioactivity of covalently bound flavins. Vertical bars show S.D.

after the injection. Twenty four hr after the injection, 2.7% of total radioactivity in the liver was found in the covalently bound flavins.[7] These results seem to indicate that riboflavin is rapidly synthesized to FAD *via* FMN and FAD thus formed combines with protein *via* covalent linkage.

EXCHANGE OF FLAVINS IN HIGHER ANIMALS

As another approach to the mode of metabolism of flavins in animal body, we studied the exchange of flavins in the whole animal.

[^{14}C]Riboflavin (80 μg) was administered *per os* daily to a mouse, and the specific radioactivity of flavins in the liver was analyzed.[8] Under this condition, half life of turnover of flavins in the liver was estimated to be 5–6 days and the radioactivity reached a plateau on 15th day, and specific radioactivity reached nearly to that of riboflavin administered (Fig. 2). Then, we stopped the administration of riboflavin by feeding the animal with riboflavin-deficient diet. The specific radioactivity gradually came down. This phenomenon means that the radioactive flavins in the liver are replaced for flavins synthesized by intestinal flora. McCormick also reported that the half life of turnover of flavins in the liver was 16 days when rat was administered with lesser amount of [^{14}C]riboflavin (55 μg of [^{14}C]riboflavin/100 g of body weight).[9] These data show that turnover of flavins in the liver depends on the amount of riboflavin administered.

As detailed in the previous section, administered riboflavin is synthesized to coenzymes and the coenzymes thus formed are exchanged for the coenzymes bound to apoenzymes in the cells. Thus, the following equilibria occur in mammals:

$$\begin{array}{ccccc} \text{Riboflavin} & \rightleftarrows & \text{FMN} & \rightleftarrows & \text{FAD} \\ & & \updownarrow{+E} & & \updownarrow{+E} \\ & & \text{E}\cdot\text{FMN} & & \text{E}\cdot\text{FAD} \end{array}$$

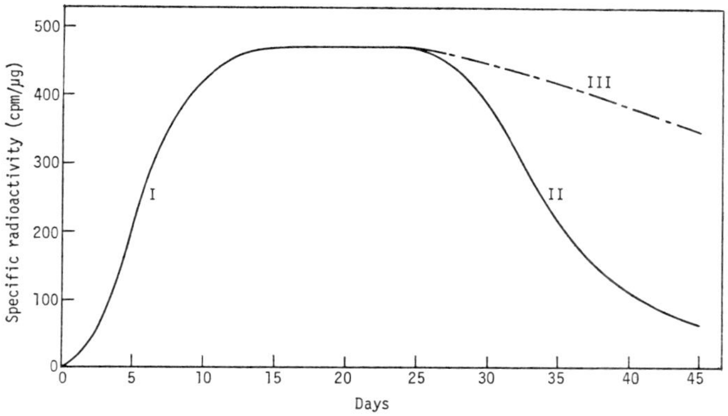

Fig. 2. Turnover of flavins in the liver of mouse administered with [^{14}C]riboflavin per os. Curve I, specific radioactivity in the liver of mouse administered with 80 μg/day of [2-^{14}C]riboflavin daily for 25 days; curve II, specific radioactivity in the liver of mouse administered with 80 μg/day of non-radioactive riboflavin daily after curve I; curve III, specific radioactivity in the liver of mouse administered with riboflavin-deficient diet after curve I.

where E represents apoenzyme. From these equilibria, it is obvious that the rate of exchange of coenzyme of individual flavin enzyme depends on the amount of free coenzyme coexisting and the rate constants of dissociation and association of flavin enzyme. Therefore, it is understandable that the administration of larger amount of riboflavin shortens the half life of turnover of flavins. Considering that covalently bound flavins are very minute compared to dissociable flavins, turnover of flavins in mammals seems to be largely regulated by association and dissociation of flavin enzyme as follows:

$$\mathrm{EF} \underset{k_2}{\overset{k_1}{\rightleftharpoons}} \mathrm{E}+\mathrm{F}$$

where E, F, and EF represent apoenzyme, flavin coenzyme, and holoenzyme, respectively. For better understanding of the regulatory mechanism of the turnover of flavin, D-amino acid oxidase and β-D-glucose oxidase were studied as model systems.[10]

The exchange of free FAD for bound FAD of D-amino acid oxidase was examined by using [^{14}C]FAD. To minimize the counting error of radioactivities of both free and bound FAD, the same amount of radioactive free FAD as that of FAD in the enzyme was added. After incubation for a definite time, the decrease of the radioactivity of free FAD was measured. It was found that the exchange reaction was very rapid ($t_{1/2}$=0.7 min at 37°). However, the exchange reaction became very slow in the presence of the substrate or the inhibitor, benzoate. If such an effect of a substrate, as seen in the case of D-amino acid oxidase, occurs in the living body, the coenzyme will be exchanged more slowly in the presence of the substrate, and *vice versa* in the deficiency of the substrate, *i.e.* on starvation.

On the other hand, the exchange reaction in β-D-glucose oxidase was found to be very slow. The rate was so slow that the effect of the substrate, β-D-glucose, or an inhibitor, *p*-chloromercuribenzoate was not clear. The values of k_1 and k_2 in these two flavin enzymes calculated from the values of half life of exchange, and dissociation constants of flavin

TABLE VI

EXCHANGE OF FREE FAD FOR BOUND FAD IN FLAVIN ENZYME

Dissociation constant for D-amino acid oxidase was obtained by fluorescence polarization at the concentration of 4×10^{-5} M.[11] Dissociation constant for β-D-glucose oxidase was obtained from equilibrium analysis.

Enzyme	*Temperature* (°C)	$t_{1/2}$	K (M)	k_1 (min^{-1})	k_2 ($M^{-1}\ min^{-1}$)
D-Amino acid oxidase	37	0.7 min	2.1×10^{-7}	5.0×10^{-1}	2.4×10^{6}
β-D-Glucose oxidase	5	400 hr	1.3×10^{-10}	1.4×10^{-5}	1.1×10^{5}

enzymes are shown in Table VI. It is of interest that the great difference in the half life between these two enzymes is mostly ascribed to the difference in k_1 values.

In conclusion, we summarize our data as follows: 1) Riboflavin administered to mammals is synthesized to FAD *via* FMN in each organ; 2) FAD and FMN injected into mammals are rapidly hydrolyzed to riboflavin and resynthesized to these coenzymes; 3) incorporation of riboflavin into covalently bound flavin is slow; 4) the rate of exchange of free flavin for flavin bound to protein depends on the amount of free flavin, the rate constants of association and dissociation, and the presence of substrate or inhibitor; 5) the rate of exchange in a whole animal depends mainly on the amount of riboflavin administered.

REFERENCES

1 K. Yagi, *J. Biochem.*, 38 (1951) 161.
2 K. Yagi, T. Nagatsu, I. Nagatsu-Ishibashi, and A. Ohashi, *J. Biochem.*, 59 (1966) 313.
3 J. Katz, G. Bonorris, S. Okuyama, and A. L. Sellers, *Am. J. Physiol.*, 212 (1967) 1255.
4 K. Yagi, K. Kato, and S. Kikuchi, *Vitamins*, 7 (1954) 128.
5 K. Yagi, S. Okuyama, and J. Okuda, *J. Nutr. Sci. Vitaminol.*, 24 (1978) 551.
6 J. Okuda, J. Nagamine, M. Okumura, and K. Yagi, *J. Nutr. Sci. Vitaminol.*, 24 (1978) 505.
7 K. Yagi, Y. Nakagawa, O. Suzuki, and N. Ohishi, *J. Biochem.*, 79 (1976) 841.
8 K. Yagi, O. Terada, M. Kobayashi, and J. Okuda, *Vitamins*, 36 (1967) 209.
9 D. B. McCormick, *J. Biol. Chem.*, 237 (1962) 959.
10 J. Okuda, J. Nagamine, and K. Yagi, *Biochim. Biophys. Acta*, 566 (1979) 245.
11 F. Tanaka and K. Yagi, Biochemistry, in press.

STRUCTURAL STUDIES OF FLAVOPROTEINS

KERRY T. YASUNOBU AND MASARU TANAKA
Department of Biochemistry-Biophysics, University of Hawaii, Honolulu, Hawaii (U.S.A.)

In 1970, Hemmerich *et al.*[1] surveyed the various flavoproteins of known function and noted that there were 45 different flavoproteins. Probably a few new flavoproteins have been discovered since that time. The various flavoproteins can be classified as oxidases, dehydrogenases, hydroxylases, or electron transferases.[2] However, very little is known about the structures of the flavoproteins with the exception of flavodoxin which have recently been under intensive investigation. An excellent review article on flavodoxin which covers the period up to 1975 by Mayhew and Ludwig has appeared.[3] The objective of this article is to review the research on flavodoxin since 1975 as well as to discuss the status of structural studies of flavoproteins, in general.

GROUP I AND GROUP II FLAVODOXINS

Group I flavodoxins cannot replace the FMN by riboflavin while the group II flavodoxins can use either FMN or riboflavin.[4] The group II flavodoxin from *Azotobacter vinelandii* is also unique in that it forms a very stable semiquinone at pH 7.0.[5] From this point onwards, let us focus our attention on the structural studies of the *A. vinelandii* flavodoxin.

AMINO ACID COMPOSITION OF *Azotobacter* FLAVODOXIN

These data are summarized in Table I and includes the amino acid composition of the other flavodoxins for comparative purposes. The molecular weights and the amino acid residues in the group I flavodoxins range from about 15,000–16,000 daltons and 137–148 amino acid residues, respectively.[6] The groupII flavodoxins have molecular weights of about 21,000 daltons and contains 179–181 amino acid residues. In keeping with the acidic nature of the flavodoxins, there are an excess of acidic (23–25%) over the basic residues (8–10%). Also, the *A. vinelandii* flavodoxin as well as some other flavodoxins contain no histidine residues which have been shown to be active site residues in hydrolytic enzymes[7] and metalloproteins.[8] Although there are 1–5 cysteine residues, they appear to be non-essential for activity. They contain 1–5 methionine residues and in some flavodoxins, one of the methionine residues is within van der Waals contact region with the isoalloxazine ring of FMN.[3] Since tyrosine and tryptophan residues are within van der Waals contact region with the isoalloxazine ring of FMN on the outer surface of flavodoxin, all flavodoxins contain 3–6 tryptophan residues and 2–8 tyrosine residues.[6] There are a slight excess of

TABLE I

AMINO ACID COMPOSITIONS OF PURIFIED FLAVODOXINS

	C.p.	*C.m.*	*P.e.*	*D.v.*	*D.g.*	*E.c.*	*S.l.*	*C.f.*	*R.r.*	*A.v.*	*A.n.*
Lys	10	10	9	4	8	7	5	12	9	12	9
Trp	4	3	4	2	1	6	3	4	3	3	6
His	0	0	0	1	0	3	1	4	1	0	0
Arg	2	2	2	7	3	3	4	4	8	5	2
Asp	18	17	15	19	17	13–14	22	28	25	20	28
Thr	4	5	8	7	9	6	8	14	16	8	8
Ser	14	8	7	8	8	4	4	11	11	15	12
Glu	19	21	17	16	18	16–17	25	22	16	21	26
Pro	4	3	5	3	6	3	4	5	7	5	3
Gly	17	14	14	18	14	11	19	25	28	20	19
Ala	14	6	18	17	15	11	15	24	20	14	12
Cys	1	3	2	4	5	3	2	5	2	1	1
Val	15	10	13	9	16	5	6	17	15	10	11
Met	4	5	5	1	2	1	1	4	2	1	1
Ile	5	15	5	9	5	9	12	9	10	6	13
Leu	12	8	7	12	14	10	12	18	22	20	13
Tyr	2	3	2	5	5	4	7	5	9	5	8
Phe	3	5	4	6	3	5	9	5	6	13	9
Total	148	138	137	148	149	122	154	216	210	179	181
Mol. wt.	14,600	16,050	15,000	16,000	16,000	14,500	17,000	22,000	22,800	23,000	21,000

C.p., *Clostridium pasteurianum*; C.m., *Clostridium MP.*; P.e., *Peptostreptococcus elsdenii;* D.v., *Desulfovibrio vulgaris*; D.g., *Desulfovibrio gigas*; E.c., *Eschericha coli*; S.l., *Synechococcus lividus*; C.f., *Chlorella fusca*; R.r., *Rhodospirillum rubrum*; A.v., *Azotobacter vinelandii*; A.n., *Anacystis nidulans.*

hydrophilic residues (over 50%) over other types of residues. The *Azotobacter* flavodoxin itself contains 179 residues and has a calculated molecular weight of about 20,800 and although the amino acid composition is similar to the other flavodoxins, it contains only one cysteine residue and one methionine residue,[9] neither of which appears to be essential.[3]

AMINO ACID SEQUENCE OF *Azotobacter* FLAVODOXIN

Figure 1 shows the amino acid sequences of all of the flavodoxins whose sequences have been determined including the *Azotobacter* flavodoxin whose sequence has just been reported.[9] Other flavodoxins sequences shown include the *Desulfovibrio vulgaris,*[10] *Clostridium MP*[11] and the *Peptostreptococcus elsdenii* flavodoxins.[12] The NH_2 terminal sequences of the *Clostridium pasteurianum,*[13,14] *Rhodospirillum rubrum*[15] and the *Anacystis nidulans* flavodoxins[16] are also shown since they contain the FMN-binding regions.

The alignment of the various proteins and the insertion of gaps were based on the crystal X-ray diffraction data of the *C. MP*[17] and the *D. vulgaris* flavodoxin[18,19] which is shown in Fig. 2 and the calculated conformation of the *A. vinelandii* flavodoxin. In general, the sequence of the flavodoxins are not nearly as constant as the sequences of cytochrome *c*,[20] ferredoxin,[21] and rubredoxin[22] from different sources. The few constant regions include residues 10–15, 19, 22, 62, 90–97, and residues 112. Residues 10–15 contain the

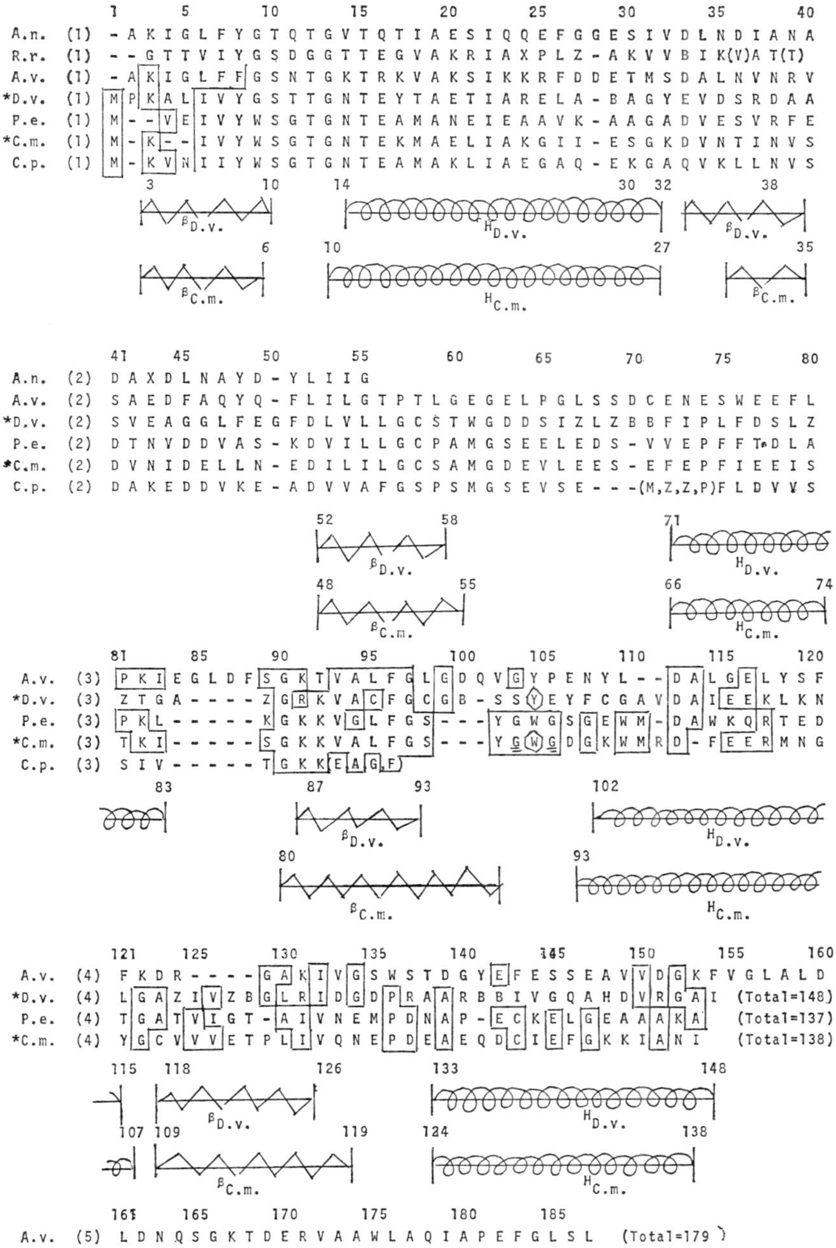

Fig. 1. A.n., R.r., A.v., D.v., P. e., C.m., and C.p. are abbreviations for *A. nidulans*, *R. rubrum*, *A. vinelandii*, *D. vulgaris*, *P. elsdenii*, *C. MP*, and *C. pasteurianum*, respectively. Also, -, stands for gaps inserted to produce maximum homology of sequences. The symbols -WWW- and -ꝏꝏ- indicate β-pleated sheet and α-helical regions determined from crystal X-ray diffraction studies.[17,19] The numbers above the secondary structures refer to actual residues numbers in the proteins. Identical sequences are blocked off.

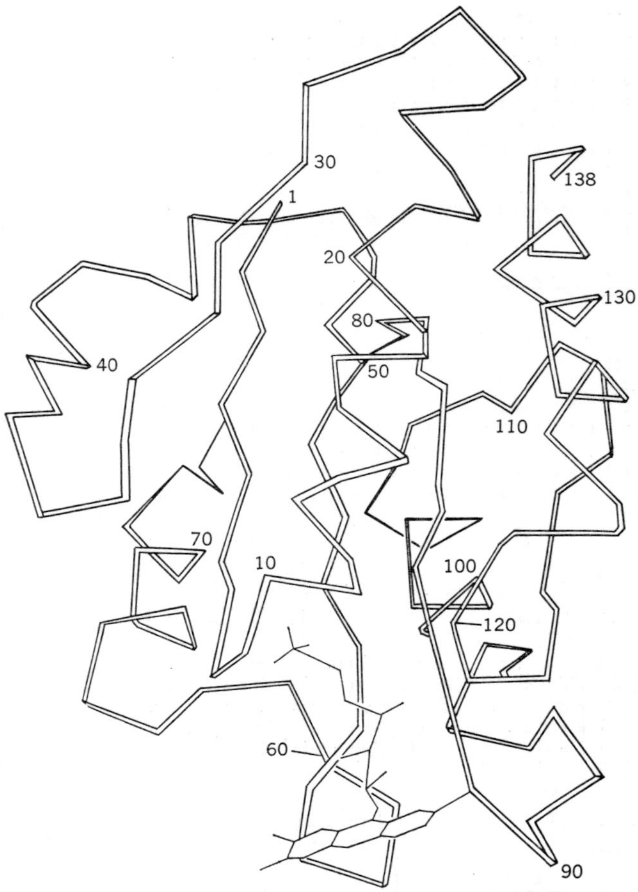

Fig. 2. The α-C configuration of the *C. MP* flavodoxin[17]. The FMN-binding site is shown at the bottom of the figure.

phosphate-binding site of FMN and residues 90–97 precedes the isoalloxazine-binding region.

As shown in Fig. 1, a number of gaps must be inserted in the NH_2-terminal regions since the phosphate-binding regions (FMN) must be in register. Gaps in the group I flavodoxins are introduced at residues 28, 50, 70, 83–87, 99–101 since the *Azotobacter* flavodoxin is longer and also to get residue 104, the residue which is possibly π-bonded to the isoalloxazine ring, in register as well as to maintain the secondary conformation constant for all the various flavodoxins. Finally a gap in the *Azotobacter* flavodoxin is inserted at residues 125–128, when the sequence is compared with the group I flavodoxins again to keep the secondary conformation of the various flavodoxins as constant as possible. The most noteworthy feature of the *Azotobacter* flavodoxin sequence is the presence of a 33–34 residue COOH-terminal extension which is absent in group I flavodoxins.

CALCULATED CONFORMATION OF THE *Azotobacter* FLAVODOXIN

A major goal of flavodoxin research is to determine the 3D structure of a group II flavodoxin of molecular weight 21,000. How does its structure differ from the *D. vulgaris*[18] and the *C. MP*[19] flavodoxin whose 3D structures have been determined? The *Azotobacter* flavodoxin, molecular weight of 20,800 daltons, has just been sequenced,[9] and we have used the Chou-Fasman procedure[23] to calculate conformation from sequence data. The predicted conformational data are shown in Table II and its comparison with the *D. vulgaris* and the *C. MP* flavodoxin is shown in Fig. 1. Starting from the NH_2-terminal end of the *A. vinelandii* flavodoxin, the β_1 and α_1 and $\beta_{b\text{-}1}$ are predicted to be nearly identical in all of the flavodoxins which have been sequenced, except for the shortening of the α_1 region by a few residues. The β_2 region starts earlier by 3–4 residues and stops earlier by 3–4 residues when compared with the *D. vulgaris* and the *C. MP* flavodoxins and is followed by $\beta_{b\text{-}2}$ which is absent in the other flavodoxins whose 3D structures are known. This area is followed by $\beta_{b\text{-}3}$ which is not present in the other two flavodoxins. The β_3 region is predicted to start several residues earlier than the *D. vulgaris* or *C. MP* flavodoxins but is predicted to end in at the same point as the *C. MP* flavodoxin. Then the $\beta_{b\text{-}4}$ and the $\beta_{b\text{-}5}$ bend regions follow which then leads to the α_2 region. (The NH_2-terminal regions of the flavodoxins are in register in all three flavodoxins. However, it is predicted that the COOH-terminal region of α_2 in the *Azotobacter* flavodoxin is 3 residues longer than the other two flavodoxins. This region is followed by $\beta_{b\text{-}4}$ which is absent in the *D. vulgaris* or *C. MP* flavodoxins). Then a $\beta_{b\text{-}6}$ bend is predicted to follow which is then

TABLE II

CALCULATED CONFORMATION OF THE *Azotobacter* FLAVODOXIN

Designation	*Residue No.*		
	α-Helical	*β-Sheets*	*β-Bends*
β_1		1–8	
$\beta_{b\text{-}1}$			9–12
α_1	13–28		
β_2		29–34	
$\beta_{b\text{-}2}$			35–38
$\beta_{b\text{-}3}$			44–47
β_3		48–57	
$\beta_{b\text{-}4}$			61–64
$\beta_{b\text{-}5}$			66–69
α_2	70–84		
$\beta_{b\text{-}6}$			85–88
β_4		89–101	
$\beta_{b\text{-}7}$			102–105
α_3	106–118		
β_5		119–125	
α_4	130–139		
β_6		140–154	
$\beta_{b\text{-}8}$			155–158
α_5	161–166		
β_7		170–179	

followed by the α_3 helical region and the conformation of all three flavodoxins under comparison are again in register. This area is then followed by the α_4 helix which is predicted to have an NH_2-terminal region which starts one residue earlier than the *D. vulgaris* and *C. MP* flavodoxin and which terminates 6–7 residues earlier than in the other two flavodoxins due to the adjacent β_6 pleated sheet region which leads then into the COOH-terminal extension region which is not present in the *D. vulgaris* and the *C. MP* flavodoxins. The predicted conformation of the COOH-terminal extension contains in order a β_{b-3} region, an α-helical α_5 region and finally a β_7 region. Thus, it is predicted that the group II flavodoxins with molecular weights of about 21,000 have conformations very similar but not identical to the *D. vulgaris* and *C. MP* flavodoxins. The three flavodoxins all have the basic structures which include 5 centrally located β-pleated sheet regions flanked by 2 α-helices on each side of this region and which contain an FMN-binding site at one side of the β-pleated sheet region.[18,19] However, there is COOH-terminal extension in the *A. vinelandii* flavodoxin which is absent in the group I flavodoxins.

ACTIVE SITE COMPARISON OF THE *Azotobacter* FLAVODOXIN

For reference purposes, the residues involved in binding of FMN (ref. 3) are summarized in Table III. The N-terminal region which is involved chiefly in H-bonding with the phosphate of FMN is underlined in Fig. 1. Ser-7 is constant in the *Azotobacter*, *D. vulgaris*, and the *C. MP* flavodoxins and the –OH group is H-bonded to the oxygen of

TABLE III
THE FMN-PROTEIN CONTACTS IN THE *C. MP* FLAVODOXIN*

FMN atom	*Protein or solvent atom*	*FMN atom*	*Protein or solvent atom*
O-I	Gly-8 NH	O′-3	W-2
	Ser-54 OH		W-3
	W-1		
O-II	Ser-7 OH	O′-4	Ser-87 OH
	Thr-12 NH		Asn-11 (NH_2,O)
	Asn-11 NH		Asn-119 (NH_2,O)
	Thr-12 OH		
	Gly-8 NH	N-1	Gly-89 NH
O-III	Thr-9 OH	O-2	Gly-91 NH
	Thr-9 OH		Gly-89 NH
	Gly-10 NH		Trp-90 NH
	Asn-11 NH		W-4
	Ser-7 OH		
	Asn-11 (NH_2,O)	N-3	Glu-59 COO^-
	Gly-8 NH		
		O-4	Glu-59 NH
O′-2	W-2		Asp-58 NH
	W-3		
		N-5	Asp-58 NH

* From Mayhew and Ludwig.[3] The O-(roman numeral) and O′stands for the phosphate oxygen atoms and the oxygen of the ribitol side chain, respectively. The N and O stands for the atoms in the isoalloxazine ring of the FMN. W stands for water.

one of the phosphate ion. Residue 8 is Asn, Thr, and Gly, respectively in the *Azotobacter*, *D. vulgaris*, and *C. MP* flavodoxins; since it is the NH– of this residue which is H-bonded to the oxygen of the phosphate of FMN, it appears that this residue can be variable. The same applies to Thr-9 and Gly-10, since its NH group is H-bonded to one of the oxygen atoms of the phosphate anion. Asn-11 in the *C. MP* and *D. vulgaris* flavodoxins is replaced by a lysine residue in the *Azotobacter* flavodoxin. It would seem that again the –NH– of this residue is also H-bonded to the phosphate oxygen. However, the presence of a positively charged ε-NH_2 group has been suggested to account for the stability of the semiquinone of the *Azotobacter* flavodoxin,[3] but we have not examined this point in the structural model of the protein. Thr-12 in all three proteins is conserved since there is a H-bond between the –OH group and the oxygen of the phosphate residue of FMN. Ser-54 is constant in the *A. vinelandii* and *C. MP* flavodoxin and the –OH group of the serine is H-bonded to the oxygen of the phosphate of FMN. Ala-55 in the *C. MP* flavodoxin is replaced by a glycine residue but this appears possible since the CO-group of this residue is again H-bonded to the oxygen of the phosphate of the FMN. The NH-group of Asp-58 is H-bonded to the oxygen atom of phosphate of FMN and is replaced by Glu in the *Azotobacter* flavodoxin. The Glu-59 $-COO^-$ is H-bonded to N-3 of the isoalloxazine ring of the FMN and its NH-group is H-bonded to one of the oxygen of the phosphate of FMN. Since this residue in the *Azotobacter* flavodoxin is proposed to be Leu, it would be predicted that the $-COO^-$ interaction is missing in the *Azotobacter* protein and therefore the FMN-binding site is different in this respect. According to the proposed alignment of sequences, Gly-89 of the *C. MP* flavodoxin is H-bonded to the N-1 of the isoalloxazine ring of the FMN-and this interaction would also be possible in the *A. vinelandii* flavodoxin. Glycine 91 in the *C. MP* flavodoxin contributes its peptide-NH group for H-bonding with N-1 of the isoalloxazine ring of the FMN. The comparable residue in the *A. vinelandii* flavodoxin is a proline residue which differs greatly because it is a secondary amine. The carbonyl and $-NH_2$ of the β-amide group of Asn-119 in the *C. MP* flavodoxin may or may not be H-bonded to the oxygen atom of C-4-OH of the ribityl side residue of FMN and is replaced by a Gly residue in the *Azotobacter* flavodoxin which is another difference in the FMN-binding site in these two proteins. Also, two residues are reported to within van der Waals radii on opposite sides of the planar isoalloxazine ring. These are residues 90 (Trp) in the *C. MP* protein and residue 98 (Tyr) in the *D. vulgaris* protein. In the *P. elsdenii* flavodoxin, a Trp residue is in an analogous position. These aromatic residues are present on the surface of the protein and may shuttle electrons into the isoalloxazine ring. The other residue which is on the opposite site, namely the interior of the protein, is a methionine residue-56 in the *C. MP* flavodoxin, the *C. pasteurianum* and *P. elsdenii* proteins, and a Trp residue in the *D. vulgaris* flavodoxin. However, this residue is predicted to be a Glu residue in the *Azotobacter* flavodoxin which may or may not account for the occurrence of the very stable semiquinone of the *A. vinelandii* flavodoxin. The comments concerning the active site and conformation of the *Azotobacter* flavodoxin are very speculative but are presented in this article without reservation since Dr. Ludwig's group at the University of Michigan have just resolved the 3D structure of *Anacystis nidulans*,[24] a group II flavodo xin of high molecular weight, to the 2.8 Å level of resolution. The *A. vinelandii* and the *A. nidulans* flavodoxins appear to be very similar structurally (see Fig. 1, Table I).

DISTRIBUTION OF HYDROPHOBIC, NEUTRAL, AND IONIC RESIDUES

Flavodoxin in its natural environment interacts with other proteins such as the NADP+ ferredoxin reductase[25] to form complexes. Armed with a knowledge of the 3D structure and the suggestion that the interaction with the reductase may be ionic,[25] we have looked for constant highly ionic regions in the sequence shown in Fig. 3. But such regions were distant from the FMN-binding site. Besides, there is the possibility that during complex formation conformational changes occur which would alter the distribution of ionic groups. Constant hydrophobic regions tended to occur in β-pleated sheet

```
             1       5         10        15        20        25        30        35       40
R.r.   (1)   - - H N N H H A H N A H H N N A H H H B B H A X H H Z - H B H H B H B H H N N
A.n.   (1)   - H B H H H H N H N N N A H N N N H H A N H N N A H H H A N H H A H N A H H N H
A.v.   (1)   - H B H H H H N H N N N H B N B B H H B N H B B B H A A A N H N A H H N H N B H
*D.v.  (1)   H H B H H H H A H N N N H N N A N N H A N H H B A H H - B H H N A H A N B A H H
P.e.   (1)   H - - H A H H A H N H N H N N A H H H N A H A H H H B - H H H H A H A N H B H A
*C.m.  (1)   H - B - - H H A H N H N H N N A B H H A H H H B H H H - A N H B A H N N H N H N
C.p.   (1)   H - B H N H H A H N H N H N N A H H H B H H H A H H N - A B H H N H B H H N H N
             |<-- β1 -->|  |<β b-1>|<----------- α1 ------------>|<β b-2>|<-- β2 -->|<β b-3-

             41    45        50        55        60        65        70        75        80
A.n.   (2)   A H X A H N H N A - N H H H H
A.v.   (2)   N H A A H H N N N - H H H H H N H N H H A H A H H H H N N A N A N A N H A A H H
*D.v.  (2)   N H A H H H H H A H H A H H H H H N N N H H A A N H Z H Z B A H H H H H A N H Z
P.e.   (2)   A N N H A A H H N - B A H H H H H N H H H H N A A H A A N - H H A H H H N A H H
*C.m.  (2)   A N N H A A H H N - A A H H H H H N N H H H A A H H A A N - A H A H H H A A H N
C.p.   (2)   A H B A A A H B A - H A H H H H H N H S H H N E H N A - - -(M,Z,Z,P)H H A H H N
             ->|               |<β b-4>|<-- β3 -->|<β b-4>|   |<-β b-5-->|<------ α2 ------

             81    85        90        95        100       105       110       115       120
A.v.   (3)   H B H A H H A H N H B N H H H H H H A N H H N H A N N H - - A H H H A H N N H
*D.v.  (3)   Z N H H - - - - Z H B B H H N H H N H B - N H N A N H N H H H A H H A A B H B N
P.e.   (3)   H B H - - - - - B H B B H H H H H N - - - N H H H N H A H H - A H H B N B N A A
*C.m.  (3)   N B H - - - - - N H B B H H H H H N - - - N H H H A H B H H B A - H A A B H N H
C.p.   (3)   N H H - - - - - N H B B (E,H,H,H)
             -->|          |<β b-6>|<------ β4 ------>|    |<β b-7>|<------ α3 ---------

             121   125       130       135       140       145       150       155       160
A.v.   (4)   H B A B - - - - H H B H H H N H N N A H N A H A N N A H H H A H B H V G L A L D
*D.v.  (4)   H H H Z H H Z B H H B H A H A H B H H B B B H H H H H B A N B H H H   (Total=148)
P.e.   (4)   N H H N H H H N - H H H N N H H A N H H - A N B A H H A A H H B H     (Total=137)
*C.m.  (4)   N H N H H H A N H H H H N N A H A A H A N A N H A H H B B H H N H     (Total=138)
             ->| |<--- β5 ------>|           |<---------- α5 ---------->|

             161   165       170       175       180       185
A.v.   (5)   H A N A N H B N A A B H H H H H H N H H H A H H H N H  (Total=179)
```

Fig. 3. The distribution of hydrophobic, ionic, and neutral residues in the various flavodoxins sequenced to date as shown in Fig. 1. H stands for hydrophobic residues; A, for acidic residues; B, for basic residues; N, for neutral residues which also includes tyrosine.

regions while the α-helical regions tended to contain ionic residues. The β-bend regions contained hydrophobic, ionic, or neutral residues.

RECENT PROGRESS WITH THE *A. nidulans* FLAVODOXIN

The *A. nidulans* flavodoxin has been crystallized and the preliminary crystal X-ray diffraction studies of the oxidized form of the protein was reported by Dr. M. Ludwig's group at the University of Michigan.[24,26] Recently, several crystalline isomorphous derivatives have been prepared and the structure of the oxidized form has been resolved to the 2.8Å level.[24] Our laboratory has determined the NH_2-terminal sequence of this protein[16] and the results of this analysis are shown in Fig. 1. It should be noted that the *A. nidulans* and *A. vinelandii* flavodoxins, both are group II flavodoxins of high molecular weight and when the crystal X-ray diffraction studies of the *A. nidulans* flavodoxin are completed, useful structural data which will also be applicable to the *A. vinelandii* flavodoxin will become available.

STRUCTURAL STUDIES OF OTHER FLAVOPROTEINS

The recent advancement in the structure determination of flavodoxin has stimulated structural studies of other flavoproteins. Ronchi *et al.*[27] have initiated sequence studies of D-amino acid oxidase, an FAD-enzyme. It was also reported that crystals suitable for X-ray diffraction studies were obtained. Our own laboratory has undertaken the sequence determination of the bovine liver monoamine oxidase (MAO). Our laboratory has recently obtained evidence that the molecular weight of MAO is about 52,000 daltons rather than 110,000 as previously reported.[28] Bovine liver monoamine oxidase contains covalently linked FAD.[29] An active center peptide was isolated by Kearney *et al.*[30,31] and was reported to have the sequence Ser-Gly-Gly-Cys(FAD)-Tyr. When the sequences of these FAD-proteins are completed, it will be very interesting to compare their structures with the FMN-proteins and with the pyridine nucleotide dehydrogenases. Active center peptides which contain cystine residues have been isolated from lipoamide dehydrogenases[32] and glutathione reductase[32] both of which are FAD-enzymes, but complete sequence studies of these proteins are probably not in progress.

CONCLUDING REMARKS

Warburg and Christian, in 1932, characterized the first FMN-protein when they characterized glucose 6-phosphate dehydrogenase.[33] In 1938, they characterized the first FAD-enzyme, D-amino acid oxidase.[34] It was not until 1973 or 41 years later that the first sequence of an FMN-protein (flavodoxin) was determined and the 3D structure solved by crystal X-ray diffraction technique.[18,19] Structure determination of FAD-proteins has only recently been initiated. In the cases of the electron transferases such as flavodoxin, regions of the protein which interact with other protein redox components remain to be elucidated. Possibly the complexes can be crystallized and the structure determined by crystal X-ray diffraction studies. It remains to be shown whether an aromatic residue, on the surafce of flavodoxin, channels electrons into the isoalloxazine ring, but thus far, there is an aromatic residue in each flavodoxin which can be postulated to have sucn a function. The isoalloxazine ring has been shown to be planar in flavodoxin while free flavins have puckered configurations in the semiquinone and reduced states.[3] It will be interesting to see if similar findings are obtained with other flavoproteins of different function. Much research remains to be done on the structure-function studies of the flavoenzymes at the molecular level.

ACKNOWLEDGMENT

The authors are grateful for the support of this research project by Grant GB 43448 from the National Science Foundation and Grant GM 22556 from the National Institutes of Health.

REFERENCES

1 P. HEMMERICH, G. NAGELSCHNEIDER, and C. VEEGER, *FEBS Lett.*, 8 (1970) 69.
2 P. D. BOYER, *The Enzymes*, Academic Press, New York, vol. 12B, 1975, p. 1.
3 S. MAYHEW and M. L. LUDWIG, *The Enzymes*, Academic Press, New York, vol. 12B, 1975, p. 57.
4 D. E. EDMONDSON and G. TOLLIN, *Biochemistry*, 10 (1971) 113.
5 G. TOLLIN and D. E. EDMONDSON, in H. KAMIN, *Flavins and Flavoproteins IIIrd, Int. Symp.*, University Park Press, Baltimore, 1971, p. 153.
6 J. L. FOX, S. S. SMITH, and J. R. BROWN, *Z. Naturforsch.*, B 27 (1972) 1096.
7 D. M. BLOW, in P. D. BOYER, *The Enzymes*, Academic Press, New York, vol. III, 1971, p. 185.
8 H. C. FREEMAN, in G. L. EICHORN, *Inorganic Biochemistry*, Elsevier, Amsterdam, vol. 1, 1973, p. 63.
9 M. TANAKA, M. HANIU, K. T. YASUNOBU, and D. C. YOCH, *Biochemistry*, 16 (1977) 3525.
10 M. DUBOURDIEU, J. LEGALL, and J. L. FOX, *Biochem. Biophys. Res. Commun.*, 52 (1973) 1418.
11 M. TANAKA, M. HANIU, K. T. YASUNOBU, and S. G. MAYHEW, *J. Biol. Chem.*, 249 (1974) 4393.
12 M. TANAKA, M. HANIU, K. T. YASUNOBU, S. G. MAYHEW, and V. MASSEY, *J. Biol. Chem.*, 249 (1974) 4399.
13 M. TANAKA, M. HANIU, G. MATSUEDA, K. T. YASUNOBU, S. G. MAYHEW, and V. MASSEY, *Biochemistry*, 10 (1971) 3041.
14 J. L. FOX, in T. P. SINGER, *Flavins and Flavoproteins*, Elsevier, Amsterdam, 1976, p. 439.
15 M. L. MACKNIGHT, W. R. GRAY, and G. TOLLIN, *Biochem. Biophys. Res. Commun.*, 59 (1974) 630.
16 M. TANAKA, M. HANIU, K. T. YASUNOBU, and M. L. LUDWIG, unpublished results.
17 R. M. BURNETT, G. D. DARLING, D. S. KENDALL, M. E. LEQUESNE, S. G. MAYHEW, W. W. SMITH, and M. L. LUDWIG, *J. Biol. Chem.*, 249 (1974) 4383.
18 K. D. WATENPAUGH, L. C. SIEKER, L. H. JENSEN, J. LEGALL, and M. DUBOURDIEU, *Proc. Natl. Acad. Sci. U.S.*, 69 (1972) 3185.
19 K. D. WATENPAUGH, L. C. SIEKER, and L. H. JENSEN, *Proc. Natl. Acad. Sci. U.S.*, 70 (1973) 3857.
20 E. MARGOLIASH and A. SCHEJTER, *Adv. Protein Chem.*, 21 (1966) 114.
21 K. T. YASUNOBU and M. TANAKA, *Handb. Biochem. Mol. Biol.*, 3 (1976) 421.
22 W. M. FITCH and K. T. YASUNOBU, *J. Mol. Evol.*, 5 (1975) 1.
23 P. Y. CHOU and G. D. FASMAN, *Biochemistry*, 13 (1974) 222.
24 M. L. LUDWIG, private communication (1977).
25 G. P. FOUST, S. G. MAYHEW, and V. MASSEY, *J. Biol. Chem.*, 244 (1969) 964.
26 W. W. SMITH, H. L. GRESPI, B. ENTSCH, M. L. LUDWIG, and C. E. NORDMAN, *J. Mol. Biol.*, 94 (1975) 123.
27 S. RONCHI, L. MINCHIOTTI, B. CURTI, and J. BRIDGEN, *Flavins and Flavoproteins*, Elsevier, Amsterdam, 1976, p. 702.

28 N. Minamiura and K. T. Yasunobu, unpublished results, 1977.
29 B. Gomes, I. Igaue, H. C. Kloepfer, and K. T. Yasunobu, *Arch. Biochem. Biophys.*, 132 (1969) 16.
30 E. B. Kearney, J. I. Salach, W. H. Walker, R. L. Seng, W. Kenney, E. Zeszotek, and T. P. Singer, *Eur. J. Biochem.*, 24 (1971) 321.
31 W. H. Walker, E. B. Kearney, R. L. Seng, and T. P. Singer, *Eur. J. Biochem.*, 24 (1971) 328.
32 C. H. Williams, Jr., L.D. Arscott, and E. T. Jones, in T. P. Singer, *Flavins and Flavoproteins*, Elsevier, Amsterdam, 1976, p. 455.
33 O. Warburg and W. Christian, *Naturwissenschaften*, 20 (1932) 288 and 290.
34 O. Warburg and W. Christian, *Biochem. Z.*, 295 (1938) 261.

METHIONINE SYNTHETASE: CHARACTERIZATION OF PROTEIN COMPONENTS AND MECHANISMS FOR ACTIVATION AND CATALYSIS

KATSUHIKO FUJII AND F. M. HUENNEKENS

Department of Biochemistry, Scripps Clinic and Research Foundation, La Jolla, California (U.S.A.)

Vitamin B_{12}, like the other B vitamins, must first be transformed into a more complex structure before it can serve as a coenzyme in various enzymatic systems (for comprehensive reviews, see refs. 1–5). One of these coenzyme forms, 5′-deoxyadenosyl-B_{12}, is required for several isomerization reactions and for the reduction of ribonucleotides. There is generalagreement that the carbon-cobalt bond breaks during catalysis and that the moving hydrogen group is carried transiently by a fragment of the coenzyme. The other form of the B_{12} coenzyme, methyl-B_{12}, participates in the biosynthesis of acetate, methane, and methionine, serving as a transient carrier of the moving methyl group. B_{12}-dependent methionine synthetase (5-methyltetrahydrofolate: homocysteine methyltransferase, EC 2.1.1.13), which catalyzes reaction (1), has been the subject of extensive investigation, since

$$\text{5-Methyltetrahydrofolate} + \text{homocysteine} \longrightarrow \text{tetrahydrofolate} + \text{methionine} \qquad (1)$$

one of its products, tetrahydrofolate, is an essential coenzyme for the synthesis of purines and pyrimidines. In addition, methionine synthetase is one of only two B_{12}-dependent enzymes yet found in mammals. The enzyme has been purified from both mammalian and bacterial sources,[6–11] but these preparations have varied considerably in purity, molecular weight, absorbance spectrum, and B_{12} content. The enzyme requires strict anaerobiosis for its catalytic action and exists in two major forms, active and inactive. As isolated, the enzyme is generally inactive. An activation process, which requires both adenosylmethionine and a reductant, is essential for initiation of reaction (1), but it is also called upon continuously as the reaction proceeds.

These properties of methionine synthetase are the result of contributions made for more than a decade by a number of distinguished investigators (reviewed in ref. 12–14). In the present investigation, the isolation of homogeneous methionine synthetase and its physiological activating system has allowed a study of the mechanism of transfer of reducing equivalents to the B_{12} enzyme and characterization of various B_{12} intermediates involved in the overall enzyme reaction.

Abbreviations: 5′-deoxyadenosyl-B_{12}, 5′-deoxyadenosylcobalamin; methyl-B_{12}, methylcobalamin; B_{12a}, aquacobalamin; B_{12r}, cob(II) alamin; B_{12s}, cob (I) alamin; AdoMet, S-adenosylmethionine; DTE, dithioerythritol; KPB, potassium phosphate buffer (pH 7.0) of indicated molarity.

METHIONINE SYNTHETASE FROM *E. coli* K-12

The methionine synthetase from *E. coli* K-12, referred to as "M protein," has been purified to homogeneity from cell-free extracts by a series of conventional techniques including fractionation with ammonium sulfate (0–50%), gel filtration on Bio-gel P-200, and ion-exchange chromatography on DEAE-cellulose, DEAE-Sephadex, and hydroxylapatite.[15] The enzyme is greatly stabilized by adenosylmethionine, and this cofactor is added routinely at all stages during the purification. Some of the properties of the *E. coli* K-12 methionine synthetase are summarized in Table I. The enzyme has a molecular weight of 186,000 as judged by: SDS polyacrylamide-gel electrophoresis, filtration through Bio-gel P-200, and 1:1 stoichiometry of the bound B_{12}-chromophore (measured after its conversion to the free dicyano derivative). The absorbance spectrum of the homogeneous protein (cf. Fig. 9 in ref. 15) exhibits a shoulder at 312 nm (ε_{mM}, 30.1) and a prominent maximum at 470 nm (ε_{mM}, 11.0), in addition to its protein peak at 278 nm (ε_{mM}, 194). The activity of the enzyme is lost gradually upon prolonged contact with oxygen, and this loss is paralleled by a concomitant change in the B_{12} spectrum to that of a B_{12a} form. These properties suggest that the chromophore on the protein as it is isolated is B_{12r}, *i.e.*, the form of vitamin B_{12} in which the central cobalt atom is in the +2 oxidation state. Although the reduction potential for this bound B_{12r} has not yet been measured directly, it may be assumed by comparison with free B_{12r},[16–18] to be *ca.* −0.7 volt, which is one of the most negative reduction potentials found in biological systems.

ACTIVATION SYSTEM IN *E. coli* K-12

Previous work with methionine synthetases had disclosed that maximum activity of these enzymes could be attained only when adenosylmethionine and a reducing system were also present.[12–14] Chemical reducing systems such as reduced flavins or dithiothreitol plus B_{12a} were generally used for this purpose, but their requirement at high concentrations obscured spectral experiments with the B_{12} enzyme. In order to overcome this and other disadvantages of chemical reducing systems, a search for a more physiological, enzymatic reducing system has been made in the *E. coli* K-12 extracts from which the synthetase itself has been purified. Fractionation of these extracts has led to the discovery of a system which consists of two flavoproteins (designated R and F) that operate in conjunction with TPNH. Both flavoproteins have been obtained in pure form.

TABLE I

PROPERTIES OF METHIONINE SYNTHETASE (M) AND THE R AND F FLAVOPROTEINS FROM *E. coli* K-12

Property	*M*	*R*	*F*
Molecular weight	186,000	27,000	19,400
Absorbance maxima (nm)	278,312 (sh), 470	274, 400, 456	274, 369, 465
Prosthetic group			
Oxidized	B_{12r}	FAD	FMN
Reduced	B_{12s}	$FADH_2$	FMNH·
E'_0 (volts)	−0.7*	−0.30	−0.29

* Estimated from value for reduction of free B_{12r} to B_{12s}.[16–18]

Homogeneity of the R and F flavoproteins (and also of M, the B_{12}-containing protein) is readily demonstrated by gel electrophoresis (cf. Figs. 5 and 6 in refs. 19 and 15). R_f values of the M, R, and F proteins are 0.41, 0.62, and 1.0, respectively. Prior to protein staining, each of the proteins is visible on the gel as a colored band, owing to its tightly bound prosthetic group. The very rapid mobility of the F flavoprotein, which causes it to appear at the front, is a result of its extreme acidity coupled with its low molecular weight. These properties, together with its bound chromophore (FMN), imply that the F protein is a type of flavodoxin.[20,21] Characteristics of the R and F flavoproteins are also summarized in Table I. R has a molecular weight of 27,000 (determined as described for M protein), and contains 1 mol of noncobalently bound FAD per mol of protein. The absorbance spectrum of the chromophore, characterized by λ_{max} at 400 (ε_{mM}, 8.3) and 456 nm (ε_{mM}, 8.0) is not typical of flavoproteins. This must be due to binding of the prosthetic group to the protein since, when the FAD is released by heat denaturation, it shows a normal absorbance spectrum. The F flavoprotein is even smaller, having a molecular weight of 19,400. It has a typical flavoprotein spectrum and contains 1 mol of noncovalently bound FMN per mol of protein. The reduction potentials of the R and F flavoproteins, determined by analyses of the spectra in equilibrium mixtures of these flavoproteins with TPNH, are -0.30 and -0.29 volt, respectively.[22]

The effectiveness of these cofactors in the enzymatic activation of methionine synthetase is shown in Table II. Nearly all of the activity of the B_{12} enzyme is lost when either the R or F flavoprotein is omitted. The requirement for TPNH can be met with DPNH provided that much higher quantities are used. K_m values for TPNH and DPNH, when these compounds are used in conjunction with R and F to activate methionine synthetase, have been calculated to be 3.8 and 68 μM, respectively.[22] The requirement for exogenous adenosylmethionine is also evident in Table II. The specific activity of the homogeneous enzyme, when assayed under optimal conditions (assay C in ref. 22) in the presence of the enzymatic reducing system and adenosylmethionine, is 5.8 μmol of methionine synthesized per min per mg of the B_{12} protein; this corresponds to a turnover number of *ca.* 1,000. Lower specific activities (by 30–50%) are obtained with chemical reducing systems. Full activation of the enzyme is obtained when these flavoproteins are used at concentrations equimolar to that of the synthetase, and this is several orders of magnitude lower than the required levels of free, reduced flavins or non-specific flavoproteins described previously[23] as reductants.

TABLE II

COFACTOR REQUIREMENTS FOR METHIONINE SYNTHETASE*

Omissions or substitutions	*Methionine (nmol)*
None	13.8
R	0.94
F	0.49
TPNH	0.99
DPNH replacing TPNH	13.9
AdoMet	0.54

* Enzyme activity was measured by Assay A (ref. 15) at 37° for 15 min with the use of 0.42 μg of methionine synthetase in a final volume of 0.25 ml. Tabulated components were used in the following amounts: R, 0.2 μg; F, 0.2 μg; TPNH, 0.025 μmol; DPNH, 2 μmol; AdoMet, 2.0 nmol.

TRANSFER OF REDUCING EQUIVALENTS

During the course of activation of the methionine synthetase, reducing equivalents are transferred by the sequence illustrated in Fig. 1. TPNH (or less efficiently, DPNH) reduces R, which reduces F, and the latter, in turn, reduces the enzyme, M. It should be noted that R is capable of reducing a variety of electron acceptors, *e.g.*, ferricyanide, dichlorophenolindophenol and cytochrome *c*. However, none of these latter compounds is able to interact with M. Several other flavoproteins that are capable of pyridinenucleotide-dependent reduction of cytochrome *c* can also be found in the *E. coli* extracts, but none of these flavoproteins can substitute for R in the reduction of F. These observations illustrate the high degree of specificity contained in the present activating system.

The R flavoprotein is reduced rapidly by TPNH. Because the reduction potential of the bound flavin is close to that of the pyridine nucleotide, addition of various increments of TPNH is seen to cause a progressive reduction of the flavin (Fig. 2). Reduction of R with excess dithionite is sluggish, but produces as a function of time, a series of spectra[22] very similar to those obtained with TPNH. In either case, the reduced prosthetic group exhibits the characteristic spectrum of the hydroquinone form of FAD.

By contrast to these results, the F flavoprotein can be reduced by TPNH only when the R flavoprotein is also present. If a catalytic amount of R is added to the system, the spectrum of F is observed to change slowly to that of a neutral blue semiquinone form of FMN, characterized by a λ_{max} at 579 nm (Fig. 3). Since the methionine synthetase appears to require only one electron for its activation, it is of interest that the F flavoprotein is reduced exclusively to the semiquinone level by its physiological reductant, TPNH, even in the presence of a large excess of the latter compound. Chemical reduction of F with dithionite, however, yields predominantly a hydroquinone form of FMN (cf. Fig. 3 in ref. 22), though the rate of reduction is very slow. The B_{12r} chromophore on the M protein cannot be reduced by treatment with TPNH plus R and F in the absence of adenosylmethionine. Inclusion of adenosylmethionine in the reaction mixture can shift the unfavorable equilibrium resulting from the tremendously low reduction potential of the B_{12} moiety. The large free energy gained by the release of the methyl group on adenosylmethionine is sufficient to overcome the free energy barrier in the reductive step. Because of the high specificity of the present activation system, it has been possible to monitor

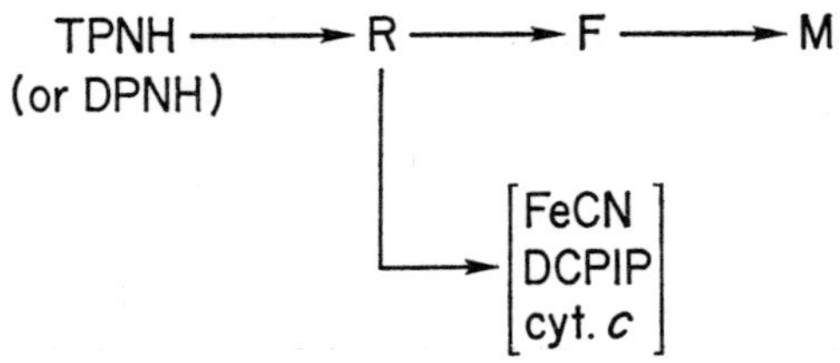

Fig. 1. Sequence of transfer of reducing equivalents during activation of methionine synthetase. FeCN, ferricyanide; DCPIP, dichlorophenolindophenol; cyt. *c*, cytochrome *c*.

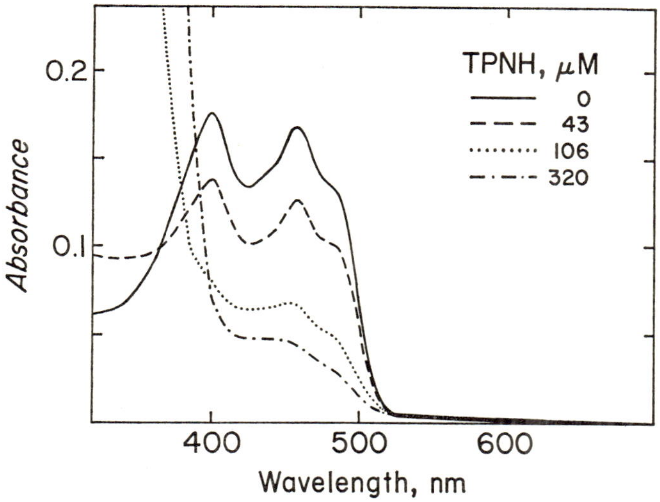

Fig. 2. Reduction of R protein by various amounts of TPNH. The main compartment of a quartz Thunberg cuvette contained 24.6 nmol of R and 120 μmol of KPB in a total volume of 1.2 ml. Various amounts of TPNH were delivered to the upper part of the cuvette as described previously[22]. After the initial spectrum had been recorded under argon at 27° (solid curve), aliquots of TPNH were added to achieve the indicated concentrations.

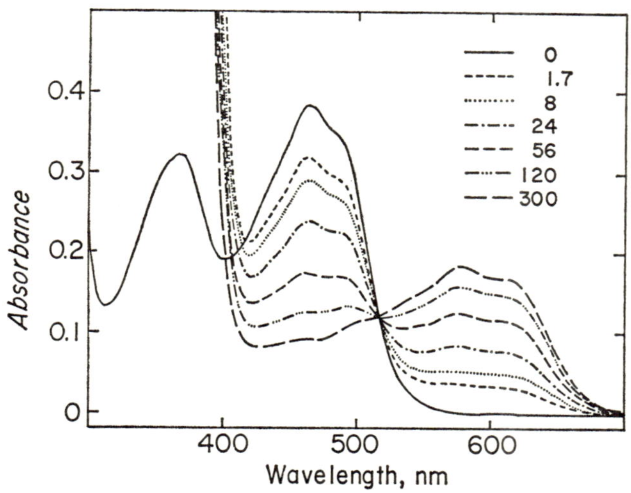

Fig. 3. Reduction of F protein by excess TPNH and a catalytic amount of R. The main compartment of a quartz Thunberg cuvette contained 50 nmol of F, 0.98 nmol of R, and 120 μmol of KPB in a total volume of 1.2 ml. A solution of TPNH (4.65 μmol in 0.085 ml) was placed in the side-arm. After the initial spectrum (zero-time) had been recorded under argon (at 37°), TPNH was added and successive spectra were recorded at 1.7, 8, 24, 56, 120, and 300 min.

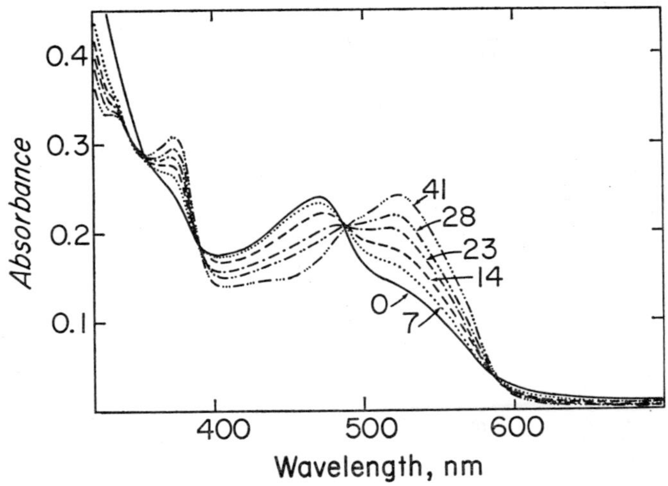

Fig. 4. Formation of methyl-B_{12} enzyme from B_{12r} enzyme. The main compartment of a quartz Thunberg cuvette contained 30 nmol of M, 1.5 nmol of R, 3.0 nmol of F, 24 μmol of DTE, and 120 μmol of KPB. TPNH (300 nmol) and AdoMet (150 nmol), each in 3.5 μl, were delivered into different positions of the side-arm. The cuvette was repeatedly evacuated and flushed with argon. After the initial spectrum had been recorded at 30° against a reference cuvette (M protein omitted), TPNH was added into both cuvettes. Successive spectra were recorded at the indicated time (min). AdoMet was added to both cuvettes at 47 min.

spectrophotometrically the course of this portion of the reaction (reductive methylation) occurring on the M protein (Fig. 4). The inactive form of the purified M protein, which contains bound B_{12r} (λ_{max} at 470 nm), is changed slowly during the course of the reaction to the active methyl-B_{12} form of the enzyme (λ_{max} at 375 and 522 nm). Under optimal conditions, activation is complete within 1 min, but in the experiment illustrated in Fig. 4, very small amounts of the activating flavoproteins were used in order to minimize spectral interference with the changes occurring in the synthetase. A kinetic plot of these results (not shown in the figure) indicates that the rate-limiting step for activation is located within the activating system. The B_{12} moiety on the M protein is converted completely to methyl-B_{12} in the absence of exogenous adenosylmethionine, and no further change in the spectrum is produced by the addition of this cofactor. However, the enzyme retains at least an equimolar quantity of the adenosylmethionine which is added as a stabilizing agent during the purification procedure. Verification that the B_{12} moiety has been transformed into methyl-B_{12} during the activation process is obtained by identifying the product released upon treatment of the enzyme with hot 80% ethanol.

The early suggestion by other investigators[24,25] that activation is required not only for the initiation of the catalytic reaction, but continuously throughout its course has been confirmed by our studies. The continuing requirement for activation is a result of the participation of B_{12s} (in which the cobalt is in the highly reactive +1 oxidation state) in the methyl transfer reaction. This labile intermediate is occasionally degraded to yield B_{12r}, the inactive form of the coenzyme. When the consumption of TPNH and adenosylmethionine are monitored during steady-state methionine synthesis, both of these cofactors are consumed at a linear rate that is $<1\%$ of the rate of methionine production.

B_{12} INTERMEDIATES OF THE CATALYTIC CYCLE

Previous workers have obtained evidence (reviewed in refs. 12–14) that enzyme-bound B_{12} serves as a transient carrier of the moving methyl group. The availability of the present purified enzyme system has made it possible to study spectrophotometrically the postulated mechanism by which B_{12s} abstracts the methyl group from 5-methyltetrahydrofolate; the resulting methyl-B_{12} then reacts with homocysteine to yield methionine and regenerate B_{12s} for another turn of the cycle.

Demethylation of activated enzyme by homocysteine, the reaction by which the catalytic cycle is initiated, has been examined by the experiment shown in Fig. 5. Activated enzyme is treated with homocysteine under anaerobic conditions in the *presence* of excess adenosylmethionine in order to prevent the latter component from becoming a limiting factor. The chromophore is converted immediately (<1 min) to B_{12s} (λ_{max} at 384 and 530 nm, with a low, broad peak centered at 680 nm). This intermediate remains stable for several minutes and then decays progressively to the native form of the enzyme (λ_{max} at 470 nm). The latter transition, characterized by isosbestic points at 354, 411, and 514 nm, is due, presumably, to oxidation of enzyme-bound B_{12s} by water.[26] When the experiment shown in Fig. 5 is repeated in the *absence* of exogenous adenosylmethionine (so that the methyl-B_{12} enzyme is formed by utilizing adenosylmethionine associated with the native

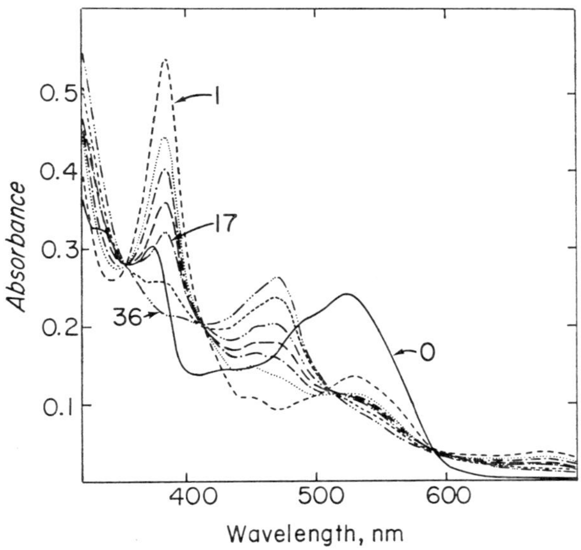

Fig. 5. Demethylation of methyl-B_{12} enzyme with homocysteine. Experimental conditions as in Fig. 4, except that the side-arm of the Thunberg cuvette also contained 6 μmol of DL-homocysteine. Methyl-B_{12} enzyme (zero-time curve) was generated as in Fig. 4, and the reaction was then initiated by the addition of homocysteine. Spectra were recorded subsequently at 1, 8.75, 11, 14, 17, 23, and 36 min. At 3 and 5.5 min, a spectrum almost identical to that shown for 1 min was observed.

enzyme), the B_{12s} intermediate is visible for a shorter period of time, and its conversion to the native form obeys pseudo first-order kinetics (data not shown). From the absorbance changes at 470 nm, a value of 6.1 min has been calculated for the half-life of enzyme-bound B_{12s} under these conditions.

Methylation of B_{12s} by 5-methyltetrahydrofolate, is more difficult, for technical reasons, to study as an isolated reaction, since the intermediate (enzyme-bound B_{12s}) cannot be generated at sufficient concentrations by the above procedures, unless the activating system and excess homocysteine are both present. In the presence of excess homocysteine, however, the catalytic reaction will prevent trapping of a methylated intermediate. The following indirect method has therefore been devised to detect this portion of the catalytic cycle: methyl-B_{12} is prepared by enzymatic activation (cf. legend for Fig. 4) except that 5-methyltetrahydrofolate (40-fold molar excess with respect to enzyme) is also present; inclusion of this substrate does not affect the rate or extent of the reductive methylation process. A small amount (1.3 molar equivalents) of homocysteine is then added to react with the adenosylmethionine-generated methyl-B_{12} and thereby allow the nascent B_{12s} to be remethylated by 5-methyltetrahydrofolate.

The spectrum of the methylated intermediate, which is generated rapidly at 30° and is stable for long periods of time, differs significantly from that of methyl-B_{12} (Fig. 6, dashed line). The spectral band of this product is rather diffuse with absorbance less than that of the original methyl-B_{12} (curve not shown) above 483 nm and greater than that of

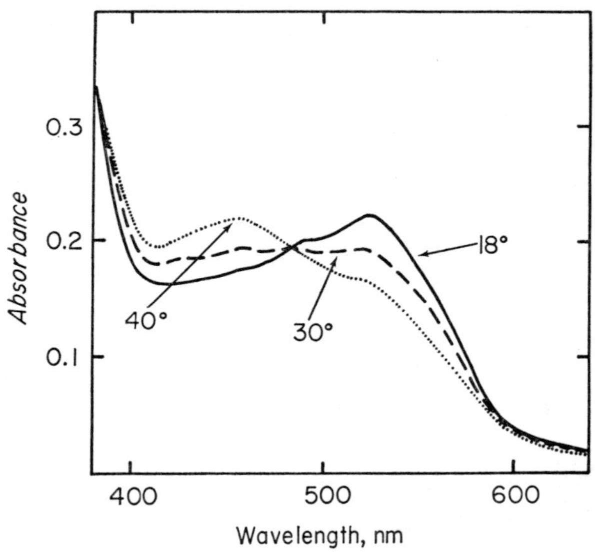

Fig. 6. Reaction of 5-methyltetrahydrofolate with B_{12s} enzyme. Contents of both the sample and reference cuvettes were the same as in Fig. 4, except for the addition of 2.4 μmol of *dl*-5-methyltetrahydrofolate to the main compartment and 80 nmol of DL-homocysteine to the side-arm. Temperature, 30°. Themethyl-B_{12} enzyme was generated as described in Fig. 4 by addition of TPNH and adenosylmethionine. Homocysteine was then added from the side-arm, and the spectrum, which was recorded 1.75 min later (---), did not change during a subsequent 40 min period. Spectra of the product are also shown at 18° (—) and 40° (···).

methyl-B_{12} below this wavelength. When the spectrum of the product is re-examined at 40°, a distinct band is observed at 455 nm with a shoulder at *ca.* 522 nm (Fig. 6). Conversely, lowering the temperature to 18° causes the 455 nm band to recede and the 522 nm peak to become more pronounced; the 18° spectrum is very similar to that of methyl-B_{12}. These spectral changes are reproducible over several temperature cycles, and maintenance of the isosbestic point at 483 nm provides evidence that no degradative side-reactions are occurring. It should be noted that methyl-B_{12}, prepared chemically or on the enzyme *via* the activation process, does *not* show these spectral changes when the temperature is altered. Thus the intermediate that is produced when the enzyme is methylated by 5-methyltetrahydrofolate (in contrast to when it is methylated by adenosylmethionine) appears to be a temperature-sensitive species of B_{12}.

Additional data similar to those shown in Fig. 6 have been used to calculate the thermodynamic constants associated with interconversion of the 18° and 40° species of B_{12}. Values of ΔF (at 37°), ΔH, and ΔS have been determined to be -0.84 kcal/mol, 44 kcal/mol, and 140 e.u., respectively.

Evidence that the temperature-sensitive B_{12} species is methylated has been obtained by examination of its reaction with homocysteine. As shown in Fig. 7, the temperature-sensitive B_{12} enzyme, $(Me\text{-}B_{12})_{ts}$, reacts with this substrate in a manner similar to that described earlier for the reaction of the methyl-B_{12} enzyme with homocysteine (cf. Fig. 5). B_{12s} with its characteristic absorbance at 384 and 680 nm is the initial product of the reaction (Fig. 7, dotted curve), but in this instance, the half-life for its conversion to the B_{12r} form is only 1.5 min.

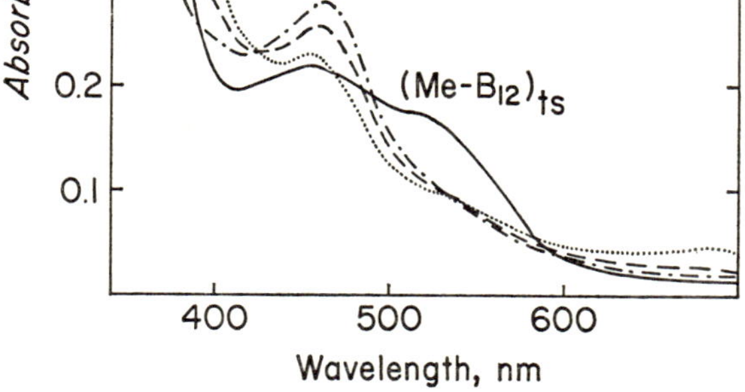

Fig. 7. Reaction of the temperature-sensitive B_{12} intermediate, $(Me\text{-}B_{12})_{ts}$, with excess homocysteine. Experiment shown in Fig. 6 was repeated at 37° and the zero-time spectrum (—) was recorded. The reaction was initiated by the addition of 3.0 μmol of DL-homocysteine from the side-arm, and successive spectra were recorded at 0.3 (···), 2.2 (---), and 12 min (-•-).

MECHANISMS FOR ACTIVATION AND CATALYSIS

The present study has provided additional information about the activation and catalysis of methionine synthetase. These mechanisms, which represent expansion and modification of the earlier extensive work in this field,[12-14] are summarized in Fig. 8. As isolated, the enzyme contains its B_{12} moiety in the B_{12r} or +2 oxidation state. In contrast to the enzymes purified by other workers,[8-10] the present preparation does not show an absorption peak in the region of 350–360 nm. Activation of the B_{12r} enzyme to its methyl-B_{12} form (step *a*) is facilitated most efficiently by adenosylmethionine and a physiological reducing system consisting of TPNH and two small flavoproteins (designated R and F). The latter system, *via* the sequence for transfer of reducing power shown in Fig. 2, provides e^- for activation (step *a*). Although the final part of the reductive sequence (F→M) could not be demonstrated directly, probably because of the unfavorable reduction potential for the enzyme-bound B_{12r}, the reaction of the reduced M protein with adenosylmethionine was readily detected as an overall reaction for activation (cf. Fig. 4). This reductive methylation (step *a*), which is facilitated by the release of the methyl group of adenosylmethionine, may proceed by a single, concerted reaction rather than in two discrete steps.

Entrance of the activated enzyme into the catalytic cycle is achieved *via* step *b* in Fig. 8. The purified preparations available in the present investigation have made it possible to follow step *b* spectrophotometrically as an isolated reaction. The absorption spectrum of the enzyme-bound B_{12s}, which is produced quantitatively, has been characterized (cf. Fig. 5). The intermediate is unstable, as observed by its facile decay to the B_{12r} form (step *e*). Longevity of B_{12s} is manipulated experimentally by the status of the activating system.

The initial portion of the catalytic cycle (step *c*) could be studied only indirectly. Reaction of the B_{12s} enzyme with 5-methyltetrahydrofolate generated a temperature-sensitive, methylated form of B_{12} which is similar to, but not identical with, the methyl-B_{12}

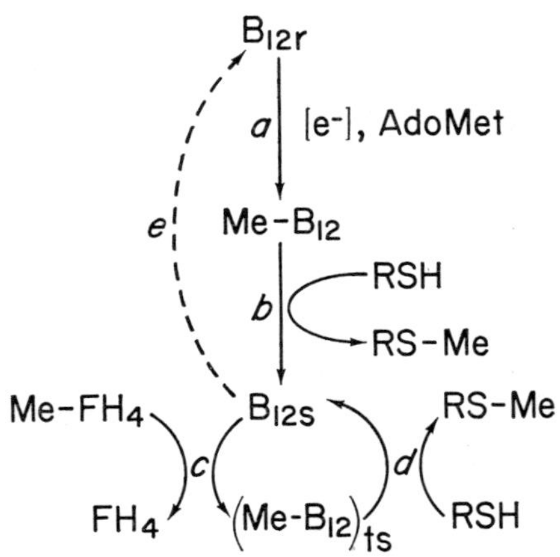

Fig. 8. Mechanisms for activation and catalysis of methionine synthetase. All B_{12} species are enzyme-bound. Me-B_{12}, methylcobalamin; RSH, L-homocysteine; RS-Me, L-methionine; Me-FH_4, *l*-5-methyltetrahydrofolate; FH_4, tetrahydrofolate. Other abbreviations are given in the text.

produced by step *a*. Its low-temperature spectrum is similar to that of the "base-on" form of methyl-B_{12}, while its high-temperature form resembles that of a "base-off" form of this compound or that of isomeric methyl-B_{12} in which the methyl group occupies the lower coordination position.[27] The temperature-dependent conversion of the bound chromophore might be facilitated by a concomitant change in apo-protein conformation; this is consistent with a rather large value of ΔS.

The temperature-sensitive species is demethylated by homocysteine (step *d*) to give methionine and B_{12s}. The cycle should then be self-perpetuating, except for the degradative side reaction (step *e*) in which B_{12s} occasionally slips from the catalytic cycle *via* its oxidation to B_{12r}. Evidence for this side-reaction includes the decay of the transient B_{12s} shown in Fig. 7 and the small but continuous operation of the activating system at the steady state. Since the rate of step *e* must be compensated by the activation rate, which is a combination of steps *a* and *b*, the overall rate of methionine synthesis would appear to be governed by the efficiency of the activating system. Kinetic studies indicate that, at the steady state, the rate constant for step *d* is at least eight times larger than that for step *c* and that 89% of the total B_{12} present in the reaction mixtures exists in the B_{12s} form (data not shown). It can be seen from these results that the mechanism of methionine synthetase is far more complex than might be envisioned. However, by working with the homogeneous enzyme and a well-defined *physiological* activating system, it has been possible to perform detailed spectrophotometric and kinetic studies of various steps in the enzyme reaction. These investigations, which have provided insight into mechanisms for activation and catalysis of methionine synthetase, may also provide clues with regard to the mechanisms of other B_{12}-dependent enzymes.

ACKNOWLEDGMENTS

The authors are indebted to Karin Vitols for her advice in the preparation of the manuscript, to Dr. J. Galivan for his collaboration in the early phase of this work and to D. S. Sampson and M. Cheng for their expert technical assistance.

These investigations have been supported by grants from the National Cancer Institute, National Institutes of Health (CA 6522 and CA 16600), the American Cancer Society (CH 31), and from the American Heart Association (69-1082). K.F. was a recipient of a Junior Fellowship from the California Division, American Cancer Society.

REFERENCES

1 H. A. Barker, *Biochem. J.*, 105 (1967) 1.
2 F. M. Huennekens, in T. P. Singer, *Biological Oxidations*, Interscience, New York, 1968, p. 439.
3 H. P. C. Hogenkamp, *Annu. Rev. Biochem.*, 37 (1968) 225.
4 H. A. Barker, *Annu. Rev. Biochem.*, 41 (1972) 55.
5 R. H. Abeles and D. Dolphin, *Acc. Chem. Res.*, 9 (1976) 114.
6 S. Takeyama and J. M. Buchanan, *J. Biochem.*, 49 (1961) 578.
7 R. E. Loughlin, H. L. Elford, and J. M. Buchanan, *J. Biol. Chem.*, 239 (1964) 2888.
8 R. T. Taylor and H. Weissbach, *J. Biol. Chem.*, 242 (1967) 1502.
9 J. Stavrianopoulos and L. Jaenicke, *Eur. J. Biochem.*, 3 (1967) 95.
10 J. H. Mangum and J. A. North, *Biochemistry*, 10 (1971) 3765.
11 J. H. Mangum, B. W. Steuart, and J. A. North, *Arch. Biochem. Biophys.*, 148 (1972) 63.
12 H. Weissbach and R. T. Taylor, *Vitam. Horm.*, 28 (1970) 415.

13 R. T. Taylor and H. Weissbach, in P. D. Boyer, *The Enzymes*, Academic Press, New York, vol. 9, 1973, p. 121.
14 H. Rüdiger and L. Jaenicke, *Mol. Cell. Biochem.*, 1 (1973) 157.
15 K. Fujii and F. M. Huennekens, *J. Biol. Chem.*, 249 (1974) 6745.
16 H. P. C. Hogenkamp and S. Holmes, *Biochemistry*, 9 (1970) 1886.
17 J. M. Pratt, *Inorganic Chemistry of Vitamin B_{12}*, Academic Press, New York, 1972, p. 109.
18 D. Lexa and J. M. Saveant, *J. Am. Chem. Soc.*, 98 (1976) 2652.
19 F. M. Huennekens, P. M. DiGirolamo, K. Fujii, D. W. Jacobsen, and K. S. Vitols, *Adv. Enzyme Regul.*, 14 (1976) 187.
20 D. C. Yoch and R. C. Valentine, *Annu. Rev. Microbiol.*, 26 (1972) 139.
21 S. G. Mayhew and M. L. Ludwig, in P. D. Boyer, *The Enzymes*, Academic Press, New York, vol. 12, 1975, p. 57.
22 K. Fujii, J. H. Galivan, and F. M. Huennekens, *Arch. Biochem. Biophys.*, 178 (1977) 662.
23 R. T. Taylor and M. L. Hanna, *Arch. Biochem. Biophys.*, 139 (1970) 149.
24 R. T. Taylor and H. Weissbach, *Arch. Biochem. Biophys.*, 129 (1969) 728.
25 R. T. Taylor and M. L. Hanna, *Arch. Biochem. Biophys.*, 137 (1970) 453.
26 S. L. Tackett, J. W. Collat, and J. C. Abbott, *Biochemistry*, 2 (1963) 919.
27 W. Friedrich and J. P. Nordmeyer, *Z. Naturforsch.*, 246 (1969) 588.

STRUCTURE-FUNCTION INTERRELATIONSHIP OF COENZYME B_{12} (ADENOSYLCOBALAMIN) IN DIOL DEHYDRASE SYSTEM

SABURO FUKUI AND TETSUO TORAYA

Laboratory of Industrial Biochemistry, Department of Industrial Chemistry, Faculty of Engineering, Kyoto University, Kyoto (Japan)

Coenzyme B_{12} (AdoCbl), discovered by Barker *et al.*,[1] is the most complex non-polymer compound in nature as well as the only naturally occurring organometallic compound (Fig. 1).[2] The most specific feature of this coenzyme is the unique Co-C bond linking the cobalt ion, the central atom of a specific tetrapyrrole macrocycle (corrin nucleus), to the 5′-carbon of 5′-deoxyadenosyl upper ligand.

As summarized in Table I, 10 kinds of rearrangement reactions (some of which are

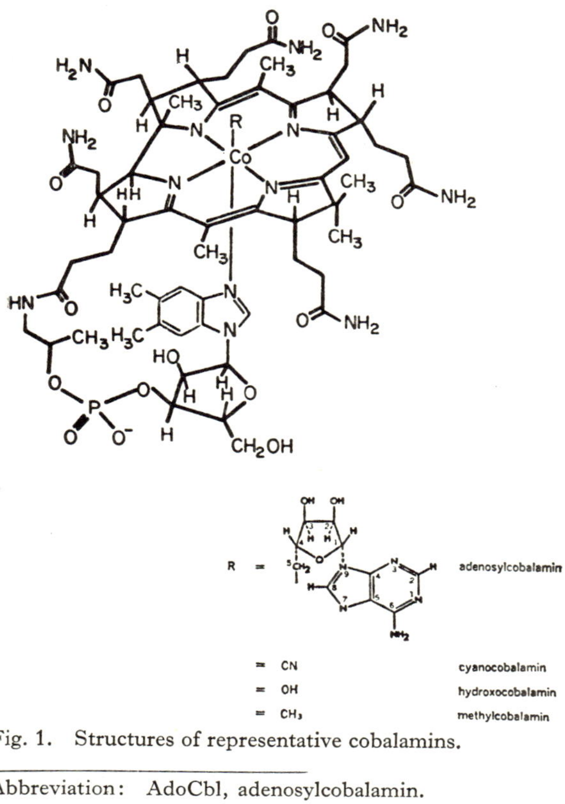

Fig. 1. Structures of representative cobalamins.

Abbreviation: AdoCbl, adenosylcobalamin.

TABLE I

COENZYME B_{12}-DEPENDENT BIOCHEMICAL REACTIONS

Reaction	Enzyme
C–C Fission	
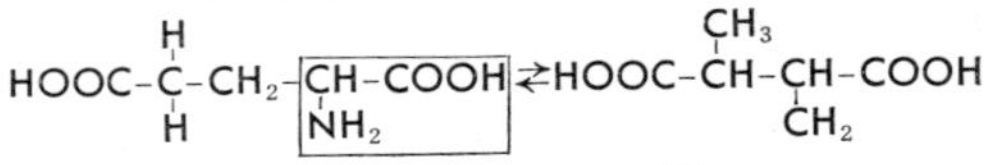	Glutamate mutase
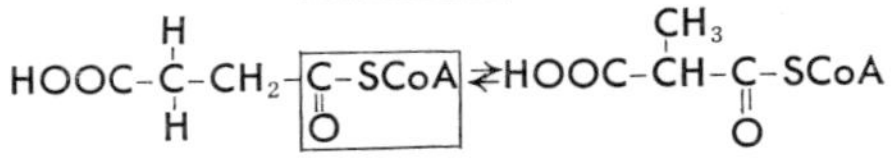	Methylmalonyl-CoA mutase
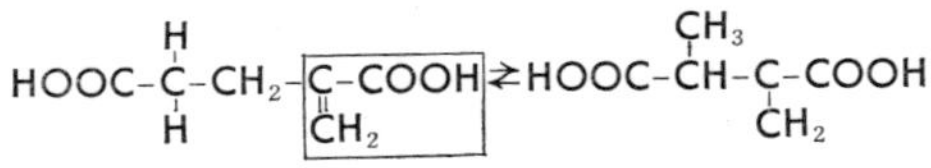	α-Methylene-glutarate mutase
C–O Fission	
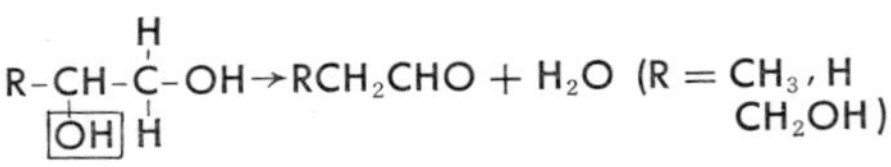	Diol dehydrase
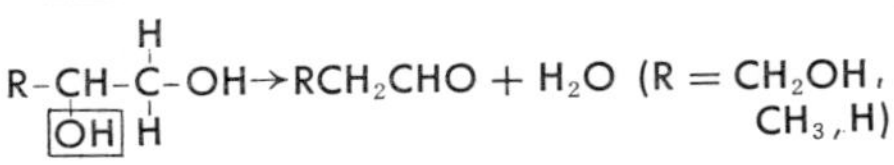	Glycerol dehydrase
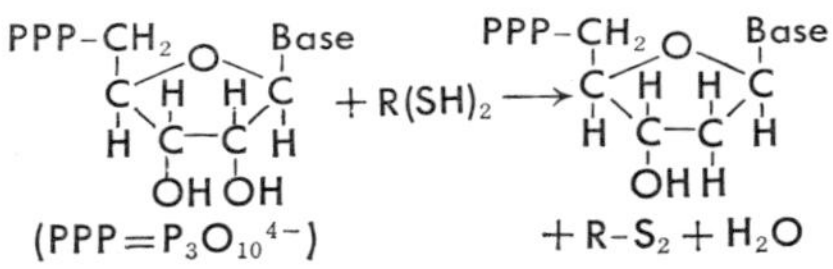	Ribonucleotide reductase
C–N Fission	
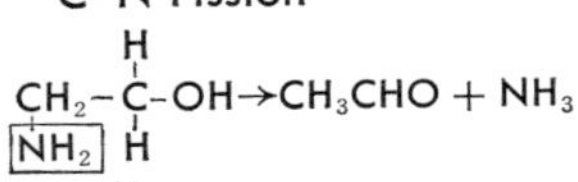	Ethanolamine ammonia-lyase
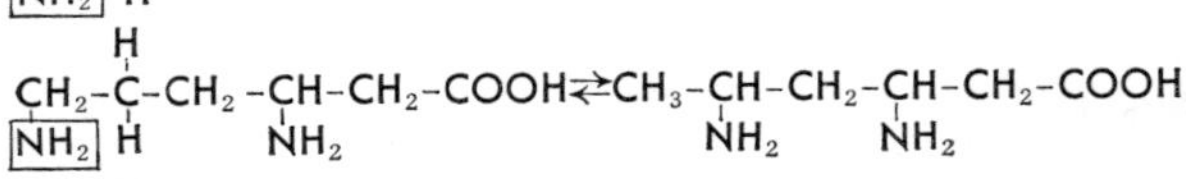	L-β-Lysine mutase
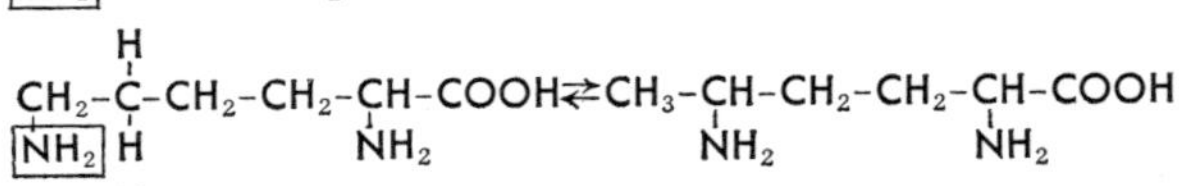	D-α-Lysine mutase
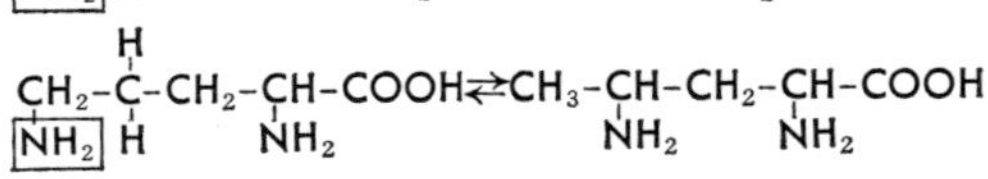	Ornithine mutase
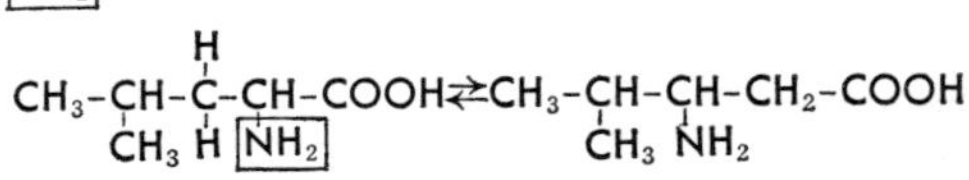	Leucine 2,3-aminomutase

accompanied by release of water or ammonia), and the reduction of ribonucleoside triphosphate to deoxyribonucleoside triphosphate, are known to be dependent upon the coenzyme.

Accumulated information indicates that the rearrangement reactions involve migra-

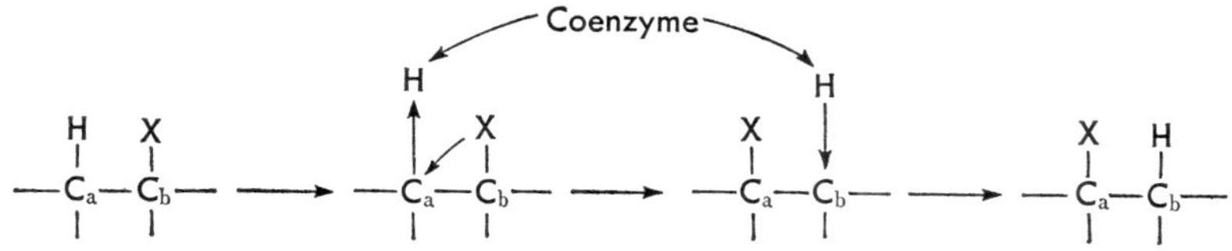

Fig. 2. Involvement of coenzyme B_{12} as the hydrogen carrier in the rearrangement reaction dependent on the coenzyme.

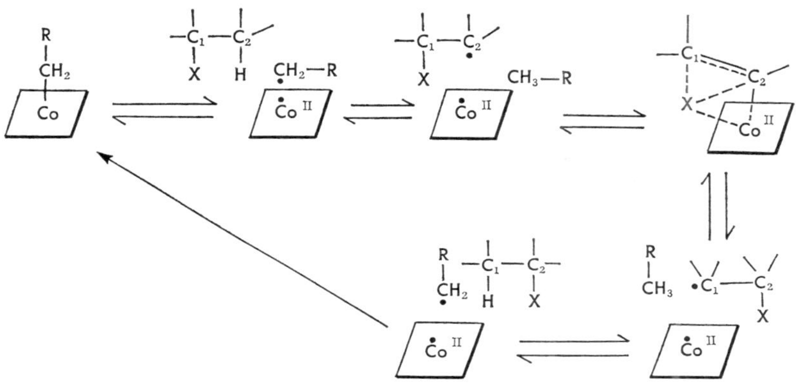

Fig. 3. Presumed reaction mechanism of the rearrangement reaction dependent on coenzyme B_{12}.

tion of a hydrogen from one carbon (C_a) of the substrate to an adjacent carbon (C_b) in exchange for a group X that moves in the opposite direction (Fig. 2). The nature of this group is alkyl, acyl or a conventional nucleophilic leaving group such as hydroxyl or amino. In these reactions, the coenzyme B_{12}-apoenzyme complex serves as an intermediate hydrogen carrier—first accepting a hydrogen from the substrate, and then, in a subsequent step, giving a hydrogen back to the product.

The elegant experiments of Abeles[3] and others have provided potent evidence which supports the hypothesis that an enzyme-catalyzed homolysis of the Co-C bond of the coenzyme leads to the appearance of cob (II) alamin (so-called, B_{12r}) and 5′-deoxyadenosyl free radical, and these active species serve as the catalytic center for abstraction and donation of hydrogen atom. The scheme shown in Fig. 3 is one example of the proposed mechanism.

However, although the hydrogen transfer mechanism is accepted in outline, many questions still remain to be solved: Is an alkyl-cobalt complex formed as an intermediate or not? What is the mechanism of intramolecular group transfer or rearrangement of molecular skeleton? Finally, the most interesting question from the biochemical viewpoint is: What force resulting from apoprotein enables the activation and cleavage of the Co-C bond of coenzyme B_{12}? In order to obtain information on the interaction of coenzyme B_{12} and apoprotein, a variety of analogs of the coenzyme (Table II) have been prepared, and the affinities of these analogs for apoprotein as well as the activities of the resulting holoenzyme species have been studied in different types of coenzyme B_{12}-dependent enzyme systems. This communication describes an outline of the structure-function relationship of coenzyme B_{12} in diol dehydrase, one of the most extensively studied enzyme in terms of the binding to coenzyme B_{12} and the reaction mechanism. The binding of co-

TABLE II
ANALOGS OF AdoCbl WHOSE COENZYME ACTIVITIES HAVE BEEN TESTED

I. Analogs with modified corrin nucleus
- a) Corrin nucleus
  - Position 10, Position 8, AdoCbl (13-*epi*)
- b) Side chains
  - *b*-, *d*-, or/and *e*-side chain(s)

II. Analogs with modified lower ligands
- a) Base moiety
- b) Ribose moiety
- c) Base moiety and ribose moiety
- d) Alkanolamine moiety

III. Analogs with modified upper ligands
- a) Adenine moiety
- b) Ribose moiety
- c) Adenine moiety and ribose moiety

enzyme B_{12} and apoprotein occurs according to "so-called induced-fit mechanism" in the presence of K^+ ion or another monovalent cation having a suitable ion radius.[4] Diol dehydrase is composed of two dissimilar protein components, designated "Component F" and "Component S," both of which are required for catalysis. Neither component alone binds coenzyme B_{12} or cyanocobalamin.[5]

The combined actions of hydrogen bond, van der Waals force, hydrophobic bond, *etc.*, at some positions of the corrin nucleus (especially its B and C rings), some of the aminocarboxyalkyl side chains, and the ribose and base moieties of the lower nucleotide ligand render the binding of coenzyme B_{12} or its analogs to apoprotein very strong and effective.[6] Incorporation of halogen at the carbon 10 position of the corrin nucleus has little influence on the affinity for apoprotein, but results in a marked loss of the activity of the resulting holoenzyme,[7] probably due to the alteration of the electronic structure of the corrin nucleus and the further electronic property of Co-C bond of the coenzyme. Adenosyl-13-epicobalamin is an analog of AdoCbl in which the adenosyl moiety in the upper coordination position is positioned differently above the corrin ring because the inverted *e*-propionamide side chain blocks its normal location above C-13. Furthermore, the lower pK_a of the "base on" $\rightleftarrows$ "base off" conversion of the analog (2.8) than that of AdoCbl (3.5) suggests that the inversion at C-13 also affects the electronic character of the cobalt atom. This coenzyme analog showed approximately 14% of the coenzyme activity of AdoCbl, while its apparent K_m value (12.7 μM) was 13 times higher than that of AdoCbl for diol dehydrase.[8] The kinetics of the reaction and the apoenzyme-adenosyl-13-epicobalamin interaction suggested a lower affinity of the enzyme for the coenzyme analog. The analog was readily dissociated even from the reacting apoenzyme-adenosyl-13-epicobalamin complex upon gel filtration. Like the native holoenzyme, the apoenzyme-coenzyme analog complex underwent inactivation by oxygen in the absence of substrate. However, the rate of inactivation was much slower than that of the native holoenzyme.[8] With respect to the function of the upper ligand, the 5′-deoxyadenosyl moiety should take the most important role in the activation of Co-C bond through interaction with the corresponding sites of apoprotein, as will be described below.

In order to obtain more detailed information on the role of each part of the coenzyme

TABLE III

STRUCTURES OF VARIOUS SEPHAROSE-BOUND COBALAMINS

L=Adenosyl, cytidyl, CH_3, CN, OH, *etc.*

No.		Partial structure
I	Cobalamin monocarboxylic-aminohexylamide-Sepharose 4B	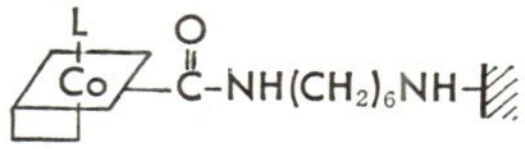
II	Cobalamin monocarboxylic-aminododecylamide-Sepharose 4B	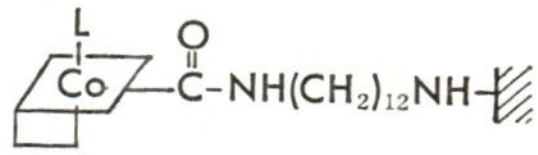
III	Nucleotide-free corrinoid monocarboxylic-aminododecylamide-Sepharose 4B	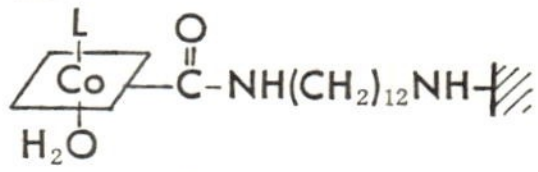
IV	Nucleotide-free corrinoid polycarboxylic-aminohexylamide-Sepharose 4B	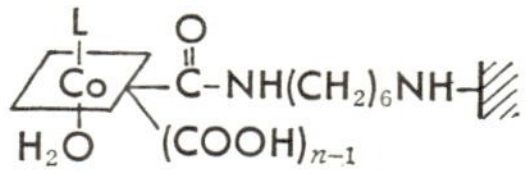
V	Cabalamin $O^{5'}$-succinic-aminohexylamide-Sepharose 4B	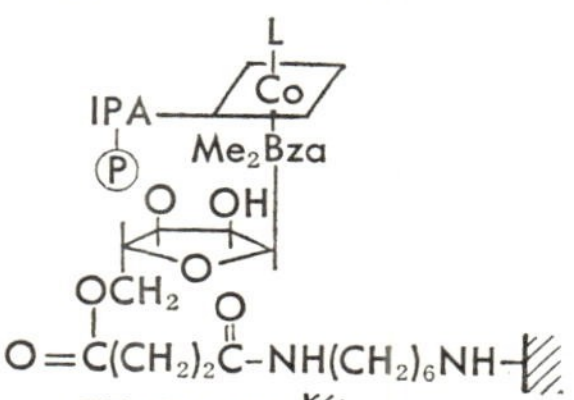
VI	Co-aminoethylcobalamin-Sepharose 4B	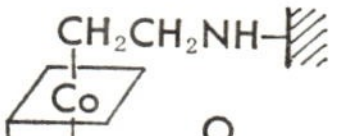
VII	Co-carboxyethylcabalamin-aminohexylamide-Sepharose 4B	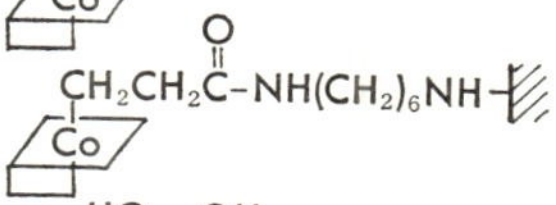
VIII	N^6-carboxymethyl-Co-adenosylcobalamin-aminohexylamide-Sepharose 4B	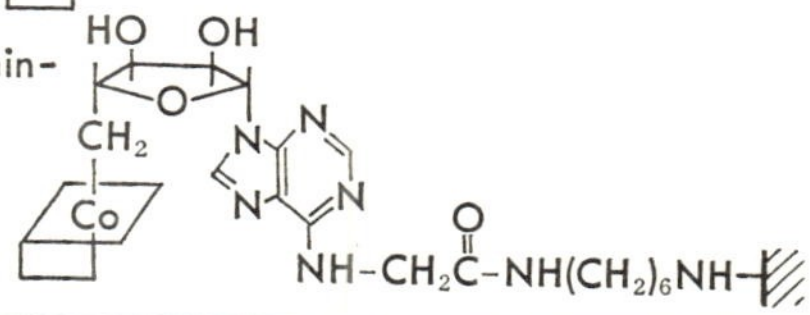

B_{12} molecule in the binding to apo-diol dehydrase, we employed an "affinity chromatography" technique by using various immobilized derivatives of vitamin B_{12}.[9] Table III shows the structure of immobilized B_{12} derivatives used. In Compounds I to IV, cobalamin links to Sepharose 4B through the carboxylic acid side chain (position *e*). Their upper ligand is adenosyl, cytidyl, methyl, cyano, or hydroxyl, *etc.*; the lower ligand is complete or replaced with H_2O. In the case of IV, the propionamide side chains of corrin nucleus are converted to free propionic acids. In Compound V, cobalamin links to Sepharose 4B at the $O^{5'}$ position of the ribose moiety of the lower nucleotide ligand. In Compounds VI and VII, cobalamin links to Sepharose through an alkyl group attached to Co atom. Cobalamin is attached at N^6-position of adenine part of the upper ligand in Compound VIII.

The principle of our affinity chromatography is based on the fact that the specific

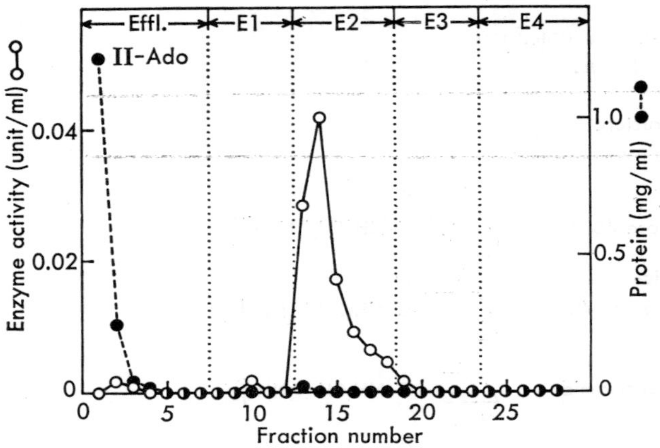

Fig. 4. Biospecific-adsorption and elution of apoprotein of diol dehydrase in affinity chromatography on Sepharose-bound AdoCbl (Compound II-type). About 1 unit of enzyme was applied to the adsorbent (1 ml of packed gel) in 0.1 M potassium phosphate buffer (pH 8) containing 2% propanediol, in a total volume of 2 ml, and affinity chromatography was carried out as described in ref. 9. Eluate 2 (E 2) was eluted with the mixture of 0.3 M Tris-HCl buffer (pH 8) and 2% propanediol. E1, with 0.5 M potassium phosphate buffer (pH 8) and 2% propanediol; E3, with 0.3 M Tris-HCl buffer (pH 8); E4, with 0.1 M acetic acid and 2% propanediol.

TABLE IV

PROPERTIES OF SEPHAROSE BOUND COBALAMINS TESTED IN THIS STUDY

No.	*Corrinoid immobilized*	*Spacer*	*Site of attachment*	*Effectiveness*
I, II	B_{12} monocarboxylic acid	$H_2N(CH_2)_{6 or 12}NH_2$	Corrin ring	○ (L=Ado, CN)
III	Nucleotide-laking corrinoid monocarboxylic acid (nucleotide-free)	$H_2N(CH_2)_{12}NH_2$	Corrin ring	○ (L=Ado), × (L=CN)
IV	Nucleotide-laking corrinoid polycarboxylic acid	$H_2N(CH_2)_6NH_2$	Corrin ring	× (L=Ado)
V	B_{12} $O^{5'}$-succinic acid	$H_2N(CH_2)_6NH_2$	Lower ligand	×
VI	Co-aminoethyl B_{12}	———	Upper ligand	×
VII	Co-carboxyethyl B_{12}	$H_2N(CH_2)_6NH_2$	Upper ligand	Unstable
VIII	N^6-carboxymethyl-Co-adenosyl B_{12}	$H_2N(CH_2)_6NH_2$	Upper ligand	×

binding of coenzyme B_{12} and apo-diol dehydrase occurs in the presence of K^+ ion; the absence of the monovalent cation caused the rapid dissociation of coenzyme due to a drastic conformational change of apoenzyme (F-S complex) and not owing to dissociation of apoprotein into F and S.[10] Hence, apoprotein bound biospecifically to immobilized B_{12} derivative should be eluted with an appropriate eluting agent in the absence of K^+ ion. Figure 4 shows a typical successful pattern of affinity chromatography: Apoprotein adsorbed on immobilized coenzyme B_{12} (Compound I, II, or III) through one carboxylic acid side chain is exclusively eluted in the fraction E-2.

Table IV summarizes the results, indicating the important roles of some of the peripheral amide side chains of corrin nucleus and the ribose moiety of the lower ligand for

TABLE V

PARTIAL STRUCTURES OF COENZYME B_{12} AND ITS ANALOGS USED IN OUR STUDY

The R group represents the nucleoside axial ligands covalently linked to the cobalt atom.

No.	Name	R	No.	Name	R
I	Adenosylcobalamin	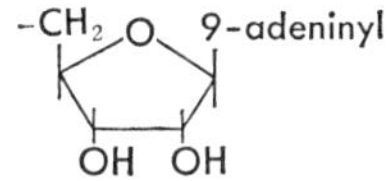	VIII	Benzimidazoleribosylcobalamin	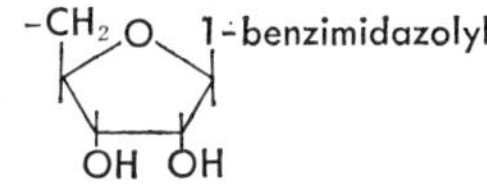
II	Ara-adenosylcobalamin	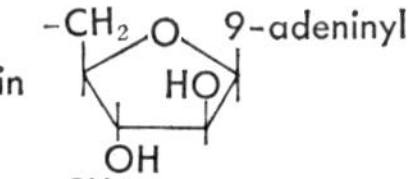	IX	L-Adenosylcobalamin	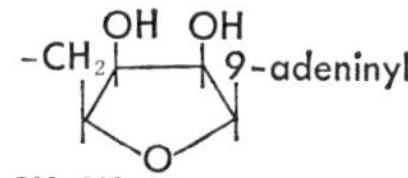
III	Aristeromycylcobalamin	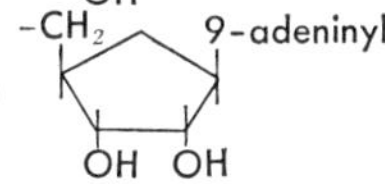	X	Adenosylethylcobalamin	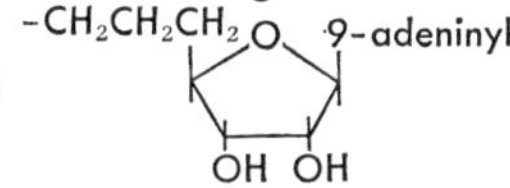
IV	3-Isoadenosylcobalamin	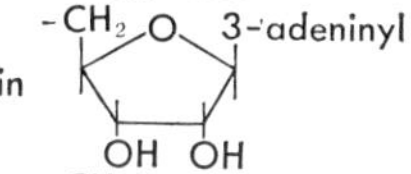	XI	Adeninylhexylcobalamin	$-(CH_2)_6-9-$adeninyl
			XII	Adeninylpentylcobalamin	$-(CH_2)_5-9-$adeninyl
V	Nebularylcobalamin	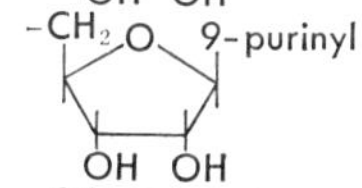	XIII	Adeninylbutylcobalamin	$-(CH_2)_4-9-$adeninyl
			XIV	Adeninylpropylcobalamin	$-(CH_2)_3-9-$adeninyl
			XV	Adeninylethylcobalamin	$-(CH_2)_2-9-$adeninyl
VI	Inosylcobalamin	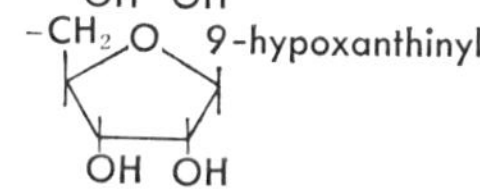	XIV	Methylcobalamin	$-CH_3$
			XVII	Cyanocobalamin	$-CN$
VII	Cytidylcobalamin	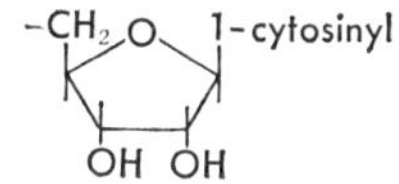			

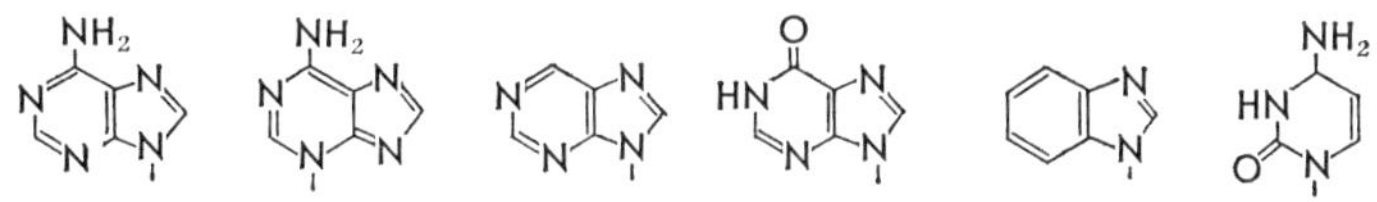

9-Adeninyl 3-Adeninyl 9-Purinyl 9-Hypoxanthinyl 1-Benzimidazolyl 1-Cytosinyl

TABLE VI

PROPERTIES OF COENZYME B_{12}-ANALOGS WITH ALTERED 5′-DEOXYADENOSYL UPPER LIGAND

Cobalamin	*Remark*	*Behavior in diol dehydrase system*	*Binding to apoenzyme*		*Properties of apoenzyme-analog complex*		
					Spectroscopic characteristics		
			Affinity	*Exchange of bound analog for AdoCbl*	*15 min (25°)*	*hν and O_2*	*Sensitivity to O_2*
Type 1	Minor change in D-ribose or adenine moiety	Active as coenzyme	High		B_{12r}*	B_{12r}* + OHB_{12}	{ Sensitive { Insensitive
Type 2	Change in adenine moiety	Weak competitive inhibitor	Low	Exchangeable	No change	B_{12r} (stabilized)	
Type 3	Change in D-ribose moiety	Strong competitive inhibitor	Very high	Not exchangeable	No change	OHB_{12}	

* The steady state concentration of B_{12r} is dependent on the coenzyme activity of the analogs.

the binding of coenzyme B_{12} to apo-diol dehydrase. As has been mentioned, the upper 5′-deoxyadenosyl ligand should play an indispensable role not only in the binding but also in the activation of Co-C bond. To obtain more precise knowledge on the function of 5′-deoxyadenosyl ligand, we studied the coenzyme action of 14 coenzyme B_{12} analogs shown in Table V, in addition to methylcobalamin and cyanocobalamin.[11] These 14 analogs have a slightly modified upper ligand. Table VI summarizes the behaviors of these analogs in the diol dehydrase system: Binding to the apoenzyme; activation of the Co-C bond leading to homolysis in the resulting holoenzyme species which was studied by absorption and ESR spectroscopy and by the sensitivity of the activated Co-C bond toward oxygen; catalytic activity of the holoenzyme species. On the basis of experimental results, we classified them into three groups. Type 1, which contains adenine or purine moiety and an intact or a slightly modified D-ribose moiety in the upper ligand, such as *ara*-adenosyl-, aristeromicyl-, 3-isoadenosyl-, and nebularylcobalamins, was able to function as coenzyme, the coenzyme activity decreasing in this order. Like the ntaive holoenzyme, complexes of these 4 analogs with apoprotein showed a cob(II)alamin (B_{12r})-like absorption peak or shoulder in the presence of substrate.

This result means that: 1) The analogs belonging to Type 1 can bind effectively to apoprotein to yield an active holoenzyme species, (2 their Co-C bond is activated by the interaction with the apoprotein, and then cleaved homolytically to yield B_{12r} and free radical species of the upper ligand when substrate comes; 3) the enzymic reaction proceeds as in the case of normal coenzyme—AdoCbl.

On the other hand, Type 2 analogs, which contain hypoxanthine, cytosine, and benzimidazole as the nucleobase moiety of the upper ligand in place of adenine, did not function as coenzyme but acted as weak competitive inhibitors against AdoCbl. Their Co-C bond was cleaved by photochemical reaction to give a B_{12r}-like spectrum which was unusually resistant toward oxidation. Type 3 analogs, in which the D-ribosyl moiety is replaced by L-ribose or by an alkyl chain of 2 to 6 carbons, were inactive as coenzyme and acted as strong competitive inhibitors. The complexes of these analogs with apoenzyme showed visible spectra similar to those of the free analogs.

In conclusion, these results give definitive evidence that both D-ribose moiety and adenine moiety of the upper ligand of AdoCbl are essential not only for the effective binding to apoprotein but also for the activation of the Co-C bond of the resulting holoenzyme.

REFERENCES

1 H. A. Barker, H. Weissbach, and R. D. Smyth, *Proc. Natl. Acad. Sci. U. S.*, 44 (1958) 1093.
2 P. G. Lenhart and D. C. Hodgkin, *Nature (London)*, 192 (1961) 937.
3 R. H. Abeles and D. Dolphin, *Acc. Chem. Res.*, 9 (1976) 114.
4 T. Toraya, T. Sugimoto, Y. Tamao, S. Shimizu, and S. Fukui, *Biochemistry*, 10 (1971) 3475.
5 T. Toraya, M. Uesaka, and S. Fukui, *Biochemistry*, 13 (1974) 3895.
6 T. Toraya, M. Kondo, Y. Isemura, and S. Fukui, *Biochemistry*, 11 (1972) 2599.
7 Y. Tamao, Y. Morikawa, S. Shimizu, and S. Fukui, *Biochem. Biophys. Res. Commun.*, 28 (1967) 692; *Biochim. Biophys. Acta*, 151 (1968) 260.
8 T. Toraya, T. Shirakashi, S. Fukui, and H. P. C. Hogenkamp, *Biochemistry*, 14 (1975) 3949.
9 T. Toraya and S. Fukui, in D. B. McCormick and L. D. Wright, *Methods in Enzymology*. (Vitamins and Coenzymes, Suppl. Ed.), Academic Press, New York, in press.
10 T. Toraya, K. Ohashi, and S. Fukui, *Biochemistry*, 14 (1975) 4255.
11 T. Toraya, K. Ushio, S. Fukui, and H. P. C. Hogenkamp, *J. Biol. Chem.*, 252 (1977) 963.

ENZYMATIC MODIFICATION OF PROTEINS BY NICOTINAMIDE ADENINE DINUCLEOTIDE

KUNIHIRO UEDA, HIROTO OKAYAMA, AND OSAMU HAYAISHI
Department of Medical Chemistry, Faculty of Medicine, Kyoto University, Kyoto (Japan)

Nicotinamide adenine dinucleotide (NAD) is the most abundant among the coenzymes derived from vitamins. Although it is well-known as a cofactor of biological oxidation/ reduction, it serves also as a precursor for protein modification. A clue to this second biological role was found in 1966 by three groups in France and in Japan including our own; the initial finding was that a portion of NAD molecule was rapidly incorporated into acid-insoluble material in the cell nucleus.[1-3]

The structure of NAD can be envisaged as the ADP-ribose moiety linked to a vitamin, nicotinamide, through a β-N-glycosidic linkage (Fig. 1). This linkage is a so-called high energy bond, since the free energy change of its hydrolysis is -8.2 kcal/mol at 25° and pH 7.0.[4] We found that the cleavage of this bond by a liver nuclear enzyme was associated with the incorporation of ADP-ribose into acid-insoluble material. Subsequent analyses revealed that the incorporated ADP-ribose took forms of monomer, oligomer, or polymer, and that all forms of ADP-ribose were bound to nuclear proteins.[5-7]

These observations opened a new era in NAD biochemistry and also in protein modification. Since then, a number of similar reactions have been discovered in various organisms, and today, ADP-ribosylation is considered to be one of the major posttranslational modifications of proteins.[8,9] Table I presents the list of those reactions. It is noteworthy that all enzymes of prokaryote origin so far found catalyze only mono-ADP-ribosylation, whereas eukaryotic enzymes catalyze oligo- or poly-ADP-ribosylation, and that the enzyme-acceptor relationship in mono-ADP-ribosylation systems is heterogeneous (encompassing different organisms) whereas it is homogeneous (within the same organism) in oligo- and poly-ADP-ribosylation systems.

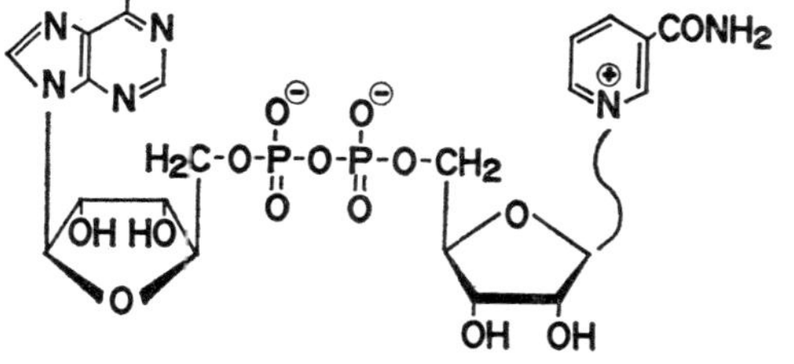

Fig. 1. Structure of NAD.

TABLE I
NATURAL DISTRIBUTION OF VARIOUS ADP-RIBOSYLATION REACTIONS

Enzyme	*Acceptor*	*ADP-ribose units*	*Reporter*
Prokaryotes			
Diphtheria toxin	Elongation factor 2	Monomer	Honjo *et al.* 1968
Pseudomonas toxin	Elongation factor 2	Monomer	Iglewski and Kabat 1975
Cholera toxin	Membrane protein	Monomer (?)	Moss *et al.* 1976
T4 phage	RNA polymerase and other *E. coli* proteins	Monomer	Goff 1974, Zillig *et al.* 1976
N4 phage	*E. coli* proteins	Monomer (?)	Pesce *et al.* 1976
Eukaryotes			
Nuclear enzyme(s)	Chromosomal proteins		
	Histones	Monomer~polymer	Nishizuka *et al.* 1968
	Non-histone proteins	Monomer~polymer	Nishizuka *et al.* 1968
	Mg^{2+}, Cd^{2+}-endonuclease	Monomer, oligomer	Yoshihara *et al.* 1974
	RNA polymerase	Polymer (?)	Müller and Zahn 1976
Mitochondrial enzyme	Mitochondrial protein	Oligomer	Kun *et al.* 1975
Cytoplasmic enzyme	Histones	Polymer (?)	Roberts *et al.* 1975

As for the nuclear system, various chromatin proteins have been reported to be modified.[8,9] The identification of the proteins, however, has been very poor, since it relies entirely on a coincidence of labeled ADP-ribose with unmodified marker proteins in chromatography or electrophoresis. These analyses may be misleading because of a change in protein behavior induced by poly-ADP-ribosylation. Characterization of poly(ADP-ribose) synthetase has also been poor, particularly in its relation to chromatin structure. In view of the importance of chromatin function, we undertook to purify and characterize the nuclear poly-ADP-ribosylation system.

Figure 2 illustrates the outline of poly-ADP-ribosylation reaction. Poly(ADP-ribose) chain is constructed on ribosyl ($1''\rightarrow2'$)-ribose linkages, and ranges in size from a monomer up to polymers of more than 100 ADP-ribosyl units. The species of acceptor protein, the mechanisms of initiation and elongation as well as the enzymes involved, the degradation pathways and responsible enzymes, and the biological significance of these findings are the subjects to be dealt with in this presentation.

The first problem studied was the properties of acceptor proteins. In order to selectively isolate poly-ADP-ribosylated proteins, we recently developed a new method.[10] A kind of affinity chromatography using a well-known interaction between a borate ion and *cis*-diols (Fig. 3). We prepared a dihydroxyboryl derivative of polyacrylamide gel. The borate residue in a negatively charged state at alkaline pH's binds a *cis*-diol compound such as ADP-ribose, and releases it upon a pH shift to neutrality. This chromatography has several advantages over other methods; for example, ADP-ribosylated material is bound and eluted essentially altogether, irrespective of the protein species and chain length, and this chromatography works in the presence of a strong dissociating agent such as guanidine-HCl. Figure 4 shows the elution profile of a 0.25 N HCl extract (or the so-called histone fraction) of rat liver nuclei preincubated with [^{14}C]NAD. Application was at pH 8.2 in morpholine buffer; 6 M guanidine-HCl was added to minimize aggregation and nonspeci-

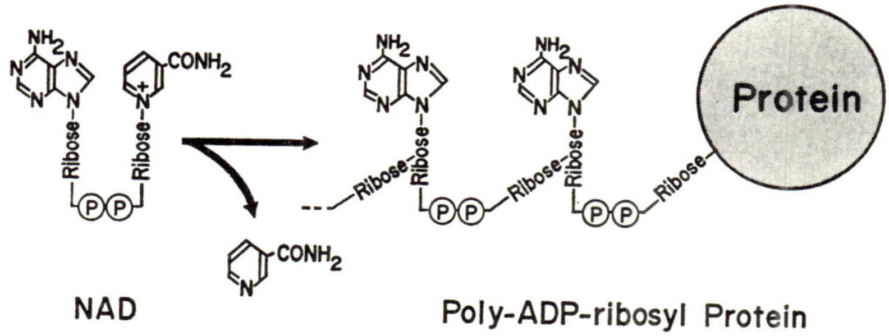

Fig. 2. Poly-ADP-ribosylation of protein in the cell nucleus.

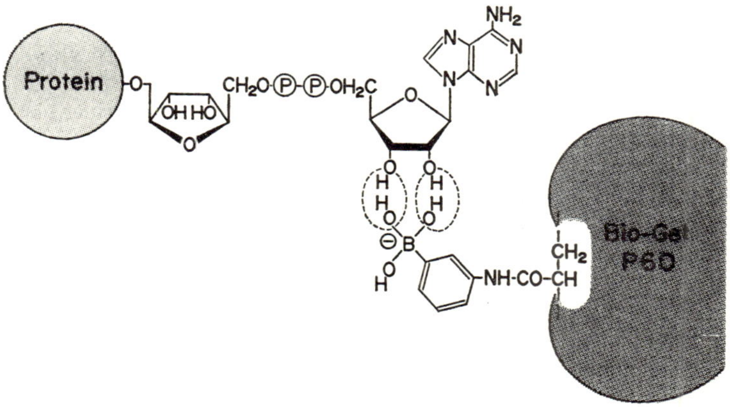

Fig. 3. Interaction of ADP-ribosyl protein with borate gel.

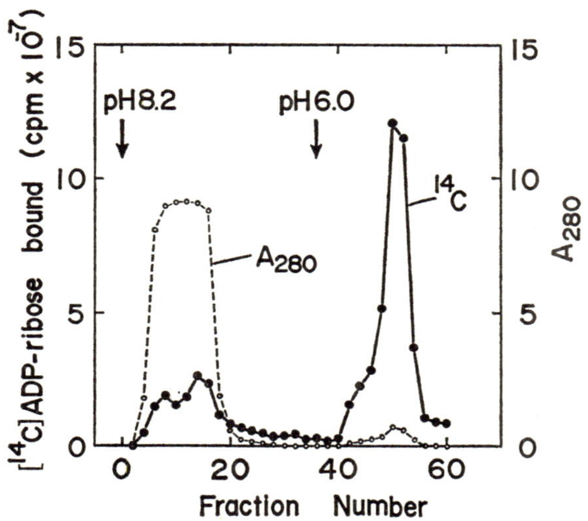

Fig. 4. Borate gel column chromatography of HCl-extracted proteins.

fic interaction of proteins. Under these conditions, most proteins passed through the column, together with a small fraction of ADP-ribose that failed to bind. The bound material was then quantitatively eluted with phosphate buffer (pH 6.0). This eluate contained most of the acid-insoluble ADP-ribose and a minute amount of protein.

The borate-bound material was then fractionated by chromatography on CM-cellulose (Fig. 5). With a gradient of KCl in phosphate buffer (pH 6.0) and 7 M urea, proteins were eluted in several peaks along with the radioactive ADP-ribose. Quantitative analysis showed that almost all ADP-ribose recovered was acid-insoluble, and at least 90% of the proteins were associated with ADP-ribose.[10] We pooled fractions (A, B, C, D) as indicated, and analyzed them by SDS-polyacrylamide gel electrophoresis.

In the electrophoretograms shown in Fig. 6, A, B, C, and D correspond to the respective CM-cellulose fractions. NC denotes total nuclear proteins of rat liver, and STD stands for proteins of molecular weight standards; BSA (bovine serum albumin), TI (soybean trypsin inhibitor), LY (egg white lysozyme), β, β', and α (*E. coli* RNA polymerase subunits). Electrophoresis was performed after the removal of ADP-ribose by a mild alkaline treatment so that the mobility of each protein was not influenced by the ADP-ribose portion. Both fractions A and B comprised a mixture of several nonhistone proteins with a wide variety of molecular weights. Fraction C gave one major band around the positions of histone H3, H2B or H2A, and a couple of minor bands. The major band was purified by preparative electrophoresis and identified as H2B by amino acid analysis. Fraction D appeared to contain almost solely H1, and, in fact, its amino acid composition coincided well with the reported value of calf thymus H1. When the alkaline pretreatment was omitted, all protein bands were found associated with ADP-ribose.[10] These results unequivocally demonstrated the (poly)ADP-ribosylation of histones H1 and H2B as well as nonhistone proteins.

In addition to these "natural" acceptors, we used another, "artificial" acceptor in our study. As described by Kun and his collaborators,[11] ADP-ribose and other ribose derivatives bind nonenzymatically to various proteins including histones in alkaline conditions. On the basis of ^{3}H incorporation upon reduction with $NaB^{3}H_4$, the linkage

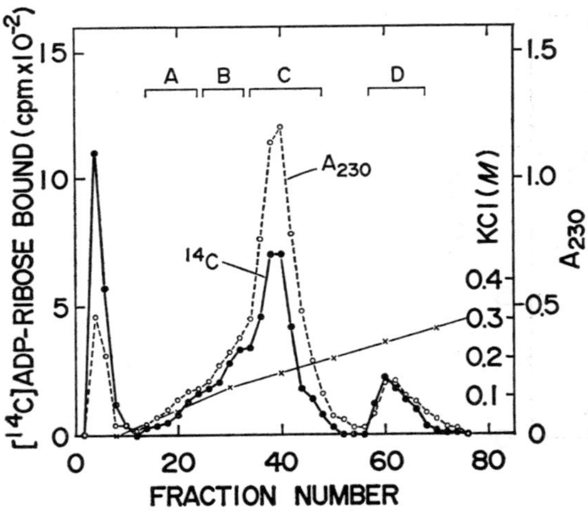

Fig. 5. CM-cellulose column chromatography of borate gel eluate.

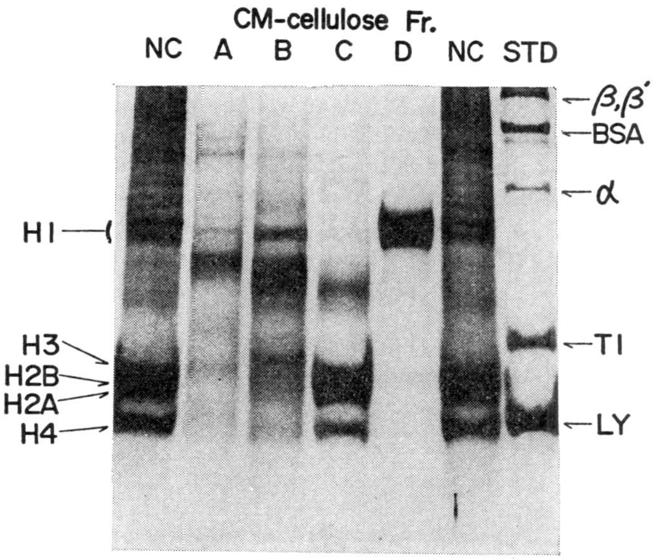

Fig. 6. SDS-gel electrophoresis of CM-cellulose fractions.

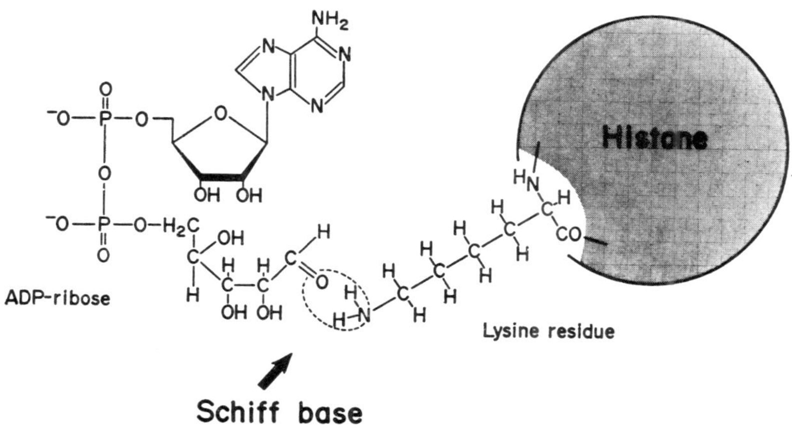

Fig. 7. Nonenzymatic formation of ADP-ribose • histone adduct.

has been reported to be a Schiff base between the aldehyde group of ribose and the ε-amino group of lysine (Fig. 7). We prepared various histone adducts, reduced them with $NaBH_4$, and employed them as ADP-ribosyl histone analogs in the following mechanism studies.

The second problem studied was the enzymatic mechanism of poly-ADP-ribosylation. The enzyme that catalyzes the ADP-ribose incorporation into acid-insoluble material is called poly(ADP-ribose) synthetase, with no reference to mono- or poly-ADP-ribosylation. We purified this enzyme about 6,000-fold from rat liver nuclei[12] and attempted to reconstitute the whole modification reaction.

The purified enzyme was unique in its almost complete dependence for activity on the presence of DNA. As shown in Table II, the addition of DNA enhanced the activity 25-fold. Further addition of histone together with DNA promoted another 4-fold stimulation, while histone alone was rather inhibitory. The latter activation by histone was once supposed to be due to a supply of acceptor sites, and the poly-ADP-ribosylation reaction to be totally reconstituted. Analyses of the reaction products, however, did not support this view; they suggested that histones did not accept ADP-ribose but acted as allosteric activators (see below).

When we compared histone H1 and chemically synthesized ADP-ribose·H1 adducts in the activation of purified synthetase, it was found that the adducts were much more potent than unmodified H1 (Fig. 8). Furthermore, the incorporated ADP-ribose was found associated with the ADP-ribose · histone adduct (Fig. 9, lower panel). With unmodified H1 and DNA, by contrast, no ADP-ribose appeared in association with the histone, but all radioactivity remained at the top of the gel where no histone was detectable (upper panel). These results suggested that the ADP-ribose portion in the adduct might accept ADP-ribose—that is, be elongated.

In order to investigate this possibility, we performed a "label transfer" experiment.[13]

TABLE II
EFFECTS OF DNA AND HISTONE ON POLY-ADP-RIBOSYLATION

Addition	*ADP-ribose incorporated (pmol)*
None	1.1
DNA	27
DNA+histone (H1)	105
Histone (H1)	0.3

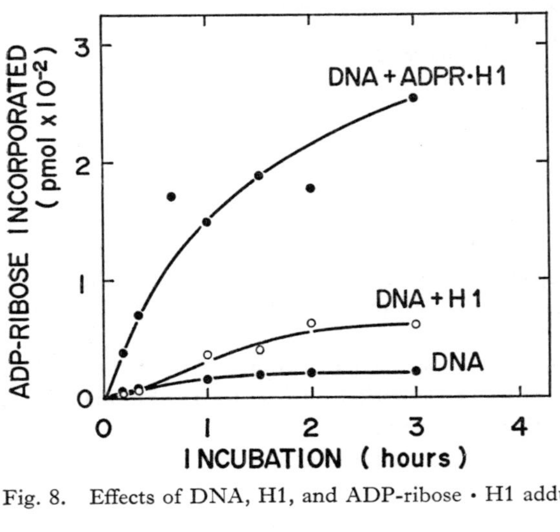

Fig. 8. Effects of DNA, H1, and ADP-ribose · H1 adduct on poly(ADP-ribose) synthesis.

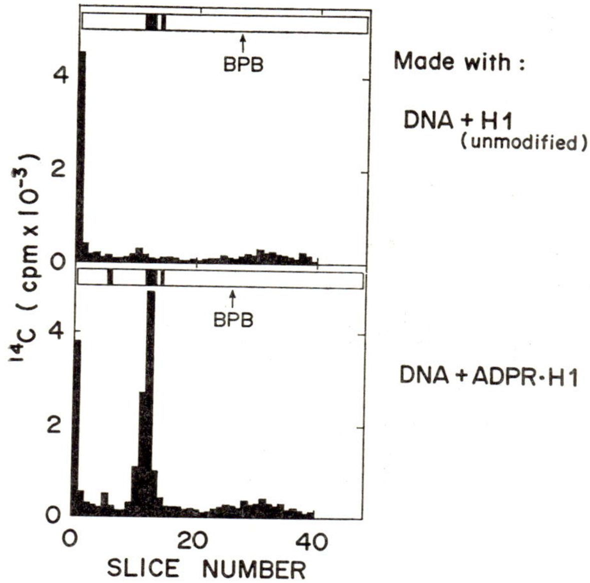

Fig. 9. SDS-gel electrophoresis of poly-ADP-ribosylated products. Poly-ADP-ribosylation was carried out with DNA plus unmodified H1 (upper) or DNA plus ADP-ribose • H1 adduct (lower).

Its principle is depicted in Fig. 10. [^{14}C]ADP-ribose labeled in the adenine portion was nonenzymatically attached to histone H1. This ADP-ribose, unless elongated, gives [^{14}C]AMP upon digestion with snake venom phosphodiesterase. If elongation takes place from this ADP-ribose and in the direction illustrated using unlabeled NAD, the phosphodiesterase treatment will give labeled *iso*ADP-ribose, a specific product from the interior of poly(ADP-ribose); the terminal AMP is no longer radioactive. The proportion of radioactivity in *iso*ADP-ribose to the total is thus a measure of elongation from the pre-attached ADP-ribose.

The experimental result is shown in Fig. 11. Analysis of digested products was performed on a Dowex 1 column. While the untreated adduct gave [^{14}C]AMP, as expected, and a small amount of adenosine (produced from AMP by contaminating phosphatases), the adduct treated with purified poly(ADP-ribose) synthetase and unlabeled NAD gave a third radioactive material in the position of *iso*ADP-ribose that preceded marker ADP-ribose. The latter material was concentrated, and was identified as *iso*ADP-ribose by paper chromatography and by conversion to ribosyl-adenosine using alkaline phosphatase. A parallel experiment using ^{3}H-labeled NAD for elongation indicated that about half of the new chains originated from the adducts and another half from an endogenous acceptor contained in the enzyme preparation (see below).

A preliminary experiment has also suggested that ADP-ribosyl histones (H1 and H2B) prepared enzymatically and isolated on borate gel (Fig. 4) also serve as good acceptors for elongation.

All these results clearly demonstrated the elongating activity of purified poly(ADP-ribose) synthetase and its action by a terminal addition mechanism. Furthermore, our successful reconstitution of the elongation step from precharged histones appeared to

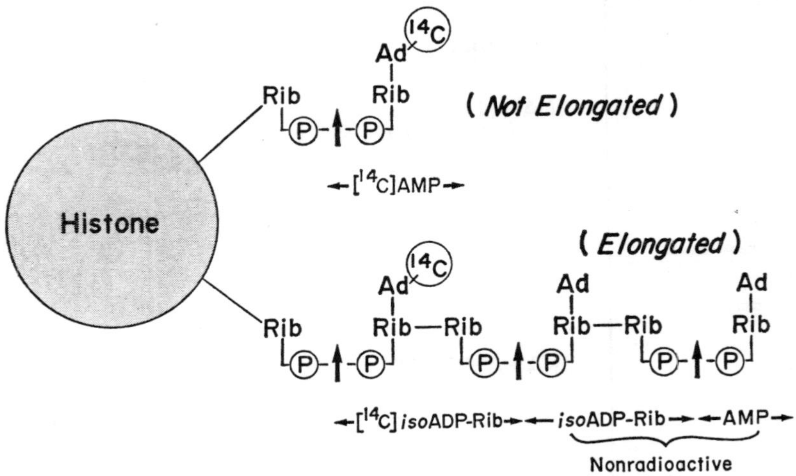

Fig. 10. Phosphodiesterase digestion of (poly)ADP-ribose • H1 adducts. Arrows indicate the linkages cleaved by phosphodiesterase.

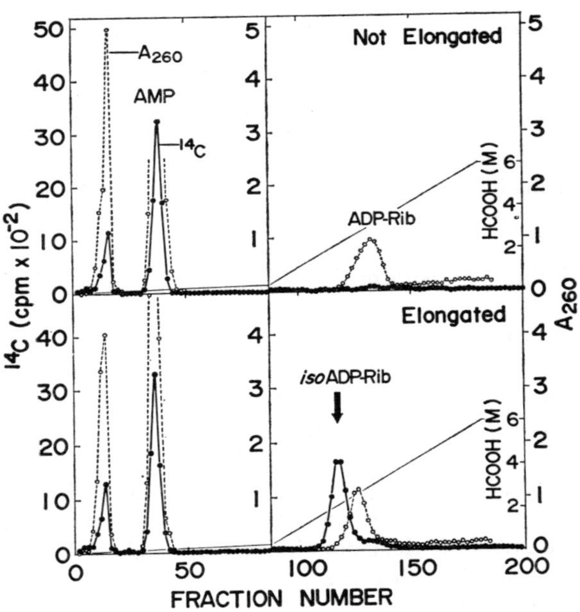

Fig. 11. Dowex 1 column chromatography of phosphodiesterase digests.

support the view that partially degraded polymer may be re-elongated *in vivo*.

During analyses of reaction products, we found that the purified synthetase did not ADP-ribosylate any of histones exogenously added.[10] As mentioned in Fig. 9 and confirmed in Fig. 12, under conditions of DNA alone, or DNA plus various histones, the

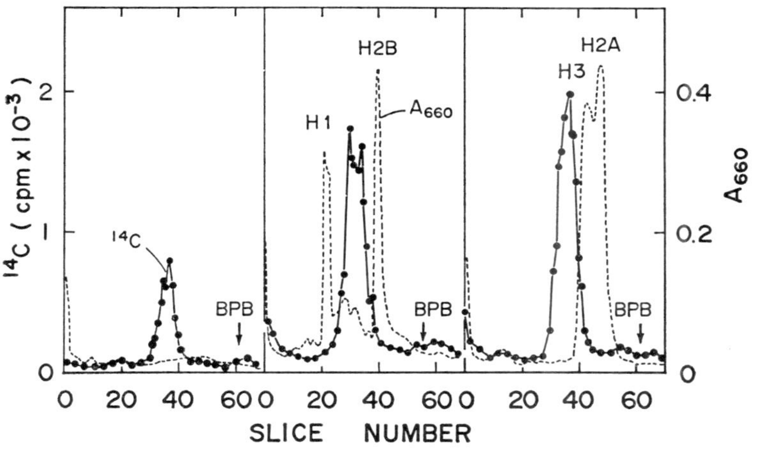

Fig. 12. SDS-gel electrophoresis of variously poly-ADP-ribosylated products. (Left) DNA alone, (middle) DNA plus histones H1 and H2B, and (right) DNA plus histones H2A and H3.

incorporated ADP-ribose did not co-migrate with histone bands; it migrated, in all cases, to a unique position with R_f 0.58 relative to a tracking dye, BPB. These results indicated that, in the reconstituted enzyme system, poly-ADP-ribosylation did not occur on histones but rather, probably, on an endogenous acceptor contained in the enzyme preparation.

The discrepancy between the histone ADP-ribosylation *in vivo* (as well as in crude nuclei) and the inability of purified enzyme to ADP-ribosylate histones led us to a tentative conclusion that our purified synthetase is an elongation enzyme and that, probably, the step of initiation is catalyzed by another, as yet unidentified, enzyme. The earlier result that the purified enzyme can modify histone once an ADP-ribose monomer is attached to the protein supports this view.

The third problem is concerned with the degradation of poly(ADP-ribose). Two pathways of degradation have so far been known. One is the cleavage of the ribosyl-ribose bond, catalyzed by poly(ADP-ribose) glycohydrolase.[14,15] This reaction produces ADP-ribose monomers and leaves the terminus as adenosine. The other pathway is the cleavage of the pyrophosphate bond by phosphodiesterase. Various lines of evidence suggest that the former glycohydrolase is mainly responsible for the polymer degradation *in vivo*, which indicates that most of partially degraded polymers have a chance to be re-elongated by the action of poly (ADP-ribose) synthetase.[14]

As for the cleavage of the linkage between ADP-ribose and protein, no enzyme has been found in spite of many researchers' efforts. Very recently, we found this enzyme activity in the nucleus and cytosol of rat liver cells.[16] The enzyme, which is assayed by liberation of ADP-ribose from mono-ADP-ribosyl histone (H1 or H2B), is distinct from poly-(ADP-ribose) glycohydrolase. As shown in Fig. 13, the two activities were clearly separated on a DEAE-cellulose column.

Figure 14 shows the time course of releasing ADP-ribose from ADP-ribosyl H2B. A is the reaction with an enzyme purified as above and B is a control without enzyme. The ADP-ribosyl H2B bond was not completely stable under the conditions employed (pH 6.0, 37°), and was gradually degraded nonenzymatically. In terms of the initial velocity, the

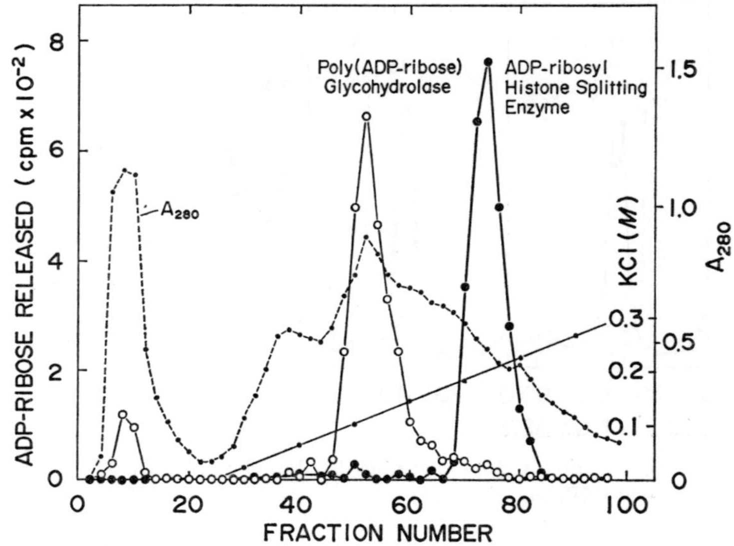

Fig. 13. Separation of poly(ADP-ribose) glycohydrolase and ADP-ribosyl histone splitting enzyme by DEAE-cellulose column chromatography.

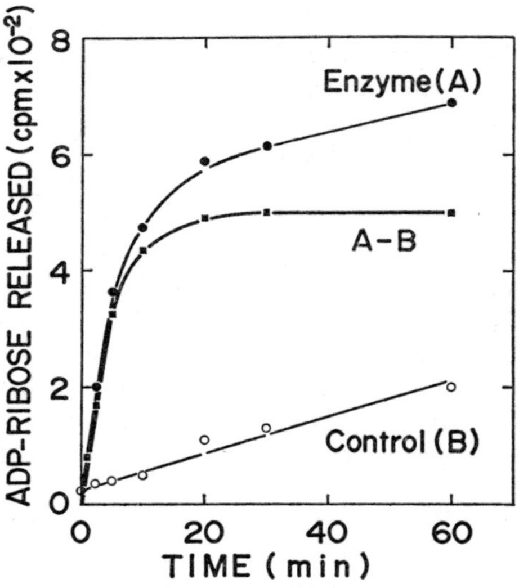

Fig. 14. Time course of ADP-ribosyl histone splitting.

addition of enzyme enhanced the net hydrolysis (A – B) at least 20-fold. The split product contained the entire portion of ADP-ribose, and it was tentatively identified as ADP-ribose by paper chromatography. Although more precise analysis is essential, this enzyme appears to be a hitherto unknown species. For this new species, we propose the tentative name "ADP-ribosyl histone splitting enzyme."

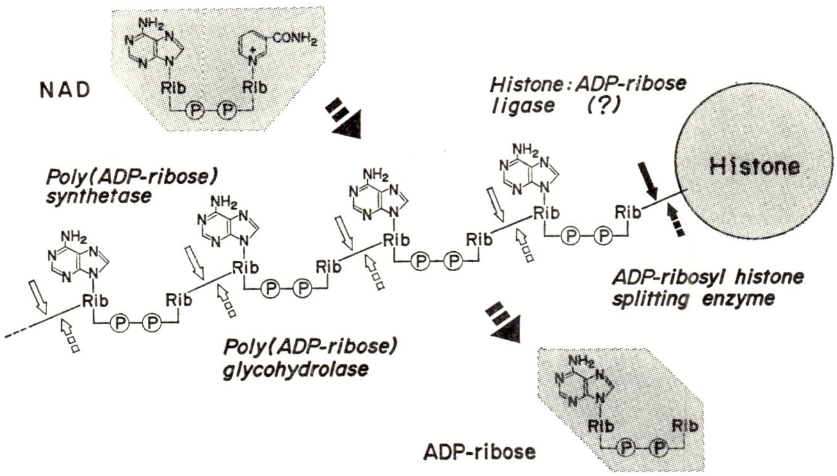

Fig. 15. Synthesis and degradation of poly-ADP-ribosyl histone.

Figure 15 summarizes our current view of poly(ADP-ribose) metabolism based on the present study. In this scheme, synthesis and degradation of poly-ADP-ribosyl histone proceed with an ADP-ribose monomer as a transfer unit, at both the ADP-ribose · protein junction and the internal ribosyl-ribose linkages. We have already found three of the four enzymes expected, and found an implication of the fourth ("histone: ADP-ribose ligase"). Although the flow of ADP-ribose appears to be energetically irreversible (*i.e.*, from NAD to polymer and further to free ADP-ribose), the polymer chain may be reversibly shortened and re-elongated *in vivo* by the actions of poly(ADP-ribose) glycohydrolase and synthetase.

The precise biological significance of poly-ADP-ribosylation has not yet been elucidated, but a number of reports suggest its close correlation with various aspects of gene expression such as DNA metabolism,[17] cell cycles,[18] differentiation,[19] transformation[20] or chromatin condensation.[21] A dynamic viewpoint of poly(ADP-ribose) metabolism such as that described above would be indispensable for biological studies of this modification.

ACKNOWLEDGMENT

This work was supported in part by Grants-in-Aid for Scientific Research and Cancer Research from the Ministry of Education, Science and Culture, Japan.

REFERENCES

1 P. Chambon, J. D. Weil, J. Doly, M. T. Strosser, and P. Mandel, *Biochem. Biophys. Res. Commun.*, 25 (1966) 638.
2 Y. Nishizuka, K. Ueda, K. Nakazawa, and O. Hayaishi, *J. Biol. Chem.*, 242 (1967) 3164.
3 T. Sugimura, S. Fujimura, S. Hasegawa, and Y. Kawamura, *Biochim. Biophys. Acta*, 138 (1967) 438.
4 L. J. Zatman, N. O. Kaplan, and S. P. Colowick, *J. Biol. Chem.*, 200 (1953) 197.
5 Y. Nishizuka, K. Ueda, T. Honjo, and O. Hayaishi, *J. Biol. Chem.*, 243 (1968) 3765.
6 H. Otake, M. Miwa, S. Fujimura, and T. Sugimura, *J. Biochem.*, 65 (1969) 145.
7 Y. Nishizuka, K. Ueda, K. Yoshihara, H. Yamamura, M. Takeda, and O. Hayaishi, *Cold Spring Harbor Symp. Quant. Biol.*, 34 (1969) 781.

8 H. Hilz and P. Stone, *Rev. Physiol. Biochem. Pharmacol.*, 76 (1976) 1.
9 O. Hayaishi and K. Ueda, *Annu. Rev. Biochem.*, 46 (1977) 95.
10 H. Okayama, K. Ueda, and O. Hayaishi, *Proc. Natl. Acad. Sci. U.S.*, 75 (1978) 1111.
11 E. Kun, A. C. Y. Chang, M. L. Sharma, A. M. Ferro, and D. Nitecki, *Proc. Natl. Acad. Sci. U.S.*, 73 (1976) 3131.
12 H. Okayama, C. M. Edson, M. Fukushima, K. Ueda, and O. Hayaishi, *J. Biol. Chem.*, 252 (1977) 7000.
13 K. Ueda, M. Kawaichi, H. Okayama, and O. Hayaishi, *J. Biol. Chem.* (1978) in press.
14 K. Ueda, J. Oka, S. Narumiya, N. Miyakawa, and O. Hayaishi, *Biochem. Biophys. Res. Commun.*, 46 (1972) 516.
15 M. Miwa, M. Tanaka, T. Matsushima, and T. Sugimura, *J. Biol. Chem.*, 249 (1974) 3475.
16 H. Okayama, M. Honda, and O. Hayaishi, *Proc. Natl. Acad. Sci. U.S.*, 75 (1978) 2254.
17 L. Burzio and S. S. Koide, *Biochem. Biophys. Res. Commun.*, 40 (1970) 1013.
18 R. A. Colyer, K. E. Burdette, and W. R. Kidwell, *Biochem. Biophys. Res. Commun.*, 53 (1973) 960.
19 A. I. Caplan and M. J. Rosenberg, *Proc. Natl. Acad. Sci. U.S.*, 72 (1975) 1852.
20 T. Sugimura, M. Miwa, Y. Kanai, K. Oda, K. Segawa, M. Tanaka, and H. Sakura, in W. E. Criss, T. Ono, and J. R. Sabine, *Control Mechanisms in Cancer*, Raven Press, New York, 1976, p. 231.
21 D. W. Mullins, Jr., C. P. Giri, and M. Smulson, *Biochemistry*, 16 (1977) 506.

VITAMIN A TRANSPORT IN PLASMA AND CONTROL OF ITS METABOLISM BY THYROXINE

M. KRISHNA BHAT, K. SREEKRISHNA, AND H. R. CAMA
Department of Biochemistry, Indian Institute of Science, Bangalore (India)

Vitamin A is an essential micronutrient for the maintenance of growth, vision, and reproduction in higher animals. Except for its role in the visual process, little information is available about the general molecular action of vitamin A. In contrast, in recent years, a better knowledge has emerged regarding its mechanism of intestinal absorption, storage and transport in blood to various target cells.

Goodman and his colleagues[1] characterized for the first time in human blood plasma a protein designated as RBP (mol. wt. $\simeq$20,000 daltons, with α-electrophoretic mobility), which specifically binds retinol (vitamin A alcohol) in 1:1 molar ratio. There onwards, it has been characterized from plasma of a variety of mammalian[2] and non-mammalian vertebrates.[3] RBP isolated from various animal species have comparable physicochemical properties,[2,3] although immunologically they are species specific.[4] Liver is the site of synthesis of RBP and is also the storage tissue for vitamin A. From liver, the retinol-RBP complex is released to blood; in the absence of RBP, retinol is not mobilized from the liver and vice versa.[5,6] In plasma retinol-RBP is generally present as an equimolar complex (*i.e.*, complexed RBP, mol. wt. $\simeq$75,000 daltons) withanother plasma protein which is characterized to be TBPA (mol. wt. $\simeq$55,000 daltons) in the case of human, monkey, rat, rabbit, and chicken.[2] We have recently[7] established the occurrence of TBPA in goat plasma, which was earlier[8] conceived to be devoid of such a protein. PA-RBP complex formation prevents the renal loss of the low mol. wt. RBP molecule and aids in the stabilization of retinol-RBP complex.[9] Very recently, employing complexed RBP preparation isolated from goat plasma, we have demonstrated as much as a 10-fold enhancement in the affinity of retinol for RBP in the presence of PA.[2]

Formation of retinol-RBP complex is of great physiological significance in the transport of vitamin A. It helps in the solubilization of the water-insoluble vitamin, stabilization of retinol molecule, prevention of tissue damage by retinol due to its non-specific surface active property[9] and in the specific delivery of the vitamin to target cells presumably through the mediation of specific cell membrane bound receptor(s).[10,11]

Apart from the RBP in plasma, specific cellular retinol- and retinoic acid-binding proteins have also been demonstrated in several tissues.[12-14] The occurrenceof these soluble intracellular receptors suggests the possibility that they may play a crucial role in mediating the vitamin action in target cells, as in the case of steroid hormones. It

Abbreviations: RBP, retinol-binding protein; TBPA, thyroxine-binding prealbumin; PA, prealbumin; PCM, protein-calorie malnutrition. T_4, thyroxine.

is quite likely that the factors which determine the availability of these binding proteins, especially that of RBP are vital in exerting a strict control over the distribution of vitamin A to target cells. For instance, protein deficiency causes an obstruction in the hepatic release of vitamin A as a consequence of impairment in the RBP synthesis.[5] Even in a normal animal, one would expect variations in the levels of these binding proteins in accordance with the needs of the animal for vitamin A. Indeed, this has been found to be true in the case of plasma RBP[15] as well as with respect to cellular retinol- and retinoic acid-binding proteins.[16]

In continuation of our work on the plasma transport of vitamin A, we have been interested in understanding the mode of vitamin A transport to the developing embryo and the mechanism of thyroidal control of vitamin A metabolism with a view to getting a better insight into the metabolic relationship that exists between vitamin A and thyroxine.[17-20]

MODE OF VITAMIN A TRANSPORT FOR EMBRYONIC DEVELOPMENT: CHARACTERIZATION OF RBP, PA, AND PA-RBP FROM DUCK EGG YOLK AND DEMONSTRATION OF THEIR IDENTITY WITH THE PLASMA COUNTER PARTS

It is clearly established that vitamin A is required for normal embryological development and in the differentiation of various tissues. In an attempt to study the manner in which vitamin A is presented and delivered for the developing embryo, we have chosen the "avian embryo model." The avian embryo is anatomically separate from the mother during its development, and its entire quota of the vitamin A must be derived from the vitamin A stores deposited in the egg; thus it offers an elegant model for the present study.

All the vitamin A reserves of the egg are solely confined to egg yolk and the major form of vitamin A present in the yolk is vitamin A alcohol "retinol"[21] as is the case with blood plasma. This made us postulate the presence of retinol-RBP complex in egg yolk as well, and we made an attempt to characterize such a complex (if present) from the yolk. Yolk was separated from egg white and mixed with five times its volume of 5 mM potassium phosphate buffer, pH 7.6 containing 0.1M NaCl and dialyzed against the same buffer for 48 hr with two changes of the buffer. The dialyzed material was centrifuged at 10,000 rpm for 1 hr and the particulate material was discarded as it was devoid of any retinol. The supernatant was subjected to DEAE-cellulose chromatography. The bound proteins were eluted with a linear gradient of 0.1 to 0.4M NaCl dissolved in the buffer same as that used for dialysis. Fractions with specific retinol fluorescence as monitored by the fluorescence intensity at 460 nm upon excitation at 330 nm were pooled and concentrated. The material that precipitated on concentrating was devoid of retinol and thus it was discarded. Polyacrylamide disc gel electrophoresis of a portion of the supernatant indicated the presence of a fluorescent band under UV light (prior to staining) characteristic of the plasma RBP. A protein with PA mobility was also detected apart from several other contaminating proteins. The supernatant fraction was subjected to the next step of purification on Sephadex G-100. This step helped in getting rid of large mol. wt. contaminants, and protein-bound retinol at this stage got eluted as a distinct peak in the 75,000 daltons mol. wt. region, which is characteristic of the plasma PA-RBP complex. This fraction was further subjected to DEAE-Sephadex A-50 chromatography which separated the protein-bound retinol from another protein, eventually shown to be free PA, which is generally present in addition to that complexed with RBP. The protein-bound retinol at

TABLE I

PROPERTIES OF DUCK YOLK PA, RBP, AND PA-RBP COMPARED WITH THEIR PLASMA COUNTERPARTS

Property	*Duck yolk*			*Chicken plasma*[2]			*Human plasma*[22]		
	RBP	*PA*	*PA-RBP*	*RBP*	*PA*	*PA-RBP*	*RBP*	*PA*	*PA-RBP*
1. Mol. wt. (daltons) (Gel-filtration)	20,000	55,000	75,000	20,000–22,000	56,000	76,000	20,000–22,000	55,000	75,000
2. Mol. wt. (daltons) (SDS electrophoresis)	20,000	14,000	—	20,000	13,000	19,000 13,000	20,000	14,000	—
3. Electrophoretic behavior	M.H.*1	—	Dissociates	M.H.	—	Dissociates	M.H.	—	Dissociates
4. Electrophoretic mobility relative to albumin	α	PA	α and PA	α	PA	α and PA	α_1, α_2	PA	α and PA
5. UV absorption max (nm)	280 330	280	280 330	280 330	280	280 330	280 330	280	280 330
6. $A_{1cm}^{1\%}$ 280 (nm)	16.2	23.4	17	19.2	22.8	20.8	17.5	—	—
7. A_{280}: A_{330}	1.6	—	3.0	0.98	—	1.76	1.0	—	2.0
8. Fluorescence									
Excitation λ_{max} (nm)	330,280	280	330,280	330,280	280	330,280	332,280	280	330,280
Emission λ_{max} (nm)	460,330	330	460,330	460,330	330	460,330	456,330	330	460,330
9. Affinity to L-T_4*2	(−)	(+)	(+)	(−)	(+)	(+)	(−)	(+)	(+)

*1 M.H., microheterogeneity.

*2 T_4, thyroxine; (+), binds; (−), does not bind.

this stage was characterized to be PA-RBP complex, based on its electro-phoretic behavior. This complex was dissociated into PA and RBP by Sephadex G-100 chromatography at low ionic strength (5 mM). This is exactly the condition under which human and chicken plasma PA-RBP are also known to dissociate.[22,23]

Properties of duck yolk RBP, PA and PA-RBP are summarized in Table I together with those of their counterparts present in chicken (homologous) and human (heterologous) plasma. It is clear that in general, they have very similar physicochemical properties. The lower content of vitamin A in the yolk RBP as indicated by a higher A_{280}:A_{330} ratio might arise due to partial dissociation of vitamin A from the protein during purification. Recently, Heller[23] has demonstrated the existence of PA and RBP in hen's egg yolk with properties similar to those present in chicken plasma. Thus, one can expect a comparable vitamin A transport system to be present in duck plasma as well.

Making use of the property that binding of either RBP or L-thyroxine to PA results in quenching of PA fluorescence at 330 nm,[24] we could demonstrate the binding of both RBP (homologous: duck egg yolk RBP, and heterologous: goat plasma RBP) and L-thyroxine to yolk PA. Further yolk PA was shown to have distinct sites for RBP and L-thyroxine, respectively. The fact that duck yolk PA can bind goat RBP suggests that RBP and PA, which were derived from distinct species, are able to recognize each other and thus their topography and conformation are similar. PA from duck yolk cross reacted with antibodies to chicken plasma PA_2.[24] Earlier, we demonstrated that of the three PAs (PA_1, PA_2, and PA_3) present in chicken plasma,[25] only PA_2 forms a specific complex with both L-thyroxine and RBP.[24] Thus, the PA purified from duck yolk is analogous to chicken plasma PA_2.

Recently, Abe *et al.*[26] have demonstrated immunoreactive RBP and PA in developing chick embryo serum, eye, and brain, while they were unable to detect any RBP in embryonic liver and defected PA only at day 13. Thus, it is quite probable that the RBP deposited in the egg yolk takes care of its requirement till the hatched chick starts synthesizing its own RBP. Further studies are necessary to understand how the retinol-RBP in egg yolk is transported across the yolk sac membrane to the developing embryo and also regarding the exact stage at which the liver starts RBP synthesis.

THYROIDAL CONTROL OF VITAMIN A METABOLISM

As pointed out earlier, the PA_2 in chicken plasma binds both thyroxine and retinol-RBP forming a quaternary complex.[2,24] But the binding of one ligand to PA_2 does not interfere with that of the other ligand[24] and hence they are independently transported. Earlier studies have shown that induction of hyperthyroidism leads to vitamin A deficiency and the onset of xerophthalmia.[17] Dosing vitamin A-deficient animals with thyroid inhibitors prolonged their lives,[18] thus indicating an inverse relationship between their plasma levels. In hyperthyroid individuals RBP and PA levels of plasma were significantly lower than normal, while the molar ratio of retinol: RBP and RBP:PA in plasma remained unaffected.[27]

The vitamin A deficiency during hyperthyroidism was believed to be due to inadequate amount of dietary vitamin A.[17] But later observations of Cama *et al.*,[19,20] with hyperthyroid rats showed that thyroxine increases intestinal conversion of carotenoids to vitamin A, its absorption and storage as vitamin A ester. From the earlier reports on increased need for all dietary essentials and negative nitrogen balance during hyperthyroidism,[28] we could anticipate an inadequacy in amino acid precursors for the synthesis of the carrier proteins of vitamin A. With this view, we have carried out an investigation of the thyroidal role in vitamin A metabolism through a study of the metabolism of its carrier proteins. By means of radioimmunoassay using specific antisera, we have measured the plasma levels of RBP and PA_2 under different conditions of treatment.

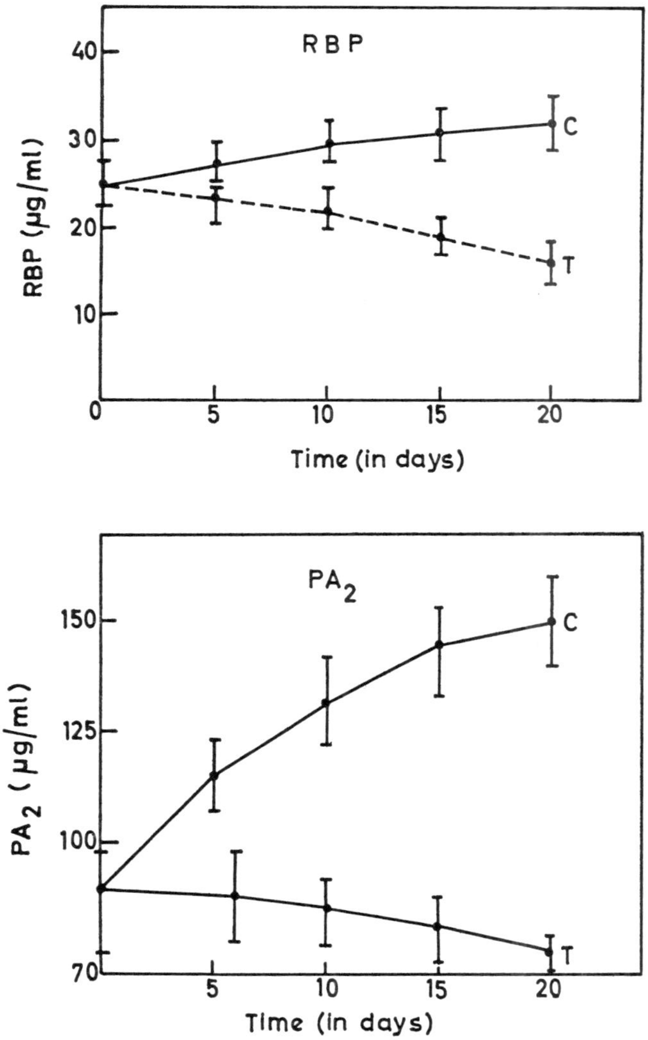

Fig. 1. Effect of thyroxine treatment on plasma levels of RBP and PA_2. Day old chicks were treated with thyroxine by intraperitoneal (i.p.) injection of L-thyroxine in phosphate buffer, pH 7.6/saline daily 25 µg/100 g body wt. for 20 days. Pair-fed control chicks were injected with the buffer alone. The RBP and PA_2 levels of plasma were measured by radioimmunoassay.

Hyperthyroidism and status of plasma vitamin A, RBP, and PA_2

The plasma levels of RBP and PA_2 declined with the progress of thyroxine treatment compared to a slight increase of their levels in the control group (Fig. 1). Concomitant with the decrease in the plasma levels of these carrier proteins in hyperthyroid chicks, a proportionate decrease in plasma level of vitamin A was also observed (Table II). The ratio of vitamin A:RBP:PA_2 was the same in the control as well as the thyroxine-treated group, thus indicating that plasma RBP level represents plasma vitamin A level during hyperthyroidism also.

Effect of amino acid supplementation along with thyroxine on RBP and PA_2 levels

The decrease in the levels of RBP and PA_2 could be due to the negative nitrogen balance caused during thyroxine treatment. To neutralize this effect amino acid supplementation was made along with thyroxine treatment. It is evident from Fig. 2 that amino acid treatment could overcome the decrease in RBP and PA_2 levels caused by thyroxine treatment. However, we do not conclude that imbalance in amino acid precursor pool alone is the cause of decrease in levels of RBP and PA_2.

Unlike the vitamin A underfed condition,[6] in all four different experimental groups (Table III), the liver levels of RBP and PA_2 were proportionate to their plasma levels, indicating no accumulation of RBP or PA_2.

Studies on the time response of increase in RBP level of plasma upon amino acid treatment of hyperthyroid chicks indicated a lag period of 6 hr (Fig. 3) presumably due to its *de novo* synthesis.

Effect of thyroxine treatment on the amino acid pool size of liver and the synthetic rates of RBP and PA_2

The steady state equilibrium that exists between the synthesis of RBP, hepatic release of retinol-RBP complex and plasma clearance under normal condition was lost during hyperthyroidism, and could be brought almost to normalcy by amino acid supplementation. The precise reason for this imbalance of the steady state during hyperthyroidism could be

TABLE II

EFFECT OF T4 AND AMINO ACID TREATMENTS ON VITAMIN A STATUS OF LIVER AND PLASMA*

The four groups of chicks were treated as described in legend to Fig. 2.

	Liver						*Plasma*	
Group	*Total vitamin A*		*Vitamin A ester*		*Vitamin A alcohol*		*Vitamin A alcohol*	
	µg/g tissue	*%*	*µg/tissue*	*%*	*µg/tissue*	*%*	*µg/100 ml*	*%*
C	333.2±32.0	100	313.2±29.6	94	20.0±2.4	6	42.0±4.5	100
	S		S		S		S	
T	659.6±25.6	198	539.8±21.0	162	119.7±4.6	36	22.0±2.5	52
	N.S.		N.S.		N.S.		N.S.	
A	346.6±26.8	104	326.6±25.2	98	20.2±1.6	6	47.25±4.2	113
	S		S		N.S.		N.S.	
A+T	493.2±24.8	148	469.8±23.4	150	22.8±1.8	7	40.7±3.5	97

* All values are mean ±S.E.M. of five chicks. S, significant at $p<0.05$; N.S., not significant at $p<0.05$.

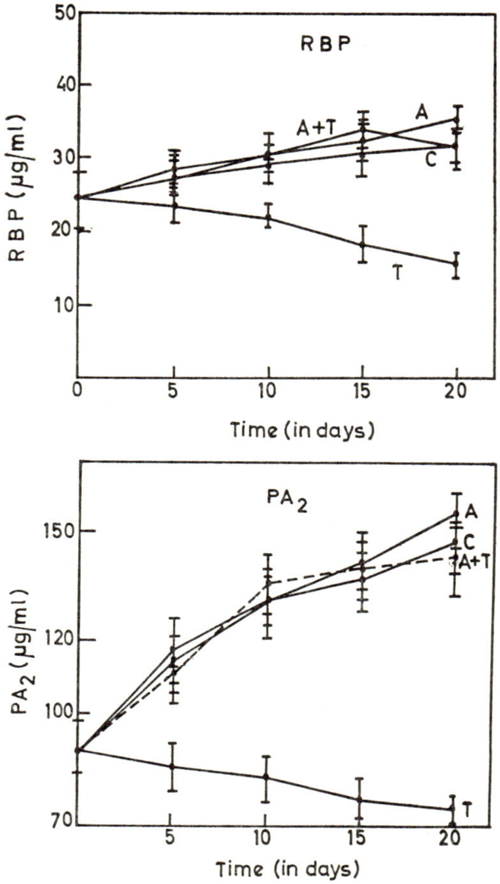

Fig. 2. Effect of T_4 and amino acid treatment on plasma levels of RBP and PA_2. Day old chicks were treated under different groups as follows. T-group, thyroxine-treated group, intra-peritoneal injection of L-T_4 in phosphate buffer, pH 7.6/saline, daily 25 μg/100 g body wt. A-group, amino acid-treated group, i.p. injection of essential amino acid mixture, daily 200 mg/100 g body wt. A+T-group, amino acid+T_4-treated group, i.p. injection of both essential amino acid mixture and T_4, daily 200 mg and 25 μg/100 g body wt., respectively. C-group, control group: pair-fed control group injected with the carrier buffer alone. The PA_2 and RBP levels were measured by radioimmunoassay.

investigated by studies on rates of synthesis and turnover of RBP and PA_2 and changes in the amino acid pool of the liver.

The relative synthetic rates of total liver protein, RBP and PA_2 in the four groups of chicks are shown in Table IV. Compared to the control group, increased rates of synthesis were seen in both thyroxine-treated groups (T- and A+T-groups). In the A+T-group the synthetic rates of RBP and PA_2 were increased about 2-fold while the T-group chicks showed only a slight increase over the control group.

As can be seen in Table V, the amino acid pool size of liver decreases upon treatment

TABLE III

EFFECT OF T_4 AND AMINO ACID TREATMENTS ON PLASMA AND LIVER LEVELS OF RBP AND PA_2*

Chicks were treated under the four groups as described in legend to Fig. 2. RBP and PA_2 levels were determined by radioimmunoassay.

Group	Level of RBP		Level of PA_2	
	Liver (μg/g protein)	*Plasma (μg/ml)*	*Liver (μg/g protein)*	*Plasma (μg/ml)*
C	410±36	32±3.7	2,070±180	170±14
	S	S	S	S
T	260±22	16±1.8	1,310±116	85± 7.5
	N.S.	N.S.	N.S.	N.S.
A	450±38.5	36±3.2	2,180±196	192±16.5
	N.S.	N.S.	N.S.	N.S.
A+T	380±33	30±2.8	1,850±162	157±14

* All values are mean±S.E.M. of five chicks.

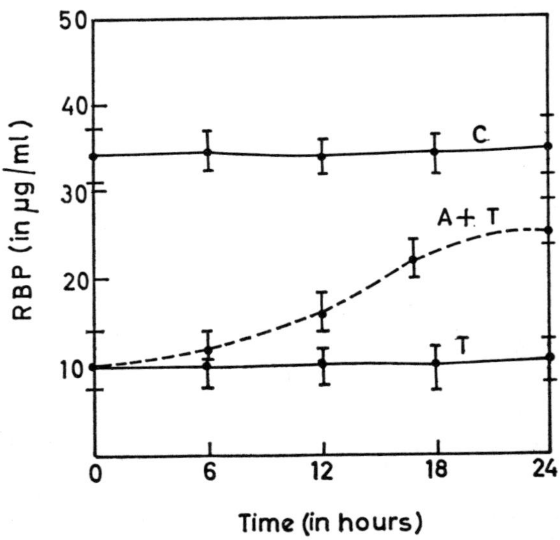

Fig. 3. Time response of RBP level of plasma of T_4-treated chicks to amino acid supplementation. Day-old chicks were treated under C- and T-group for 20 days as described in legend to Fig. 2. T_4-treated chicks were supplemented with essential amino acid mixture (200 mg/100 g body wt.) by i.p. injection and RBP level was measured at different time intervals.

with thyroxine. However, the major change might be due to decrease of the essential amino acid content, as is evident from the decrease in tryptophan content while alanine content remains almost the same.

From the analysis of amino acid pool size and rates of synthesis of RBP and PA_2, it is clear that thyroxine has a great tendency to increase the rates of synthesis of these proteins. But the amino acid pool size in the livers of T-group chicks was considerably decreased due to decrease of the essential amino acid; hence the synthetic rate could not cope

TABLE IV

EFFECT OF T_4 AND AMINO ACID TREATMENTS ON SYNTHETIC RATES OF TOTAL LIVER PROTEIN, RBP, AND PA_2*

Chicks were treated under the four different groups as described in legend to Fig. 2. 50 μCi of ^{3}H-leucine was injected (i.p.) and incorporation of leucine radioactivity in liver was measured after 1 hr.

Group	*Total protein*		*RBP*		*PA_2*	
	cpm/mg	*%*	*cpm/100 mg*	*%*	*cpm/100 mg*	*%*
C	5,844±425	100	542±32	100	1,562± 98	100
	N.S.		S		S	
T	7,480±364	128	786±88	145	2,124±120	136
	N.S.		N.S.		N.S.	
A	6,492±340	111	609±46	112	1,797±110	115
	S		S		S	
A+T	9,476±447	162	1,080±52	190	3,906±233	250

* All values are mean±S.E.M. of three chicks.

TABLE V

AMINO ACID POOL OF LIVER*

Group	*Alanine (μg/g protein)*	*Tryptophan (μg/g protein)*	*Total amino acid content (OD of ninhydrin residues at 570 /mg protein)*
C	94.2±12.7	9.7 ±0.7	0.195±0.01
	N.S.	S	S
T	91.3±12.4	6.1 ±0.45	0.122±0.005
	N.S.	N.S.	N.S.
A	96.7±13.9	11.25±1.25	0.24 ±0.01
	N.S.	N.S.	N.S.
A+T	93.7±10.9	10.25±1.15	0.21 ±0.008

* All values are mean±S.E.M. of five chicks.

up with the catabolic rate. As shown in Table IV, a mixture of essential amino acids was supplied along with thyroxine, there was substantial increase in rates of synthesis of RBP and PA_2 leading to maintenance of their normal plasma levels.

Turnover studies on RBP and PA_2

Studies on rates of plasma clearance of ^{125}I-labeled proteins in the various groups of chicks indicated the thyroxine treatment causes substantial increase in turnover rates of RBP and PA_2. The half-life ($T_{1/2}$) (Table VI) of RBP was 6.6 hr in control group and that of PA_2 was 5.2 hr, while the half-life of both the proteins were decreased by about 3-fold in case of T- and A+T-groups, indicating that T_4 treatment markedly increases the catabolic rates irrespective of aminoacid treatment.

From the above studies it is clear that the loss of steady state is mainly due to the inability in the rate of synthesis of these proteins to cope up with the excessive catabolic rate upon thyroxine treatment. The main reason for this imbalance is mot likely to be the decrease of the amino acid precursors for the synthesis of these proteins.

TABLE VI

EFFECT OF T_4 AND AMINO ACID TREATMENTS ON TURNOVER RATES OF RBP AND PA_2*

Disappearance of ^{125}I-radioactivity from plasma of the four groups of chicks, injected (i.p.) with ^{125}I-labeled proteins (10^{12} cpm)+100 μg of cold proteins were measured by taking blood samples at different time intervals.

Group	*RBP*		*PA_2*	
	Half-life ($T_{1/2}$) (hr)	*Turnover rate (hr^{-1})*	*Half-life ($T_{1/2}$) (hr)*	*Turnover rate (hr^{-1})*
C	6.6 ±0.45	0.103±0.005	5.26±0.48	0.132±0.006
	S	S	S	S
T	2.9 ±0.28	0.245±0.023	2.07±0.18	0.34 ±0.015
	N.S.	N.S.	N.S.	N.S.
A	6.2 ±0.4	0.11 ±0.005	4.93±0.45	0.142±0.007
	S	S	S	S
A+T	2.83±0.26	0.252±0.022	2.1 ±0.17	0.33 ±0.033

* All values are mean±S.E.M. of four chicks.

Vitamin A status of liver and plasma—control of hepatic release of retinol

Table II shows the results of analysis of vitamin A ester and alcohol content of liver and retinol content of plasma. Compared to the control chicks in the T-group, the plasma level of vitamin A was decreased proportionate to that of RBP level; and this corroborates the observations of earlier workes.[5] In the amino acid-supplemented group (A+T-group), however, vitamin A level of plasma could be maintained almost in the normal range. Total vitamin A content of liver was increased in the case of thyroxine-treated group. Further, an increase in the vitamin A alcohol content of liver by about 6-fold could be seen over the control group.

Earlier studies have indicated an increase in the retinyl palmitate hydrolase activity during thyroxine treatment.[29] This might also be one of the factors which increases the accumulation of vitamin A alcohol in the liver, apart from the obstruction in mobilization due to the impairment in RBP synthesis. But in the A+T-group we could not find accumulation of alcohol form compared to C-group, although ester form was slightly above the normal level observed in the C-group. This might be due to the increased absorption of vitamin A by thyroxine treatment as pointed out earlier by Cama and Goodwin.[20]

It is clear from the studies on vitamin A metabolism under the three conditions—*viz.*, a) PCM (refs. 5, 30) b) vitamin A underfed condition[6]; and c) hyperthyroidism—that the hepatic release of vitamin A to plasma is under the controlling steps depicted in Fig. 4.

In the vitamin A underfed condition[6] the inadequate supply of vitamin A leads to accumulation of its specific carrier protein (*viz.*, RBP) in liver, and apo-RBP alone is not secreted. Thus, the limiting steps are No. 1 and No. 2.

During PCM,[5,30] the synthesis of RBP is decreased and esterase activity goes down. Here vitamin A ester is not mobilized; hence availability of both the components of holo-RBP complex are limiting steps. Thus, the controlling steps are No. 1 and No. 3. During hyperthyroidism, steps 2 and 3 are limiting. Although there is increase in rate of synthesis of RBP, it is inadequate to cope up with the catabolic rate, and thus vitamin A alcohol accumulates.

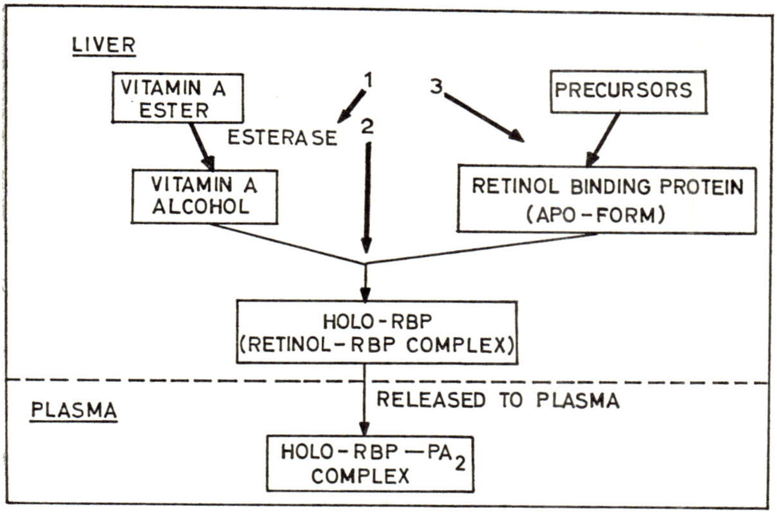

Fig. 4. Control of hepatic release of vitamin A. Pathological condition: (I) protein calorie malnutrition (PCM), controlling step 1 and 3; (II) vitamin A deficiency, 1 and 2; (III) hyperthyroidism, 2 and 3.

ACKNOWLEDGMENT

The authors wish to thank the Council of Scientific and Industrial Research, India, for financial support. The assistance rendered by Mr. C. Venkateshan and Miss V. Seetha is also gratefully acknowledged.

REFERENCES

1 M. Kanai, A. Raz, and D. S. Goodman, *J. Clin. Invest.*, 47 (1968) 2025.
2 K. Sreekrishna, M. Krishna Bhat, S. K. Podder, and H. R. Cama, *World Rev. Nutr. Diet.*, 31 (1978) 52.
3 Y. Muto, *World Rev. Nutr. Diet.*, Karger, Basel, 31 (1978) 45.
4 Y. Muto, F. R. Smith and D. S. Goodman, *J. Lipid Res.*, 14 (1973) 525.
5 P. A. Peterson, S. F. Nilson, L. Ostberg, L. Rask, and A. Vahlquist, *Vitam. Horm.*, 32 (1974) 181.
6 Y. Muto, J. E. Smith, P. O. Milch, and D. S. Goodman, *J. Biol. Chem.*, 247 (1972) 2542.
7 K. Sreekrishna, S. K. Podder, and H. R. Cama, unpublished results.
8 L. S. Farer, J. Robbins, B. S. Blumberg, and J. E. Rall, *Endocrinology*, 70 (1962) 686.
9 D. S. Goodman, *Vitam. Horm.*, 32 (1974) 167.
10 L. Rask, *World Rev. Nutr. Diet.*, Karger, Basel, 31 (1978) 71.
11 J. Heller, *World Rev. Nutr. Diet.*, Karger, Basel, 31 (1978) 42.
12 F. Chytil, *World Rev. Nutr. Diet.*, Karger, Basel, 31 (1978) 27.
13 B. Wiggert, D. R. Bergsma, R. J. Helmsen, J. Alligood, M. Lewis, and G. J. Chader, *Biochim. Biophys. Acta*, 491 (1977) 104.
14 D. R. Bergsma, B. Wiggert, M. Funahashi, T. Kuwabara, and G. J. Chader, *Nature*, 265 (1977) 66.

15 J. GLOVER, *World Rev. Nutr. Diet.*, Karger, Basel, 31 (1978) 21.
16 D. E. ONG and F. CHYTIL, *Proc. Natl. Acad. Sci. U. S.*, 73 (1976) 3976.
17 B. SURE and K. S. BUCHANAN, *J. Nutr.*, 13 (1937) 521.
18 C. E. WEISE, J. W. MEHL, and H. J. DEUEL, *J. Biol. Chem.*, 175 (1948) 21.
19 H. R. CAMA, N. C. PILLAI, P. R. SUNDARESAN, and C. VENKATESHAN, *J. Nutr.*, 63 (1957) 571.
20 H. R. CAMA and T. W. GOODWIN, *Biochem. J.*, 45 (1949) 236.
21 A. W. NEFF, D. B. PARRISH, J. S. HUGHES, and L. F. PAYNE, *Arch. Biochem.*, 21 (1949) 315.
22 J. GLOVER, *Vitam. Horm.*, 31 (1973) 1.
23 J. HELLER, *Dev. Biol.*. 51 (1976) 1.
24 M. K. BHAT, K. SREEKRISHNA, and H. R. CAMA, *Ind. J. Biochem. Biophys.*, 14 (1977) 125.
25 C. M. A. BAKER, C. MANWELL, R. F. LABISKY, and J. A. HAPER, *Comp. Biochem. Physiol.*, 17 (1966) 467.
26 T. ABE, Y. MUTO, and N. HOSOYA, *Life Sci.*, 17 (1975) 1579.
27 F. R. SMITH and D. S. GOODMAN, *J. Invest.*, 50 (1971) 2426.
28 J. MEITOR and M. M. NELSON, *Vitam. Horm.*, 18 (1960) 205.
29 G. S. KISHORE, A. S. PERUMAL, and H. R. CAMA, *Int. J. Vitam. Nutr. Res.*, 41 (1971) 171.
30 M. S. SUREKHARAO, K. THYAGARAJAN, and H. R. CAMA, *Int. J. Vitam. Nutr. Res.*, 44 (1974) 151.

THE METABOLISM AND MECHANISM OF ACTION OF VITAMIN D

H. F. DELUCA

Department of Biochemistry, College of Agricultural and Life Sciences, University of Wisconsin-Madison, Madison, Wisconsin (U.S.A.)

Since its discovery in 1919–1922[1,2] and for almost five decades it has been believed that vitamin D functions as a vitamin which requires no further metabolic alteration. With the preparation of radioactive vitamin D compounds of high specific activity and the development of chromatographic procedures powerful enough to separate vitamin D from its metabolites, it could be demonstrated that vitamin D is converted to biologically active metabolites.[3-5] This led to the isolation and identification of the active forms of vitamin D overturning the concept that vitamin D functions without metabolic alteration.[5,6] A pursuit of this investigation has led to the discovery that vitamin D is the precursor of a hormone, 1,25-$(OH)_2D_3$ which then functions to regulate calcium and phosphorus metabolism.[7-9]

In children where there is rapid growth of the bones, failure of mineralization because of vitamin D deficiency leaves the elaborated collagen matrix without cement support in the form of hydroxyapatite and as a result the skeleton becomes soft, bent, and twisted giving rise to the overt symptoms of rickets. In the vitamin D-deficient adult, there is failure to mineralize newly formed bone which results from the remodeling process. This gives rise to large osteoid seams, weak bones, and severe bone pain. This disease is called osteomalacia and both it and rickets can be characterized by a failure of the mineralization process. Although it has been believed that vitamin D functions directly in the mineralization process, support for this concept is lacking. Instead the failure of mineralization in rickets and osteomalacia appears to result from an insufficient supply of calcium and phosphorus to the mineralization sites. In essence, vitamin D through its metabolites functions to elevate plasma calcium and phosphorus concentration.

Another important concept of vitamin D function is that it plays an essential role in preventing hypocalcemic tetany. It is well known that a major function of calcium in the extracellular fluid is to support normal muscle contraction and normal neurotransmission. In the absence of sufficient amounts of calcium in the extracellular fluid, the neuromuscular junction fails to operate properly giving rise to continuous excitation of the skeletal system resulting in convulsions and the disease tetany. Vitamin D and the parathyroid hormone function jointly in preventing hypocalcemic tetany. However, this must be regarded as a major function of vitamin D. Finally, it should be noted that vitamin D plays an important role in permitting the intestine to adapt its efficiency of absorption of calcium to the needs

---

Abbreviations: 1,25$(OH)_2D_3$, 1,25-dihydroxyvitamin D_3; 25-OH-D_3, 25-hydroxyvitamin D_3; 24,25-$(OH)_2D_3$, 24,25-dihydroxyvitamin D_3; PTH, parathyroid hormone.

of the organism.[10] For example, an animal placed on a low calcium diet will develop a highly efficient intestinal absorption of calcium as compared to animals placed on a normal or high calcium diet. This ability to adapt the intestine to calcium needs requires the presence of vitamin D[10]. Nicolaysen[11] who discovered this vitamine D dependence attributed the ability to adjust to an endogenous hormonal factor secreted from the bone which would inform the intestine of skeletal needs.[10] It now seems clear that the messenger that the intestine receives is 1,25-$(OH)_2D_3$ and that the need for calcium indirectly stimulates production of this hormone which is responsible for elevating intestinal calcium absorption. The ability of the intestine to adapt and to absorb calcium when it is needed protects the skeleton against mobilization which occurs to prevent hypocalcemic tetany. In this manner, vitamin D must certainly function to help prevent bone erosion and which probably helps prevent the appearance of osteopenia or osteoporosis.

THE ORIGIN OF VITAMIN D IN SKIN

In 1919 Huldshinsky demonstrated that rachitic children could be cured by exposing them to ultraviolet light either from sunlight or artificial means.[12] The biochemical mechanism of this healing remained unknown until Steenbock and Black demonstrated that ultraviolet light activates an inactive sterol present in food and skin to the active antirachitic substance.[13,14] The discovery by Steenbock and Black which was confirmed quickly by Hess *et al.*[15] undoubtedly resulted in the isolation and identification of vitamin D_3 from ergosterol irradiation mixtures.[16,17] Discovery of vitamin D_3 came as a result of a synthetic effort to prepare analogs of vitamin D_2. Windaus's group was successful in preparing the sterol 7-dehydrocholesterol and upon photolysis it yielded a new form of vitamin D termed vitamin D_3.[18] It was not until an abundant quantity of 7-dehydrocholesterol was identified in skin that it was realized that vitamin D_3 was probably the naturally produced form of vitamin D upon ultraviolet irradiation.[19] However, it has only been in the last year that the antirachitic substance produced in the skin *in vivo* by ultraviolet irradiation has been isolated in pure form and its structure clearly identified as vitamin D_3 (ref. 20) by mass spectrometry and ultraviolet absorption spectra. Undoubtedly previtamin D is the initial reaction product of photolysis 7-dehydrocholesterol in skin as suggested by Holick *et al.*[21] We have not been able to demonstrate any enzymes or proteins which play a role in the photolysis of 7-dehydrocholesterol in skin, despite many efforts (Esvelt and DeLuca, unpublished results). It is our belief that this reaction is strictly a chemical photolysis of 7-dehydrocholesterol without participation of enzymes or regulatory factors. This conversion, therefore, does not appear to be a regulated process.

THE METABOLISM OF VITAMIN D TO ITS ACTIVE HORMONE 1,25-$(OH)_2D_3$ (FIG. 1)

Vitamin D administered by the intravenous route or by the oral route rapidly accumulates in the liver.[22,23] Vitamin D_3 is rapidly cleared from the blood and circulates at a low concentration of less than 5 ng/ml (Shepard and DeLuca, unpublished results). In the liver vitamin D_3 undergoes hydroxylation on carbon-25 to give rise to the major circulating form of vitamin D; namely, (25-OH-D_3) (ref. 5). This reaction is microsomal, it requires NADPH, molecular oxygen and magnesium ions.[24,25] It is not known whether this is a mixed function mono-oxygenase requiring cytochrome P-450 or not. In birds, some 25-hydroxylation of vitamin D_3 occurs in the intestine[26] whereas

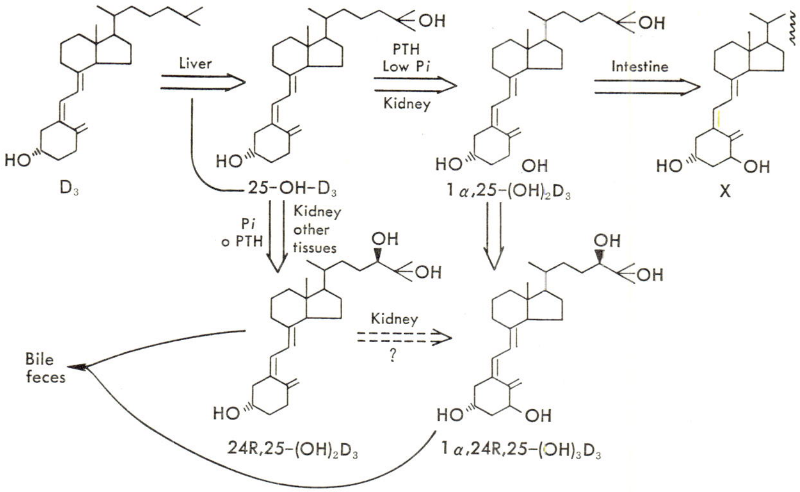

Fig. 1. Metabolism of vitamin D_3 to its metabolically active form 1α-25-$(OH)_2D_3$ and further to 1,24,25-$(OH)_2D_3$ and to the unknown compound X. Heavy arrows are major pathways. The organ in which the reactions take place is indicated over the respective arrow and the stimulatory factors are also presented over the arrows. The actual excretion forms of vitamin D remain unknown.

this 25-hydroxylation in mammals appears to be almost entirely of hepatic origin.[23,27] The cells which carry out the 25-hydroxylation are still unknown, however. The product 25-OH-D_3 in the hepatic cell brings about a suppression of the 25-hydroxylase.[24] The suppression of the 25-hydroxylase by the hepatic 25-OH-D_3 is of limited capacity and the administration of large amounts of vitamin D results in large amounts of 25-OH-D_3 appearing in the circulation.[28] 25-OH-D_3 circulates at a level of about 30 ng/ml in normal man[28,29] and it circulates bound to an α-globulin of 52,000 mol. wt. which has been isolated in pure form from human plasma[30,31] and rat plasma.[32] However 25-OH-D_3 does not act directly at physiologic doses but must be metabolically further altered before it can function. The kidney is the site of the second hydroxylation in which an hydroxyl is inserted on carbon 1 of 25-OH-D_3.[6,33] This enzyme functions only on vitamin D molecules which have a 25-hydroxyl function.[34] The 25-OH-D_3-1α-hydroxylase is entirely mitochondrial and in our group it has been possible to solubilize this hydroxylase and reconstitute it.[35,36] It is composed of a renal ferredoxin reductase which is a flavoprotein, an iron sulfur protein called renal ferredoxin and a cytochrome P-450 which is the specific enzyme recognizing 25-OH-D_3. With oxygen-18 it had been clearly demonstrated that the oxygen on carbon-1 arises from molecular oxygen.[37] Thus the mechanism of the 1-hydroxylation of 25-OH-D_3 is shown in Fig. 2. It is striking that this hydroxylase is almost identical in mechanism to the steroidogenesis system found in the adrenal glands providing additional evidence, therefore, that the vitamin D system is an analogous endocrine system to the steroid systems of the adrenals. 1,25-$(OH)_2D_3$ formed in the mitochondria is then transported to the target tissues where it carries out its functions. The essentiality of 1- and 25-hydroxylation can be easily demonstrated using a nephrectomized animal which is unable to carry out the 1-hydroxylation.[38] Nephrectomized animals do not respond in terms of intestinal calcium transport,[38,39] bone calcium mobilization,[40] and intestinal

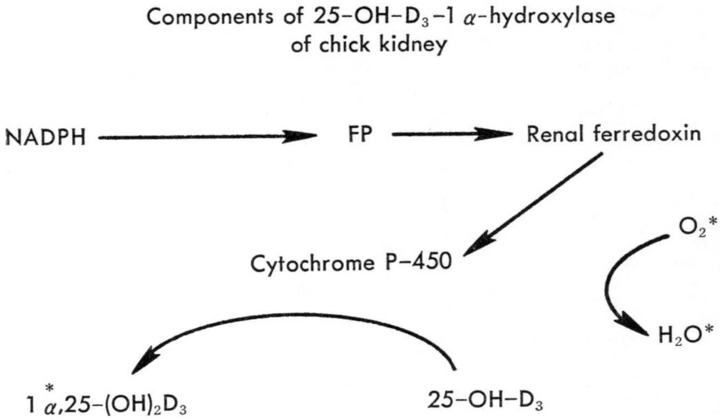

Fig. 2. Mechanism of 1-hydroxylation of 25-OH-D_3 to 1α,25-$(OH)_2D_3$.

phosphate transport[41] to 25-OH-D_3 administered at physiologic doses. On the other hand, these nephrectomized animals respond quite normally to 1,25-$(OH)_2D_3$ whether kidneys are present or not. Because rats made uremic by ureteric ligation but still possessing renal tissue will respond to 25-OH-D_3 it can be concluded that the absence of renal tissue prevents 25-OH-D_3 from functioning not uremia. It is on this basis, therefore, that one can conclude that 1,25-$(OH)_2D_3$ or a further metabolite is the metabolically active form of vitamin D and must be regarded as a hormone.[7]

24-HYDROXYLATION AND ITS SIGNIFICANCE (FIG. 1)

In normal animals or man, 25-OH-D_3 is rapidly hydroxylated to another product which has been isolated in pure form and identified as 24,25-dihydroxy-vitamin D_3 (24,25-$(OH)_2D_3$).[42] On the other hand rachitic animals do not possess the capability of 24-hydroxylation.[43] The reason for this is that 1,25-$(OH)_2D_3$ has among its functions the induction of the 25-OH-D_3-24-hydroxylase.[44] This hydroxylase which has been located in isolated kidney mitocondria from chickens given vitamin D and a high calcium diet requires a vitamin D molecule with a 25-hydroxyl group for a substrate.[45] Therefore, both 25-OH-D_3 and 1,25-$(OH)_2D_3$ are 24-hydroxylated.[46] The 24-hydroxyl in both compounds is in the *R* configuration.[46,47] The true products of the 24-hydroxylase are the 24*R*,25-$(OH)_2D_3$ and 1,24*R*,25-$(OH)_3D_3$. Of special interest is the fact that 24-hydroxylation of 1,25-$(OH)_2D_3$ is not eliminated by nephrectomy.[46] Thus the 24-hydroxylase is obviously not restricted to renal sites. A search for this additional site of 24-hydroxylation has resulted in our demonstrating that 24-hydroxylation of 1,25-$(OH)_2D_3$ and 24,25-$(OH)_2D_3$ occurs in intestinal homogenates supported by NADPH and molecular oxygen.[47] In addition to this, a report has appeared that cartilage cells possess the ability to 24-hydroxylate 25-OH-D_3 in culture.[48]

There is still considerable controversy regarding the importance of the 24-hydroxylation reaction. It is known that 24*R*,25-$(OH)_2D_3$ has no effect in nephrectomized animals and must be given to animals with intact kidneys before it can function.[49] 24*R*,25-$(OH)_2D_3$ therefore must be 1-hydroxylated before it can stimulate intestine and bone. Although there have been reports that 24*R*,25-$(OH)_2D_3$ has unusual calcification properties[50] or functions in man without kidneys,[51] these have not been verified by adequate experimental evidence. In our laboratory, 24-hydroxylation of vitamin D compounds always reduces biological activity below that of the substrate, thus, 1,24R,25-$(OH)_3D_3$ is much less active than the 1,25-$(OH)_2D_3$ in both mammals[52] and birds.[53] On this basis 24-hydroxylation is likely an excretory pathway.[53] However there may be some specialized and unknown function of the 24-hydroxylated vitamins. An interesting idea has been put forth by Capen *et al.* that 24R,25-$(OH)_2D_3$ plays some role in the suppression of PTH secretion.[54] However, because 24,25-$(OH)_2D_3$ production is favored by the absence of PTH, this concept does not appear to make physiologic sense. Furthermore, convincing evidence that 24,25-$(OH)_2D_3$ at physiologic concentration affects PTH secretion is lacking.

REGULATION OF 1,25-$(OH)_2D_3$ PRODUCTION

In 1971 Boyle *et al.*[55] demonstrated that the accumulation of 1,25-$(OH)_2D_3$ in plasma and in the target tissues of intestine and bone is related in an inverse fashion with dietary calcium intake and plasma calcium concentration.[56] Thus under conditions of hypocalcemia 1,25-$(OH)_2D_3$ accumulation is markedly increased whereas under conditions of hypercalcemia its appearance in plasma is markedly diminished and instead, 24,25-$(OH)_2D_3$ appears. Omdahl *et al.*[57] demonstrated that this was the result of an alteration in the 25-OH-D_3-1-hydroxylase level of the kidney by direct *in vitro* measurements. These observations were subsequently confirmed in 1974.[58] Thus the need for calcium as established by hypocalcemia stimulates 1,25-$(OH)_2D_3$ production. Garabedian *et al.*[59] provided clear evidence that the parathyroid glands mediated this regulation. The absence of the parathyroid glands prevented increased production of 1,25-$(OH)_2D_3$ under conditions of hypocalcemia. Production of 1,25-$(OH)_2D_3$ could be restored by the administration of exogenous PTH. Fraser and Kodicek demonstrated that in the bird injections of PTH could increase the 25-$(OH)_2D_3$-1-hydroxylase.[60]

Boyle *et al.*[56] were the first to recognize that 1,25-$(OH)_2D_3$ might represent the Nicolaysen endogenous factor responsible for intestinal calcium absorption adaptation to dietary calcium, since increased plasma and intestinal accumulation of 1,25-$(OH)_2D_3$ could be observed in rats on a low calcium diet *versus* those on a high calcium diet. Ribovich and DeLuca[61] and Omdahl and DeLuca[62] have both provided evidence in the rat and chick respectively that the administration of exogenous sources of 1,25-$(OH)_2D_3$ to animals eliminates their ability to adapt their intestine to dietary calcium. Ribovich and DeLuca[63] have also demonstrated that parathyroidectomy together with constant exogenous sources of PTH eliminates the ability of the intestine to adapt to dietary calcium levels. These results provide strong support for the idea that the parathyroid hormone-vitamin D endocrine system in the kidney is essentially the endogenous factor of Nicolaysen and is responsible for intestinal adaptation to dietary calcium.

Because of this finding we have examined the question of whether patients suffering from osteoporosis have low levels of 1,25-$(OH)_2D_3$ commensurate with their low rates of intestinal calcium absorption. Together with Drs. Gallagher and Riggs at the Mayo Clinic we have been able to analyze plasma smaples taken from postmenopausal, osteoporotic patients and their age-matched controls. Patients suffering from osteoporosis have significantly lower levels of 1,25-$(OH)_2D_3$. This coupled with the demonstration that they are unable to adapt their intestines to meet calcium needs suggest that a factor involved in the genesis of osteoporosis is the inability to absorb sufficient amounts of calcium when demanded by the body. Therefore, it appears that 1,25-$(OH)_2D_3$ or one of its analogs might be useful in preventing bone deterioration which results in osteoporosis.

In examining extraordinary demands for calcium exerted during egg shell formation we have studied the control of the 25-OH-D_3-1-hydroxylase in the egg-laying birds. During the active process of egg production, birds have higher levels of circulating 1,25-$(OH)_2D_3$ and demonstrate increased levels of 25-OH-D_3-1-hydroxylase.[65,66] However, unlike the conclusion of Kenny,[67] we were unable to demonstrate that the 1,25-$(OH)_2D_3$ production was related to the position of the egg in the oviduct. Instead, it appears that the 25-OH-D_3-1-hydroxylase is markedly regulated during the egg-laying cycle and the major stimulatory factors are the sex hormones.[65,66] Estradiol when administered to intact mature male birds will markedly stimulate 25-OH-D_3-1-hydroxylase and suppress the 24-hydroxylase as illustrated in Fig. 3. When this is tested in the immature or castrate mature male birds or immature female birds no response is found. However, when testosterone is given together with the estradiol, the response is found in castrate males or immature birds. Furthermore, a combination of estradiol, testosterone, and progesterone produce the most marked elevation in the 25-OH-D_3-1-hydroxylase. The relationship of progesterone levels to the stimulation of the 1-hydroxylase is shown in Fig. 4. In this experiment castrate male birds were given 5 mg of estradiol per kg, 5 mg testosterone per kg, and the indicated dose of progesterone. Notice that marked stimulations are observed at a progesterone level of 12.5 mg/kg. Thus the sex hormones clearly exert a regulatory influence on the 25-OH-D_3-1-hydroxylase in the egg-laying birds. Presumably this relates to the abnormal calcium metabolism which must occur in the formation of calcium carbonate shells. More recent evidence in man and in rats have indicated that the sex hormones in these species do exert a regulatory influence on the 25-OH-D_3-1-hydroxylase. It must be emphasized, however, that the sex hormones could function through the parathyroid glands in producing the stimulation of the 1-hydroxylase. In any case, under circumstances of abnormally high demands for calcium such as in the egg-laying process it appears that other endocrine systems may satisfy such a need by stimulating the 1-hydroxylase to provide the most potent calcium mobilizing hormone, 1,25-$(OH)_2D_3$.

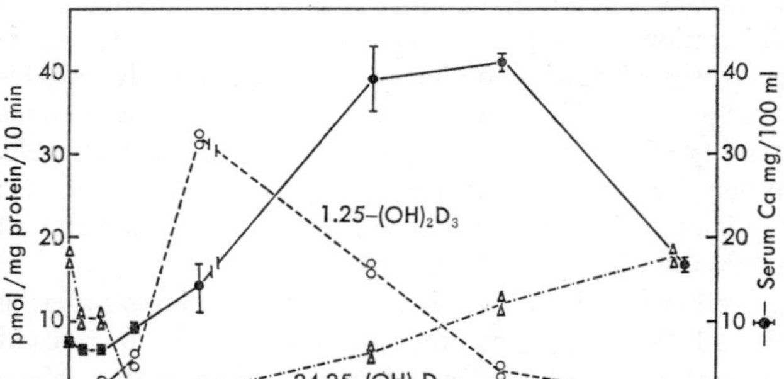

Fig. 3. The response of the renal 25-OH-D_3-24-hydroxylase (△), the renal 25-OH-D_3-1-hydroxylase (○), and serum calcium concentration (●) in adult male Japanese Quail to a single dose of 5 mg of estradiol valerate.

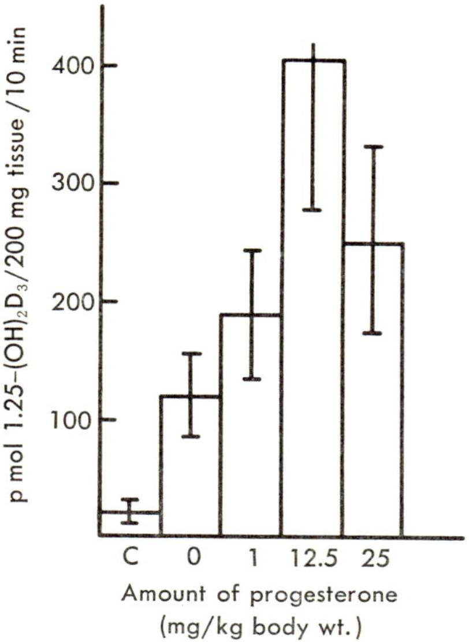

Fig. 4. The stimulation of chick kidney mitochondrial 25-OH-D_3-1-hydroxylase by the administration of progesterone to castrate adult male birds who have recieved 5 mg/kg of estradiol valerate and 12 mg/kg testosterone. Control birds received no sex hormones whereas zero animals received the testosterone and estradiol valerate.

In addition to the sex hormones, regulation by prolactin,[68] growth hormone,[68] and plasma phosphate[69] levels have been reported. Stimulation by prolactin and growth hormone are certainly a reasonable expectation because of the unusual demands for calcium during growth and during lactation. In the case of phosphate stimulation, there has been something of a controversy as to whether the elevated plasma levels of 1,25-$(OH)_2D_3$ which result from phosphate depletion result from increased biogenesis of 1,25-$(OH)_2D_3$, increased accumulation in the plasma and target tissues or decrease destruction.[61,70] All three factors appear to operate. Certainly there is a 2–5-fold stimulation in the renal 25-OH-D_3-1-hydroxylase of birds in extreme phosphate depletion.[71] Ribovich and DeLuca[72] have provided evidence that there is increased accumulation of injected radioactive 1,25-$(OH)_2D_3$ in intestine and plasma of phosphate-depleted rats. There is also evidence that there is decreased destruction of the 1,25-$(OH)_2D_3$. In any case, phosphate depletion results in marked accumulations of 1,25-$(OH)_2D_3$ in the target tissues resulting in elevated phosphate and calcium transport reactions.

Feedback regulation of the 1-hydroxylase by 1,25-$(OH)_2D_3$ is well known.[43,44] There is some controversy, however, as to the mechanism. Suda and his colleagues[73] have provided evidence that suppression of the 1-hydroxylase by 1,25-$(OH)_2D_3$ is the result of suppression of parathyroid secretion. On the other hand, Tanaka and DeLuca[43] and MacIntyre and his colleagues[74] believe that 1,25-$(OH)_2D_3$ causes the induction of a regulatory substance which then suppresses 1,25-$(OH)_2D_3$ production. To some extent both are likely to be correct inasmuch as animals on a low phosphate diet in which there is minimal parathyroid hormone secretion anyway, do show a suppression of 1-hydroxylation by the administration of 1,25-$(OH)_2D_3$.[43] It would appear unlikely that the PTH mediates this suppression by the 1,25-$(OH)_2D_3$.

The mechanism whereby the regulation of the 1-hydroxylase occurs in response to parathyroid hormone, phosphate depletion, sex hormonal stimulation or prolactin stimulation remains unknown. Many attempts have been made using ionic manipulations to elucidate the mechanism of this regulation.[75] However, regulation *in vivo* requires many hours following stimulation and it seems lilely that the regulation involves new protein synthesis and/or protein degradation. Likely the ionic manipulation experiments *in vitro* with kidney tubules or mitochondria have little significance regarding *in vivo* regulation. There has been a contention that there are two forms of regulation. One is ionic and the other is the longer range, *in vivo* regulation. However, there is no evidence to support the idea that there are rapid adjustments of the 1-hydroxylase, consistent with ionic regulation.

MECHANISM OF ACTION OF 1,25-$(OH)_2D_3$

The only target tissue which has undergone extensive investigation regarding the mechanism of action of 1,25-$(OH)_2D_3$ is the intestine. As might be expected, since 1,25-$(OH)_2D_3$ is a secosteroid, it would be expected to function by a steroid hormone mechanism; namely, interaction with a receptor, transfer to the nucleus and stimulation of transcription of DNA which codes for the transport proteins.[76] Brumbaugh and Haussler[77] were the first to demonstrate the existence of a 3.7 S cytosol receptor in rachitic chick intestinal mucosa. Although we were unable to confirm this work initially we learned that extensive washing of mucosa which eliminates many of the digestive protyolytic enzymes was very useful in preventing degradation of the receptor.[78] We can therefore, show in rachitic chick intestinal mucosa a 3.7 S cytosol receptor. This has limited capacity and high affinity [(k_d) of 2×10^{-11} M] and has all of the characteristics that might be expected of a receptor. It is highly specific for 1,25-$(OH)_2D_3$ as shown in displacement analyses.[79,80] At least a factor of 10 is required of the nearest competitor to compete for the binding site on the 3.7 S cytosol receptor. Several laboratories have looked for receptors in the intestine of mammals, especially rats and have failed to detect a specific 1,25-$(OH)_2D_3$ binding protein. Using our newly synthesized 80 Ci/mmol 1,25-$(OH)_2D_3$ prepared by Dr. Sachiko Yamada in our group it was possible to demonstrate 3.2 S cytosol receptor, specific for 1,25-$(OH)_2D_3$ in rat intestine.[81] Both high salt and the presence of dithiothreitol played an important part in this demonstration. In addition, the presence of a 6 S binding complex added difficulty to this demonstration. The 6 S binding complex was reported by Haddad and Birge[82] to be very wide spread, a point which we could easily confirm. We have learned that the 6 S cytosol binder crossreacts with an antibody directed to the plasma transport protein (4.1 S) whereas the 3.2 S 1,25-$(OH)_2D_3$ binder did not. When intestinal villus cells are prepared by the method of Kimmich[83] and washed carefully to eliminate all plasma, no 6 S binder could be detected. Furthermore, if one adds 4.1 S plasma transport protein or serum to homogenate of intestinal mucosa, no 4.1 S appears, but instead a 6 S complex appears in increasing amounts (Kream and DeLuca, unpublished results). Van Baelen *et al.* have provided additional evidence that the 6 S binding complex is an artifact of combination of the 4.1 S plasma transport protein with a non-vitamin D-related cytosol protein. They are able to dissociate this complex by heating it to 60°, regenerating the 4.1 S plasma transport protein. These results make it unlikely that the 6 S complex reported by Haddad and Birge[82] has any physiologic significance in terms of a receptor function. Thus the 3.2 S protein appears to be the specific receptor protein for 1,25-$(OH)_2D_3$ in the mammalian species. The 3.2 S cytosol receptor has also been found in embryonic bone from rats and chicks[84] and more recently in rachitic rat and chick bone. The presence therefore of a specific 1,25-$(OH)_2D_3$-binding protein believed to be a receptor can easily be demonstrated in cytosol of target tissues.

The ultimate nuclear location of 1,25-$(OH)_2D_3$ prior to initiation of intestinal calcium transport has been the subject of considerable debate. There is no doubt that by biochemical means the nuclear-debris fraction contains 80% of the intestinal mucosal homogenate quantity of 1,25-$(OH)_2D_3$.[85] Impure chromatin also contains this high level of the homogenate 1,25-$(OH)_2D_3$.[86] Pure chromatin and pure nuclei however, do not appear to account for all of the radioactivity found in the nuclear fratcion.[85] However, the methods of preparing pure chromatin and pure nuclei leave much to be desired for intestine since low yields are obtained.[87] Recently with the chemical synthetic efforts of Dr. Sachiko Yamada, high specific activity 1,25-$(OH)_2[23,24\text{-}^3H]D_3$ was prepared and it was possible to carry out autoradiography studies with truly physiologic doses of 1,25-$(OH)_2[23,24\text{-}^3H]D_3$. Using the frozen section technique we could eliminate the possible translocation of the label and furthermore could remove the chances of loss of this lipid soluble material during the imbedding and fixation procedures. Using this technique a clear nuclear location of 1,25-$(OH)_2D_3$ could be demonstrated in the villus and crypt cells of intestinal mucosa.[88] No specific localization could be found in muscle, liver, parathyroid tissue, and some parts of the kidney. Specific nuclear location has also been found in osteoblasts and osteocytes (Mathews and DeLuca, unpublished). Some specific localization in nuclei has been found in renal tissue. In any case, in regard to the intestine, there is no question that 1,25-$(OH)_2D_3$ ultimately becomes associated with the nucleus.

Brumbaugh and Haussler[89] have edmonstrated the transfer of radioactive 1,25-$(OH)_2D_3$ from cytosol to nuclei. Brumbaugh and Haussler[90] and Lawson and Wilson[91] reported that the binding protein in the nucleus is similar to the binding protein found in the cytosol which has lead to the belief that the 1,25-$(OH)_2D_3$-receptor complex is transferred to the nucleus. Increased template activity of chromatin in response to vitamin D or 1,25-$(OH)_2D_3$ has also been reported but so far the messengers which are made in response to 1,25-$(OH)_2D_3$ have not been characterized. Furthermore, we do not know the nature of the transport substances made in response to 1,25-$(OH)_2D_3$. Only one protein has been identified, that is the calcium-binding protein of Wasserman and Taylor.[92] However, there is evidence that this protein is not present in intestinal tissue at the time transport is initiated in response to 1,25-$(OH)_2D_3$.[93,94] Furthermore, when the transport subsides in response to a single dose of 1,25-$(OH)_2D_3$, the calcium binding protein level remains high. It is evident that 1,25$(OH)_2D_3$ must induce factors in addition to or other than calcium-binding protein to initiate calcium transport. These are being studied but so far, they have not been clearly shown.

Finally, it should be mentioned that the metabolites of vitamin D and their analogs are of great interest to clinical medicine because they are being used to treat renal osteodystrophy, hypoparathyroidism, pseudohypoparathyroidism, and steroid induced osteoporosis.[95] They are also being tried in the case of postmenopausal and senile osteoporosis. Likely these compounds will be of major medical significance and will also be of major biochemical interest in regard to mechanism of action and further metabolism.

ACKNOWLEDGMENTS

This work was supported by a program grant AM-14881 from the U.S.P.H.S., a contract from the U.S. Energy Research and Development Administration ♯ EY-76-S-02-1668 and the Harry Steenbock Research Fund.

REFERENCES

1 E. Mellanby, *Lancet*, i (1919) 407.
2 E. V. McCollum, N. Simmonds, J. E. Becker, and P. G. Shipley, *J. Biol. Chem.*, 53 (1922) 293.
3 J. Lund and H. F. DeLuca, *J. Lipid Res.*, 7 (1966) 739.
4 H. Morii, J. Lund, P. F. Neville, and H. F. DeLuca, *Arch. Biochem. Biophys.*, 120 (1967) 508.
5 J. W. Blunt, H. F. DeLuca, and H. K. Schnoes, *Biochemistry*, 7 (1968) 3317.
6 M. F. Holick, H. K. Schnoes, H. F. DeLuca, T. Suda, and R. J. Cousins, *Biochemistry*, 10 (1971) 2799.
7 H. F. DeLuca, *Fed. Proc.*, 33 (1974) 2211.
8 E. Kodicek, *Lancet*, i (1974) 325.
9 H. F. DeLuca and H. K. Schnoes, *Annu. Rev. Biochem.*, 45 (1976) 631.
10 R. Nicolaysen, N. Eeg-Larsen, and O. J. Malm, *Physiol. Rev.*, 33 (1953) 424.
11 R. Nicolaysen, *Acta Physiol. Scand.*, 6 (1943) 201.
12 K. Huldshinsky, *Dtsch. Med. Wochenschr.*, 45 (1919) 712.
13 H. Steenbock and A. Black, *J. Biol. Chem.*, 61 (1924) 405.
14 H. Steenbock and A. Black, *J. Biol. Chem.*, 64 (1925) 263.
15 A. F. Hess, M. Weinstock, and F. D. Helman, *J. Biol. Chem.*, 63 (1925) 305.
16 F. A. Askew, R. B. Bourdillon, H. M. Bruce, R. G. C. Jenkins, and T. A. Webster, *Proc. Roy. Soc.*, B107 (1931) 76.
17 A. Windaus and A. Lüttringhaus, *Hoppe Zeyler's Z. Physiol. Chem.*, 203 (1931) 70.
18 A. Windaus, F. Schenck, and F. von Werder, *Hoppe Zeyler's Z. Physiol. Chem.*, 241 (1936) 100.
19 D. R. Idler and C. A. Baumann, *J. Biol. Chem.*, 195 (1952) 623.
20 R. P. Esvelt, H. K. Schnoes, and H. F. DeLuca, *Arch. Biochem. Biophys.*, 188 (1978) 282.
21 M. F. Holick, J. Frommer, S. McNeill, N. Richt, J. Henley, and J. T. Potts, Jr., *Biochem. Biophys. Res. Commun.*, 76 (1977) 107.
22 G. Ponchon and H. F. DeLuca, *J. Clin. Invest.*, 48 (1969) 1273.
23 E. B. Olsen, Jr., J. C. Knutson, M. H. Bhattacharyya, and H. F. DeLuca, *J. Clin. Invest.*, 57 (1976) 1213.
24 M. Horsting and H. F. DeLuca, *Biochem. Biophys. Res. Commun.*, 36 (1969) 251.
25 M. Bhattacharyya and H. F. DeLuca, *Arch. Biochem. Biophys.*, 160 (1974) 58.
26 G. Tucker, III, R. E. Gagnon, and M. R. Haussler, *Arch. Biochem. Biophys.*, 155 (1973) 47.
27 M. H. Bhattacharyya and H. F. DeLuca, *J. Biol. Chem.*, 248 (1973) 2969.
28 J. G. Haddad and T. C. B. Stamp, *Am. J. Med.*, 57 (1974) 57.
29 J. A. Eisman, R. M. Shepard, and H. F. DeLuca, *Anal. Biochem.*, 80 (1977) 298.
30 M. Imawari, K. Kida, and D. S. Goodman, *J. Clin. Invest.*, 58 (1976) 514.
31 J. G. Haddad and J. Walgate, *J. Biol. Chem.*, 251 (1976) 4803.
32 K. M. Botham, J. G. Ghazarian, B. E. Kream, and H. F. DeLuca, *Biochemistry*, 15 (1976) 2130.
33 D. R. Fraser and E. Kodicek, *Nature*, 228 (1970) 764.
34 R. W. Gray, J. L. Omdahl, J. G. Ghazarian, and H. F. DeLuca, *J. Biol. Chem.*, 247 (1972) 7528.

35 J. G. Ghazarian, C. R. Jefcoate, J. C. Knutson, W. H. Orme-Johnson, and H. F. DeLuca, *J. Biol. Chem.*, 249 (1974) 3026.
36 J. I. Pedersen, J. G. Ghazarian, N. R. Orme-Johnson, and H. F. DeLuca, *J. Biol. Chem.*, 251 (1976) 3933.
37 J. G. Ghazarian, H. K. Schnoes, and H. F. DeLuca, *Biochemistry*, 12 (1973) 2555.
38 I. T. Boyle, L. Miravet, R. W. Gray, M. F. Holick, and H. F. DeLuca, *Endocrinology*, 90 (1972) 605.
39 R. G. Wong, A. W. Norman, C. R. Reddy, and J. W. Coburn, *J. Clin. Invest.*, 51 (1972) 1287.
40 M. F. Holick, M. Garabedian, and H. F. DeLuca, *Science*, 176 (1972) 1146.
41 T. C. Chen, L. Castillo, M. Korycka-Dahl, and H. F. DeLuca, *J. Nutr.*, 104 (1974) 1056.
42 M. F. Holick, H. K. Schnoes, H. F. DeLuca, R. W. Gray, I. T. Boyle, and T. Suda, *Biochemistry*, 11 (1972) 4251.
43 Y. Tanaka and H. F. DeLuca, *Science*, 183 (1974) 1198.
44 Y. Tanaka, R. S. Lorenc, and H. F. DeLuca, *Arch. Biochem. Biophys.*, 171 (1975) 521.
45 J. C. Knutson and H. F. DeLuca, *Biochemistry*, 13 (1974) 1543.
46 Y. Tanaka, L. Castillo, H. F. DeLuca, and N. Ikekawa, *J. Biol. Chem.*, 252 (1977) 1421.
47 Y. Tanaka, H. F. DeLuca, N. Ikekawa, M. Morisaka, and N. Koizumi, *Arch. Biochem. Biophys.*, 170 (1975) 620.
48 M. Garabedian, M. T. Corvol, M. Bailly du Bois, M. Liederherr, and S. Balsan, *Proc. of the 6th Parathyroid Conference*, Excerpta Medica, Amsterdam, 1977, in press.
49 I. T. Boyle, J. L. Omdahl, R. W. Gray, and H. F. DeLuca, *J. Biol. Chem.*, 248 (1973) 4174.
50 P. Bordier, A. Ryckwaert, P. Marie, L. Miravet, A. Norman, and H. Rasmussen, in A. W. Norman, K. Schaefer, J. W. Coburn, H. F. DeLuca, D. Fraser, H. G. Grigoleit, and D. v. Herrath, *Vitamin D: Biochemical, Chemical and Clinical Aspects Related to Calcium Metabolism*, Walter de Gruyter, New York, 1977, p. 897.
51 J. A. Kanis, G. Heynen, R. G. G. Russell, R. Smith, R. J. Walton, and G. T. Warner, in A. W. Norman, K. Schaefer, J. W. Coburn, H. F. DeLuca, D. Fraser, H. G. Grigoleit, D. v. Herrath, *Vitamin D: Biochemical, Chemical and Clinical Aspects Related to Calcium Metabolism*, Walter de Gruyter, New York, 1977, p. 793.
52 M. F. Holick, A. Kleiner-Bossaller, H. K. Schnoes, P. M. Kasten, I. T. Boyle, and H. F. DeLuca, *J. Biol. Chem.*, 248 (1973) 6691.
53 M. F. Holick, L. A. Baxter, P. K. Schraufrogel, T. E. Tavela, and H. F. DeLuca, *J. Biol. Chem.*, 251 (1976) 397.
54 C. C. Capen, H. L. Henry, and A. W. Norman, in A. W. Norman, K. Schaefer, J. W. Coburn, H. F. DeLuca, D. Fraser, H. G. Grigoleit, and D. v. Herrath, *Vitamin D: Biochemical, Chemical and Clinical Aspects Related to Calcium Metabolism*, Walter de Gruyter, New York, 1977, p. 101.
55 I. T. Boyle, R. W. Gray, and H. F. DeLuca, *Proc. Natl. Acad. Sci. U.S.*, 68 (1971) 2131.
56 I. T. Boyle, R. W. Gray, J. L. Omdahl, and H. F. DeLuca, in S. Taylor, *Endocrinology* 1971, Wm. Heinemann Medical Books, Ltd., London, 1972, p. 468.
57 J. L. Omdahl, R. W. Gray, I. T. Boyle, J. Knutson, and H. F. DeLuca, *Nature New Biol.*, 237 (1972) 63.
58 H. L. Henry, R. J. Midgett, and A. W. Norman, *J. Biol. Chem.*, 249 (1974) 7584.
59 M. Garabedian, M. F. Holick, H. F. DeLuca, and I. T. Boyle, *Proc. Natl. Acad. Sci. U.S.*, 69 (1972) 1673.
60 D. R. Fraser and D. Kodicek, *Nature New Biol.*, 241 (1973) 163.
61 M. L. Ribovich and H. F. DeLuca, *Arch. Biochem. Biophys.*, 170 (1975) 529.
62 J. L. Omdahl and H. F. DeLuca, *J. Nutr.*, 107 (1977) 1975.
63 M. L. Ribovich and H. F. DeLuca, *Arch. Biochem. Biophys.*, 175 (1976) 256.
64 C. Gallagher, L. Riggs, J. Eisman, S. Arnaud, and H. F. DeLuca, *Clin. Res.*, 24 (1976) 360A.
65 Y. Tanaka, L. Castillo, and H. F. DeLuca, *Proc. Natl. Acad. Sci. U.S.*, 73 (1976) 2701.

66 L. Castillo, Y. Tanaka, H. F. DeLuca, and M. L. Sunde, *Arch. Biochem. Biophys.*, 179 (1977) 211.
67 A. D. Kenny, J. Lamb, N. R. David, and T. A. Losty, *Fed. Proc.*, 33 (1974) 679 (abstr.).
68 E. Spanos and I. MacIntyre, *Lancet*, i (1977) 840.
69 Y. Tanaka and H. F. DeLuca, *Arch. Biochem. Biophys.*, 154 (1973) 566.
70 A. W. Norman, E. J. Friedlander, and H. L. Henry, in S. G. Massry and E. Ritz, *Phosphate Metabolism*, Plenum Press, New York, 1977, p. 211.
71 L. A. Baxter and H. F. DeLuca, *J. Biol. Chem.*, 251 (1976) 3158.
72 M. L. Ribovich and H. F. DeLuca, *Fed. Proc.*, 36 (1977) 1096 (abstr.).
73 N. Horiuchi, T. Suda, S. Sasaki, H. Takahashi, E. Shimazawa, and E. Ogata, *Biochem. Biophys. Res. Commun.*, 73 (1976) 869.
74 R. G. Larkins, S. J. MacAuley, and I. MacIntyre, *Nature*, 252 (1974) 412.
75 H. F. DeLuca, *Life Sci.*, 17 (1975) 1351.
76 B. W. O'Malley and A. R. Means, *Science*, 183 (1974) 610.
77 P. F. Brumbaugh and M. R. Haussler, *Life Sci.*, 13 (1973) 1737.
78 B. E. Kream, R. D. Reynolds, J. C. Knutson, J. A. Eisman, and H. F. DeLuca, *Arch. Biochem. Biophys.*, 176 (1976) 779.
79 B. E. Kream, M. J. L. Jose, and H. F. DeLuca, *Arch. Biochem. Biophys.*, 179 (1977) 462.
80 J. A. Eisman and H. F. DeLuca, *Steroids* (1977) in press.
81 B. E. Kream, S. Yamada, H. K. Schnoes, and H. F. DeLuca, *J. Biol. Chem.*, 252 (1977) 4501.
82 J. G. Haddad and S. J. Birge, *J. Biol. Chem.*, 250 (1975) 299.
83 G. A. Kimmich, *Biochemistry*, 9 (1970) 3669.
84 B. E. Kream, M. Jose, S. Yamada, and H. F. DeLuca, *Science*, 197 (1977) 1086.
85 T. C. Chen and H. F. DeLuca, *J. Biol. Chem.*, 248 (1973) 4890.
86 H. C. Tsai, R. G. Wong, and A. W. Norman, *J. Biol. Chem.*, 247 (1972) 5511.
87 T. C. Chen, J. C. Weber, and H. F. DeLuca, *J. Biol. Chem.*, 245 (1970) 3776.
88 M. Zile, E. C. Bunge, L. Barsness, S. Yamada, H. K. Schnoes, and H. F. DeLuca, *Arch. Biochem. Bipohys.* (1977) in press.
89 P. F. Brumbaugh and M. R. Haussler, *J. Biol. Chem.*, 249 (1974) 1258.
90 P. F. Brumbaugh and M. R. Haussler, *Life Sci.*, 16 (1975) 353.
91 D. E. M. Lawson and P. W. Wilson, *Biochem. J.*, 144 (1974) 573.
92 R. H. Wasserman and A. N. Taylor, *Science*, 152 (1966) 791.
93 R. Spencer, M. Charman, P. Wilson, and E. Lawson, *Nature*, 263 (1976) 161.
94 J. Harmeyer and H. F. DeLuca, *Arch. Biochem. Biophys.*, 133 (1969) 247.
95 H. F. DeLuca, Ann. Royal College of Physicians and Surgeons of Canada, Annals, 1977, p. 216.

POSSIBLE ROLE OF VITAMIN D IN CALCIUM ABSORPTION IN INTESTINE

SACHIKO MORIUCHI AND NORIMASA HOSOYA
Faculty of Medicine, University of Tokyo, Tokyo (Japan)

Vitamin D_3 is required for intestinal Ca absorption. It is well known that vitamin D_3 is first metabolized to hydroxylated products, 1,25-$(OH)_2D_3$, before it acts on the aprocess of intestinal Ca absorption. However, the role of 1,25-$(OH)_2D_3$ in intestinal Ca bsorption is still not clarified. 1,25-$(OH)_2D_3$ is now regarded as a hormone which is secreted from kidney and accumulated specifically in the nuclei of the target tissues, such as intestine and bone, *via* specific cytoplasmic receptor for 1,25-$(OH)_2D_3$. Therefore, it is suggested that 1,25-$(OH)_2D_3$ stimulates the synthesis of specific proteins *via* receptor mechanism.[1]

With respect to the specific proteins induced by 1,25-$(OH)_2D_3$, two kinds have been demonstrated. One is a soluble CaBP and the others are proteins associated with microvillus membrane.

CaBP was first identified in chick duodenal cytosol. It was followed by the demonstration of similar soluble proteins in intestine and some other tissues (kidney, shell gland, brain, *etc.*) of various vertebrate species. Two CaBPs differing in molecular size have been shown. One is of molecular size *ca.* 28,000 and is mainly found in chick tissues; the other is *ca.* 10,000 and is mainly found in mammalian tissues.[2]

However, it is interesting to note that two kinds of CaBPs have been demonstrated in rat intestine using ^{45}Ca-equilibrated Sephadex G-200 column chromatography for ^{45}Ca binding assay.[3] The larger CaBP, found predominantly in the jejunum and ileum, had a mol. wt. of 27,000. On the other hand, the smaller CaBP, which was associated mainly with duodenum and jejunum, had a mol. wt. of 12,500. Both CaBPs were vitamin D-dependent, but the smaller showed higher vitamin D dependency than the larger. ^{45}Ca binding activity of the smaller CaBP was easily detected by chelex 100 assay, but that of the larger CaBP was not so sensitive to the chelex 100 assay (Figs. 1, 2).[3] The difference in electrophoretic mobility and Ca binding properties was also observed between the larger and smaller CaBP.[4] Furthermore, deprivation of Ca from diet decreased the Ca binding activity of smaller CaBP in jejunum a little, but did not change that of the larger CaBP in jejunum. Cd feeding did not influence Ca binding activity of the larger CaBP, but that of the smaller CaBP was almost completely abolished.[5] The differences between the two CaBPs is summarized in Table I. The smaller CaBP is much more influenced by dietary factors.

Ca absorption in the duodenum is predominantly dependent on active transport, whereas in the distal intestine, it is rather dependent on simple diffusion. Therefore, the

Abbreviations: 1,25-$(OH)_2D_3$, 1,25-dihydroxyvitamin D_3; CaBP, calcium-binding protein.

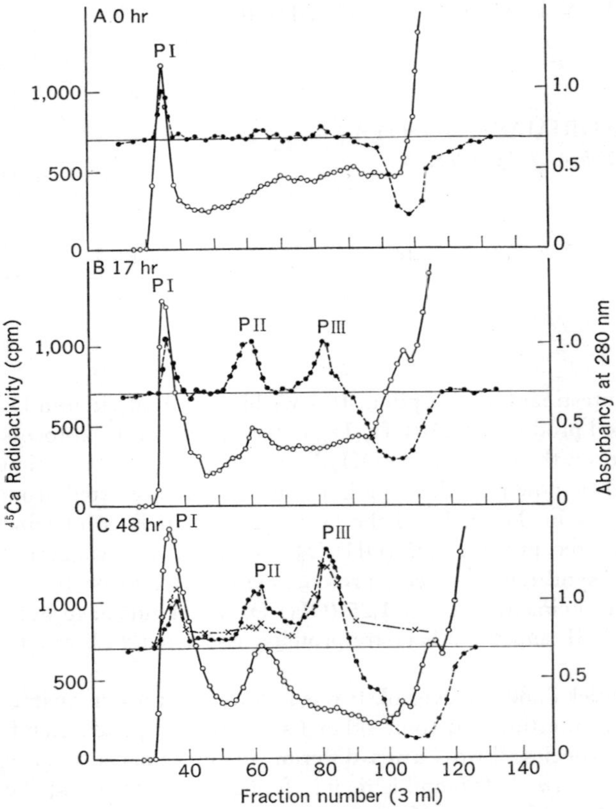

Fig. 1. Elution profiles of ^{45}Ca binding activity and absorbancy at 280 nm of proteins from small intestinal mucosa. Heat-treated supernatants from the mucosa of vitamin D-deficient and vitamin D_3-repleted rats were eluted from Sephadex G-100 column equilibrated with ^{45}Ca. A, vitamin D-deficient controls. B, vitamin D_3-repleted mucosa, 17 hr after administration of 2,000 IU of vitamin D_3 to the animals. C, vitamin D_3-repleted mucosa, 48 hr after administration of 2,000 IU of vitamin D_3 to the animals. ○ absorbancy at 280 nm; ● radioactivity eluted; × radioactivity remaining in supernatant after chelex assay[3].

presence of CaBPs differing in tissue distribution and Ca binding properties might be ascribed to the difference in the molecular mechanism of Ca absorption.

CaBP has been found mainly in the tissues transporting Ca. However, the role of CaBP in the intestinal Ca absorption is still not clear. A definitive demonstration of intracellular localization of CaBP will be necessary for an understanding of the role of CaBP in intestinal Ca absorption. However, regarding the intracellular localization of CaBP, there are some discrepancies among investigators. Taylor and Wasserman[6] demonstrated histochemically that CaBP was found on brush border membranes and in goblet cells in chick duodenum, indicating that CaBP is involved in intestinal Ca absorption. The other finding is that chick duodenal CaBP is located neither on brush border membranes nor in goblet cells, but rather located inside the intestinal epithelial cells.[7]

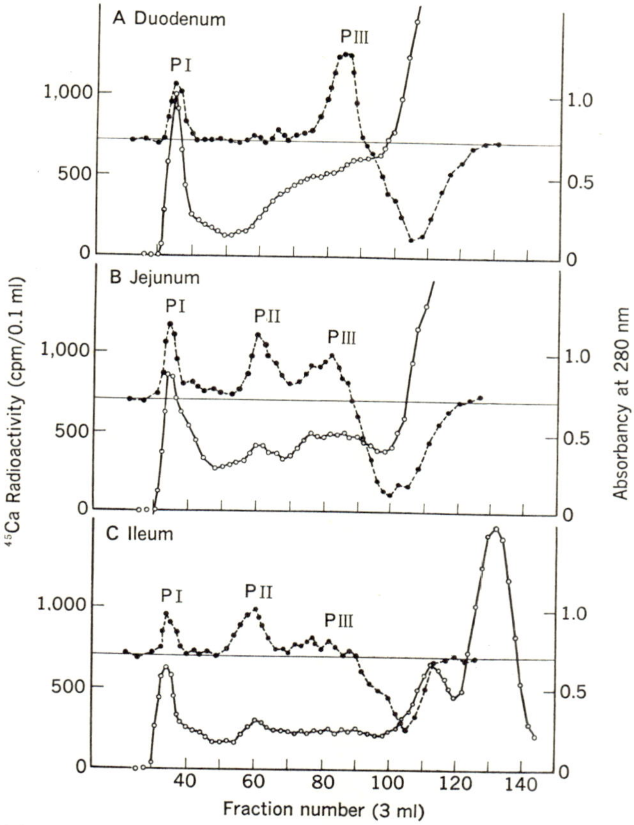

Fig. 2. Elution profiles of ^{45}Ca binding activity and absorbancy at 280 nm of mucosal proteins from various sections of small intestine. Heat-treated supernatants from the mucosa were eluted from Sephadex G-100 column equilibrated with ^{45}Ca. The animals were vitamin D-deficient rats given 2,000 IU vitamin D_3 48 hr before sacrifice. ○ absorbancy at 280 nm; ● radioactivity.[3]

TABLE I

COMPARISON OF TWO CaBPs IN RAT INTESTINAL MUCOSA

		Large CaBP	*Smaller CaBP*
Molecular weight		27,000	12,500
Tissue distribution		Jejunum, ileum	Duodenum, jejunum
Vitamin D dependency		+	++
Electrophoretic mobility pH 8.3		Fast	Slow
Affinity constant (k_i) M^{-1}	a	1.2×10^6	2.5×10^5
	b	2.2×10^4	
Binding site (n)	a	3.6	1
	b	85	
Response to dietary Ca			
Normal		++	++
Low		++	+
Sensitivity to Cd		±	++

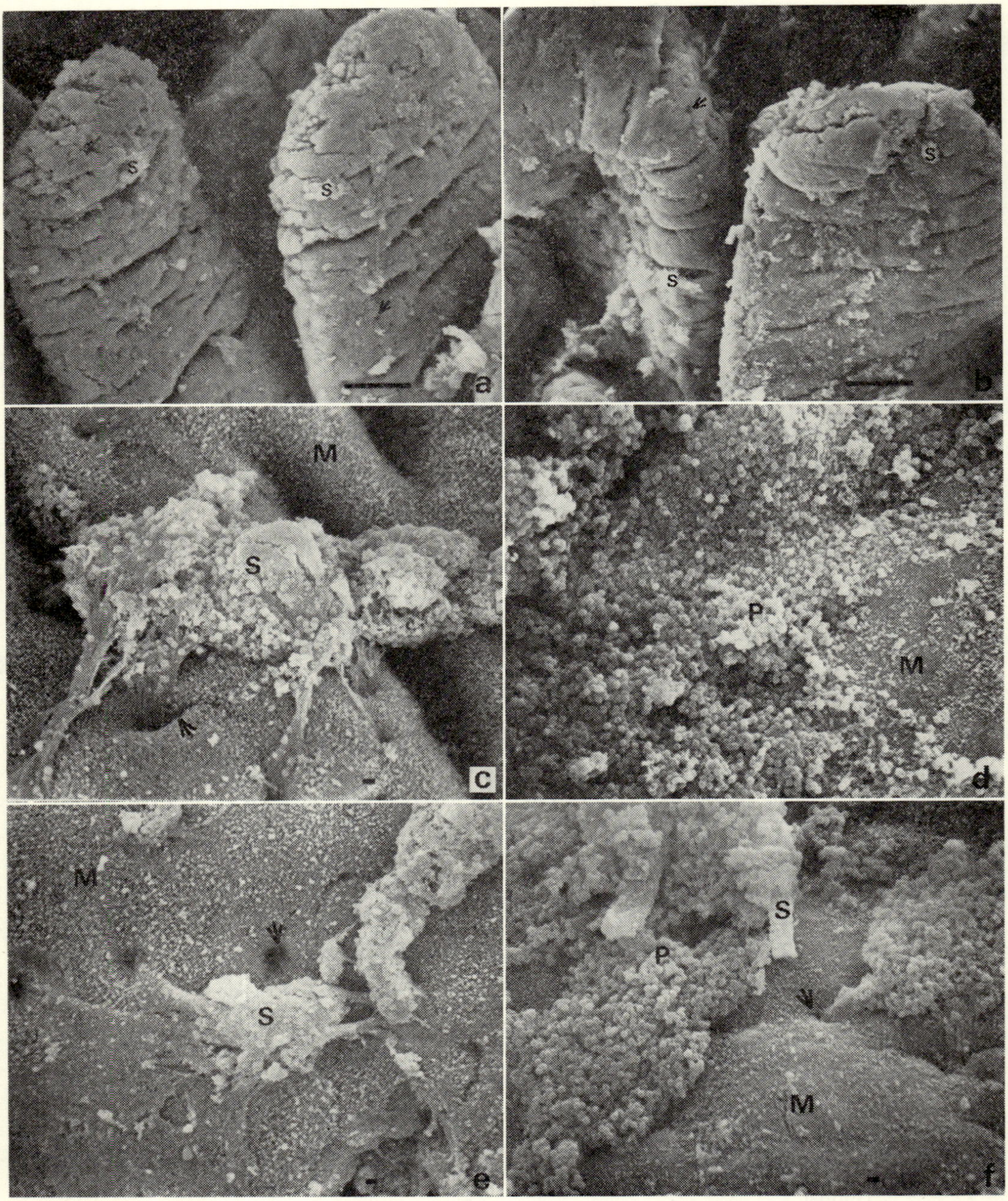
s
s
a
s
s
b
M
S
c
P
M
d
M
S
e
S
P
M
f

Immuno-scanning electron microscopy techniques have been developed for the visualization of antigen exposed to the cell surface.[8] If CaBP is located on brush border as reported by Taylor and Wasserman, this method can be applied for the visualization of CaBP in the intestine. In this method, polystylene latex is used as a marker of CaBP. As shown in Fig. 3, polystylene latex particles were observed on the secretory substances of goblet cells and the microvilli in vitamin D_3-treated chick duodena, when the doudena were fixed without rinsing their surface, however, very few in the vitamin D-deficient chicks (Fig. 3-c, d). On the other hand, the polystylene latex particles were not observed on the microvilli of vitamin D_3-treated chick, when the doudenal surface was well rinsed by phosphate buffer before fixation of tissues. In this case, the polytsylene latex particles were only observed on the secretory substances of goblet cells in the vitamin D_3-treated chick duodenal villi (Fig. 3-e). This suggestes that CaBP is contained in the secretory substances of goblet cells and covers the intestinal surface.

On the other hand, recent evidence suggests that the appearance of CaBP is not closely related to the initial stimulation of Ca absorption by 1,25-$(OH)_2D_3$. Therefore,

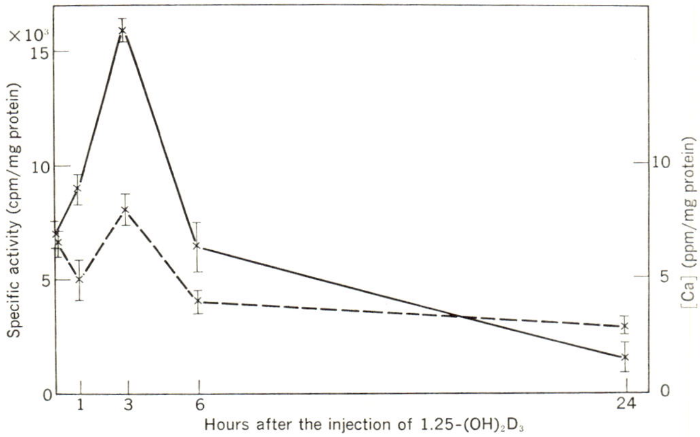

Fig. 4. Effect of 1,25-$(OH)_2D_3$ on sialic acid incorporation and Ca content in chick intestinal microsomes. Each point represents the average of four to five chicks ± S.E. Vitamin D-deficient chicks were dosed with either 325 pmol of 1,25-$(OH)_2D_3$ in 50 μl of 95% ethanol or 50 μl of 95% ethanol intravenously *via* wing vein at various hours before sacrifice. —×— sialic acid incorporation; ···×··· Ca content.[15]

←

Fig. 3. Immuno-scanning electron micrograph of duodenal villi from vitamin D-deficient (a, c, e) and vitamin D_3-treated (b, d, f) chick. Either 50 μl of 95% ethanol or 2,000 IU of vitamin D_3 in 50 μl of 95% ethanol was dosed to vitamin D-deficient chicks 48 hr before sacrifice intravenously. Duodena were fixed in 10% formalin in phosphate buffer (pH 7.4) either immediately (a, b, c, and d) or after being well rinsed with ice-cold phosphate buffer (pH 7.4) (e and f), incubated with anti-CaBP rabbit γ-globulin followed by the incubation with polystylene latex bound anti-rabbit goat γ-globulin. The tissues were fixed with glutaraldehyde and prepared for the scanning electron microscopy. a and b, observation of duodenal villi at low magnification. Black bar denotes 50 μm. c, d, e, and f, observation of duodenal villi at higher magnification. Black bar denotes 1 μm. The apices of goblet cell (arrows) appeared as depression within the coat of microvilli (M) or were covered with their secretory substances(S). P, denotes polystylene latex particles.[13]

TABLE II

TIME COURSE OF INTESTINAL RESPONSES TO 1,25-$(OH)_2D_3$

Vitamin D-deficient chicks were dosed with 125 ng of 1,25-$(OH)_2D_3$ at various hours before sacrifice.

Responses	*Time after 1,25-$(OH)_2D_3$*			
	0	*3*	*6*	*24 hr*
Ca absorption	−	±	++	++
CaBP (Chelex assay)	−	−	−	+
(Immunoassay)	−	−	+	++
Alkaline phosphatase	−	−	±	+
Brush border protein change in mobility	−	±	+	+
Alkaline phosphatase isozyme change	−	±	+	+
Sialyltransferase	+++	++++	++	+
Microsomal Ca	+++	++++	++	+

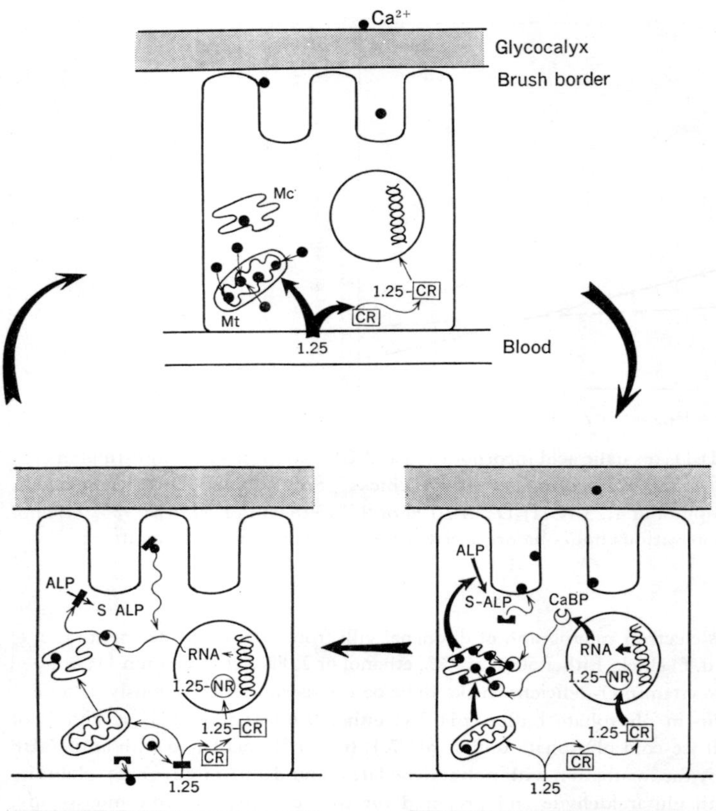

Fig. 5. Suggested mechanism of action of 1,25-$(OH)_2D_3$ in the intestine and its effects on intestinal calcium translocation. 1,25, 1,25-$(OH)_2D_3$; CR, cytosol receptor for 1,25-$(OH)_2D_3$; NR, nuclear receptor for 1,25-$(OH)_2$ D_3; Mc, microsome; Mt, mitochondria; ALPase, alkaline phosphatase (desialoenzyme); S-ALPase, sialo-alkaline phosphatase (sialoenzyme).

CaBP may be necessary but not sufficient to account for the intestinal response to 1,25-$(OH)_2D_3$.

Recently, vitamin D induced changes in the proteins associated with microvillus membranes are reported, *viz.*, an increase in alkaline phosphatase activity,[10] Ca-ATPase activity[11]: the stimulation of membrane protein synthesis which molecular size is 150,000, 84,000, and 45,000 respectively, especially 45,000 protein responds to 1,25-$(OH)_2D_3$ very rapidly[12]: the modulation of membrane protein which has alkaline phosphatase activity.[13]

An increase of alkaline phosphatase activity shows a similar pattern as CaBP after the dose of 1,25-$(OH)_2D_3$, but the modulation of alkaline phosphatase occurs more rapidly in good correlation with the initial stimulation of Ca absorption by 1,25-$(OH)_2D_3$.[13]

The *n*-butanol-solubilized alkaline phosphatase from chick duodenum has been resolved into three groups of molecules. The two isozymes show fast-moving bands on electrophoresis differing in their association with sialic acid.[14] Polyacrylamide disc gel electrophoresis of *n*-butanol-solubilized alkaline phosphatase from chick duodenum revealed that the change of alkaline phosphatase induced by 1,25-$(OH)_2D_3$ involved the transformation of desialoenzyme to sialoenzyme. The initial stimulation by 1,25-$(OH)_2D_3$ of the incorporation of sialic acid into duodenal microsomes corresponded with the initial increase in Ca absorption. After this initial stimulation, there was a rapid decline in sialic acid incorporation into microsomes decreasing below control levels at 24 hr after the dose of 125 ng of 1,25-$(OH)_2D_3$. Ca concentration in the microsomes followed a pattern similar to the incorporation of sialic acid into microsomes (Fig. 4). The depressed sialic acid incorporation was reversed by the addition of Ca *in vitro*.[15]

At present time, it is not possible to propose definitive role of vitamin D in intestinal Ca absorption. Therefore, it will be better to leave it blank which you can write as you like. However, finally, we would like to propose a possible role of vitamin D in intestinal Ca absorption mainly from our observations as summarized in time course of intestinal responses induced by 1,25-$(OH)_2D_3$ (Table II).

The initial action of 1,25-$(OH)_2D_3$ would be to change the membrane permeability to Ca and to change the subcellular distribution of Ca in the small intestine. The accumulated Ca in the microsomes then stimulates the sialic acid incorporation into desialoenzyme. This results in the changes of isozyme pattern of alkaline phosphatase, *viz.*, the transformation of desialoenzyme to sialoenzyme. The transformed alkaline phosphatase might be one of the factors involved more directly in the regulation of Ca absorption in intestine.

On the other hand, nuclear 1,25-$(OH)_2D_3$, which was transported to nuclei by cytosol receptor mechanism, as the mechanism elucidated for steroid hormone, may induce CaBP, although it appears after the stimulation of Ca transport. The function of the induced CaBP is not clear, but it could be to sequester Ca from microsomes so as to regulate or terminate the action of 1,25-$(OH)_2D_3$ (Fig. 5).

REFERENCES

1 H. F. DeLuca, this volume, p. 219.
2 R. H. Wasserman, R. A. Corradino, C. S. Fullmer, and A. N. Taylor, *Vitam. Horm.* (*New York*), 32 (1974) 299.
3 S. Moriuchi, T. Yamanouchi, and N. Hosoya, *J. Nutr. Sci. Vitaminol.*, 21 (1975) 251.
4 T. Yamanouchi, S. Moriuchi, and N. Hosoya, *Vitamins* (*Japan*), 51 (1977) 221.

5 T. YAMANOUCHI, F. TSURUKI, S. MORIUCHI, and N. HOSOYA, *Bone Metab. (Japan)*, 11 (1978) 383.
6 A. N. TAYLOR and R. H. WASSERMAN, *J. Histochem. Cytochem.*, 18 (1970) 107.
7 R. L. MORRISSEY, D. T. ZOLOCK, D. D. BIKLE, and P. W. MELLICK, *Fed. Proc.*, 36 (1977) 1097.
8 J. J. RINEHART, S. P. BALCERZAK, and A. F. LO BUGLIO, *J. Lab. Clin. Med.*, 78 (1971) 167.
9 S. NODA, K. KUBOTA, S. MORIUCHI, S. YOSHIZAWA, and N. HOSOYA, *J. Nutr. Sci. Vitaminol.*, 24 (1978) 331.
10 A. W. NORMAN, A. K. MIRCHEFF, R. H. ADAMS, and A. SPIELVOGEL, *Biochim. Biophys. Acta*, 215 (1971) 348.
11 M. J. MELANCON and H. F. DELUCA, *Biochemistry*, 9 (1970) 1958.
12 P. W. WILSON and D. E. M. LAWSON, *Biochim. Biophys. Acta*, 497 (1977) 805.
13 S. MORIUCHI and H. F. DELUCA, *Arch. Biochem. Biophys.*, 174 (1976) 367.
14 C.-H. CHANG and F. MOOG, *Biochim. Biophys. Acta*, 258 (1972) 154.
15 S. MORIUCHI, S. YOSHIZAWA, and N. HOSOYA, *J. Nutr. Sci. Vitaminol.*, 23(1977) 497.